Atlas of
INFECTIOUS DISEASES

Volume VII

INTRA-ABDOMINAL INFECTIONS, HEPATITIS, AND GASTROENTERITIS

Atlas of
INFECTIOUS DISEASES

Volume VII
INTRA-ABDOMINAL INFECTIONS, HEPATITIS, AND GASTROENTERITIS

Editor-in-Chief

Gerald L. Mandell, MD

Professor of Medicine
Owen R. Cheatham Professor of the Sciences
Chief, Division of Infectious Diseases
University of Virginia Health Sciences Center
Charlottesville, Virginia

Editor

Bennett Lorber, MD

Thomas M. Durant Professor of Medicine
Chief, Section of Infectious Diseases
Temple University Health Sciences Center
Philadelphia, Pennsylvania

With 10 contributors

**Churchill
Livingstone**

DEVELOPED BY CURRENT MEDICINE, INC.
PHILADELPHIA

96-195

CURRENT MEDICINE
400 MARKET STREET, SUITE 700
PHILADELPHIA, PA 19106

Library of Congress Cataloging-in-Publication Data

Intra-abdominal infections, hepatitis, and gastroenteritis/editor-in-chief, Gerald L. Mandell; editor, Bennett Lorber; developed by Current Medicine.
      p. cm.–(Atlas of infectious diseases; v. 7)
  Includes bibliographical references and index.
  ISBN 0-443-07730-4 (hardcover)
  1. Gastrointestinal system–Infections–Atlases. 2. Hepatitis, Viral–Atlases.
3. Abdomen–Infections–Atlases. I. Mandell, Gerald L. II. Lorber, Bennett 1943– .
III. Current Medicine, Inc. IV. Series.
  [DNLM: 1. Gastroenteritis–diagnosis–atlases. 2. Hepatitis–diagnosis–atlases.
3. Abdomen–pathology–atlases. 4. Bacterial Infections–pathology–atlases.
WI 17 I61 1996]
RC830.I56 1996
616.3'307–dc20
DNLM/DLC
for Library of Congress   96-13984
                                                 CIP

Development Editors:	Lee Tevebaugh and Michael Bokulich
Editorial Assistant:	Elena Coler
Art Director:	Paul Fennessy
Design and Layout:	Patrick Ward and Lisa Weischedel
Illustration Director:	Ann Saydlowski
Illustrators:	Elizabeth Carrozza, Ann Saydlowski, and Gary Welch
Production:	David Myers and Lori Holland
Managing Editor:	Lori J. Bainbridge
Indexer:	Ann Cassar

Printed in Hong Kong by Paramount Printing Group Limited.

10 9 8 7 6 5 4 3 2 1

PREFACE

The diagnosis and management of patients with infectious diseases are based in large part on visual clues. Skin and mucous membrane lesions, eye findings, imaging studies, Gram stains, culture plates, insect vectors, preparations of blood, urine, pus, cerebrospinal fluid, and biopsy specimens are studied to establish the proper diagnosis and to choose the most effective therapy. The *Atlas of Infectious Diseases* is a modern, complete collection of these images. Current Medicine, with its capability of superb color reproduction and its state-of-the-art computer imaging facilities, is the ideal publisher for the atlas. Infectious diseases physicians, scientists, microbiologists, and pathologists frequently teach other health-care professionals, and this comprehensive atlas with available slides is an effective teaching tool.

Dr. Bennett Lorber is a superb clinician-teacher-investigator with a wealth of insight into the complex problems related to gastrointestinal infections. He has organized a volume that covers the field in both a broad and detailed fashion and has recruited distinguished authors for the chapters. This volume is extremely useful for clinicians, educators, and researchers who are concerned with the broad field of intra-abdominal infections, hepatitis, and gastroenteritis.

Gerald L. Mandell, MD
Charlottesville, Virginia

CONTRIBUTORS

Helen Buckley, PhD
Professor, Microbiology and Immunology
Temple University School of Medicine
Director, Clinical Mycology Laboratory
Temple University Hospital
Philadelphia, Pennsylvania

Sydney M. Finegold, MD
Professor, Departments of Medicine and Microbiology
  and Immunology
University of California at Los Angeles School of Medicine
Staff Physician, Infectious Disease Section
Veterans Affairs Medical Center West Los Angeles
Los Angeles, California

Robert A. Gatenby, MD
Professor of Radiology
Diagnostic Imaging
Temple University School of Medicine
Section Chief, Abdominal Imaging
Department of Diagnostic Imaging
Temple University Hospital
Philadelphia, Pennsylvania

Robert M. Genta, MD
Professor of Pathology, Medicine, Microbiology, and
  Immunology
Baylor College of Medicine
Pathologist, Departments of Pathology and Medicine
Veterans Affairs Medical Center
Houston, Texas

David Y. Graham, MD
Professor of Medicine and Molecular Virology
Chief, Gastroenterology
Baylor College of Medicine
Chief, Digestive Disease Section
Veterans Affairs Medical Center
Houston, Texas

Richard L. Guerrant, MD
Thomas H. Hunter Professor of International Medicine
University of Virginia
Chief, Division of Geographic and International Medicine
University of Virginia Hospital
Charlottesville, Virginia

Lionel Rabin, MD, CM
Clinical Associate Professor
Division of Hepatic Pathology
Veterans Administration Special Reference Laboratory for
  Pathology
Department of Hepatic and Gastrointestinal Pathology
Armed Forces Institute of Pathology
Washington, DC

Robert D. Shaw, MD
Assistant Professor of Medicine
State University of New York at Stony Brook
Stony Brook, New York
Staff Physician, Gastroenterology
Northport Veterans Affairs Medical Center
Northport, New York

Rosemary Soave, MD
Associate Professor of Medicine and Public Health
Cornell University Medical College
Associate Attending Physician
New York Hospital-Cornell Medical Center
New York City, New York

Samuel E. Wilson
Professor and Chair
Department of Surgery
University of California at Irvine College of Medicine
Irvine, California

CONTENTS

CHAPTER 1

Intra-abdominal Infections and Abscesses

Sydney M. Finegold
Samuel E. Wilson

NORMAL FLORA OF THE GASTROINTESTINAL TRACT

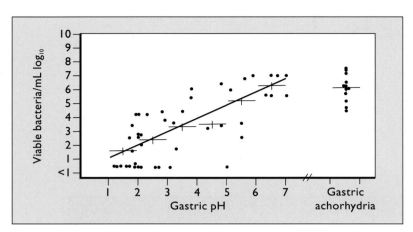

FIGURE 1-1 Relationship between gastric pH and bacterial counts in the stomach. In the normal state, with the usual low pH, bacterial counts in fasting persons are extremely low (< 100–1000 organisms/mL of gastric contents). Patients with achlorhydria, related to either pathology or medication, have much higher counts of organisms. Should such patients aspirate gastric contents, the organisms present would play an important role in the subsequent aspiration pneumonia. Similarly, if such subjects have perforation of a peptic ulcer or undergo gastric surgery, the high bacterial count in the stomach may lead to contamination with bacterial peritonitis and/or postoperative wound infection. Gastric acid is part of our normal defense mechanisms that prevent invasion by pathogenic bacteria into the bowel. (*Adapted from* Draser and Hill [1].)

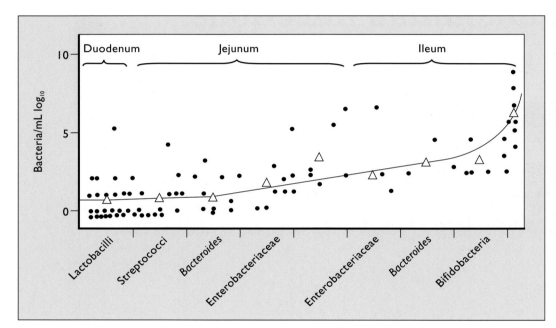

FIGURE 1-2 Bacterial flora at different levels of the small bowel. Increased numbers and variety of bacteria encountered as one traverses from the upper small bowel to the ileum. In the duodenum and upper jejunum, counts are low (usually 100–1000/mL of contents), and the organisms seen are primarily transients from the oral flora—lactobacilli and streptococci. In the distal jejunum and particularly in the ileum, counts are higher and one begins to see Enterobacteriaceae and *Bacteroides*. Counts in the distal ileum approach those seen in the colon, and a greater variety of anaerobes is encountered. The implications are that with trauma or surgery involving the distal small bowel or large bowel (where counts are still higher), the risk of contamination and subsequent intra-abdominal or wound infection is significantly greater than when the upper small bowel is involved. (*Adapted from* Draser and Hill [1].)

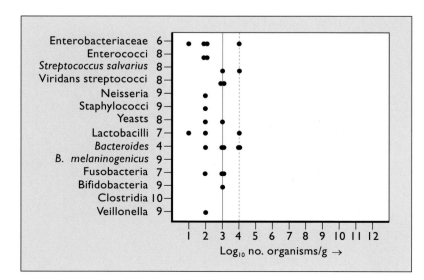

FIGURE 1-3 Jejunal flora in patients with achlorhydria. Achlorhydric subjects may have significant counts of certain organisms in the jejunum, which demonstrates that the normal gastric acid content minimizes passage of bacteria into the small bowel. Enterobacteriaceae and *Bacteroides* are the organisms most commonly found. *Bacteroides melaninogenicus* has been reclassified as other species of *Bacteroides*, *Prevotella*, and *Porphyromonas*.

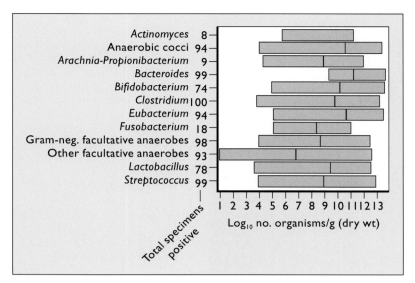

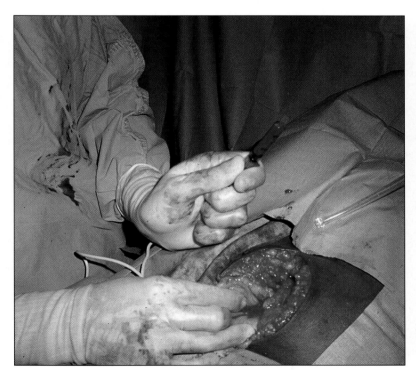

Figure 1-4 Normal fecal flora. Data on the frequency and mean counts of various microorganisms found in human feces are presented. As such, it reflects the bacteriology of the distal colon. Note that *Bacteroides* were found in virtually all subjects of this large study group and that the counts of this organism exceeded those of all other organisms encountered. Clostridia, eubacteria, and anaerobic cocci were found in the vast majority of subjects, and counts of these other anaerobes were also very high. Also, anaerobes outnumbered nonanaerobes, such as Enterobacteriaceae, by a factor of 100 to 1000:1. Interactions between these organisms and potential pathogens may determine whether or not intestinal infection ensues. Short-chain fatty acids produced by the anaerobes are often inhibitory to such pathogens as *Shigella*. In the figure, the length of the *bar* represents the range of the counts measured; the median is indicated by the *vertical line* within each bar.

COLLECTION AND TRANSPORT OF SPECIMENS

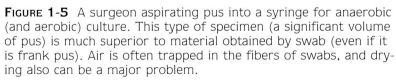

Figure 1-5 A surgeon aspirating pus into a syringe for anaerobic (and aerobic) culture. This type of specimen (a significant volume of pus) is much superior to material obtained by swab (even if it is frank pus). Air is often trapped in the fibers of swabs, and drying also can be a major problem.

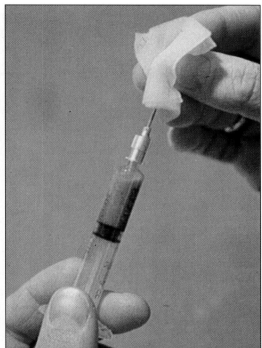

Figure 1-6 Specimen collection for anaerobes. It is necessary to push out all bubbles of air or gas that may have entered the syringe and the needle in which the pus is collected. This step ensures a solid column of pus or other fluid, which in turn ensures that anaerobic conditions will be obtained and that no air will be introduced into the transport container along with the specimen.

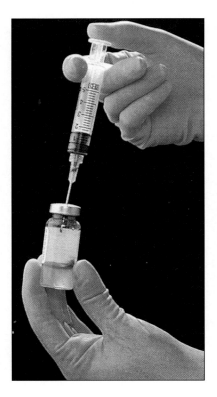

FIGURE 1-7 Injection of the specimen into an anaerobic transport vial. The agar in the bottom of the vial is nonnutritive and contains an oxidation-reduction indicator, such as methylene blue or, preferably, resazurin. Care should be taken not to inject air inadvertently along with the specimen. The specimen should be injected slowly so that it remains on top of the agar. Specimens remain anaerobic in such containers for at least 72 hours, but obviously it is advantageous for the laboratory to culture the material as soon as possible. (*From* Finegold *et al.* [2]; with permission.)

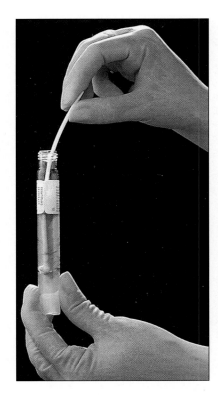

FIGURE 1-8 Anaerobic transport tube with agar deep for transporting swabs when no other specimen can be obtained. This tube contains a deep column of nonnutritive agar (with oxidation-reduction indicator) into which a swab may be placed if it is not feasible to obtain tissue or pus for culture. Ideally, the swab should be maintained under anaerobic conditions prior to obtaining the specimen, and its stick should be scored near the top to facilitate breaking. The agar contains reducing substances to help ensure anaerobic conditions. The cap should be replaced immediately after the swab is placed into the tube. Transport containers such as this one, which are not truly gas-tight, should not be refrigerated because oxygen diffuses better at lower temperatures.

POSTTRAUMATIC INFECTION

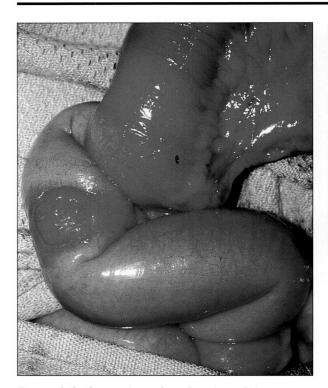

FIGURE 1-9 Gross view of perforation of the jejunum secondary to trauma. After such trauma, the peritoneal cavity is contaminated with bowel contents. Knowledge of the usual flora of the bowel at this level and how it might have been modified by previous pathology or antimicrobial therapy permits early institution of the most appropriate antibiotic regimen. Gram stain of the bowel contents or peritoneal exudate may also influence the decision as to the best antimicrobial regimen. Subsequently, results of the aerobic culture and preliminary anaerobic culture data may dictate a change in regimen.

Bacteriology of 50 intra-abdominal abscesses after trauma

Aerobes (90%)	Patients, *n*	Anaerobes (48%)	Patients, *n*
Enterococcus	29	*Peptococcus*	10
Staphylococcus aureus	2 (2 MR)	*Peptostreptococcus*	4
Streptococcus	3	*Bacteroides*	14
Escherichia coli	26	*Clostridium*	11
Enterobacter	10	*Fusobacterium*	2
Pseudomonas	5	*Eubacterium*	2
Klebsiella	4		
Proteus	4		

MR—methicillin-resistant.

FIGURE 1-10 Bacteriology of 50 intra-abdominal abscesses after trauma. (*From* Jones [3].)

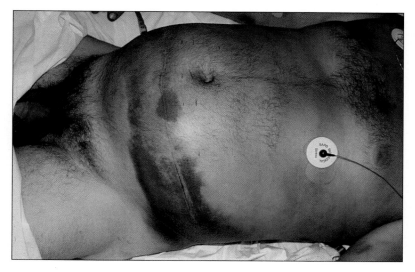

FIGURE 1-11 Severe crush injury of the anterior abdominal wall (truck loading dock injury) that led to mesenteric infarction. Interference with the mesenteric circulation affects a large segment of bowel and thus is an extremely critical event. The superior mesenteric artery supplies all of the small bowel below the ligament of Treitz and the proximal half of the colon. Therefore, a huge bacterial load is released as the affected bowel becomes ischemic and then necrotic. Early definitive surgery plus systemic antimicrobial therapy are crucial, but the prognosis is poor in any case. In this situation, optimal coverage of all anticipated bowel flora is required. In a community-situated accident, such as occurred in this patient, appropriate regimens include a carbapenem, or a β-lactam/β-lactamase-inhibitor combination such as ticarcillin/clavulanic acid, or metronidazole plus ampicillin, plus an aminoglycoside such as gentamicin. In the hospital setting, one would need to be concerned also about nosocomial pathogens, such as various gram-negative aerobic and facultative bacteria, including *Pseudomonas aeruginosa*, and *Staphylococcus aureus*.

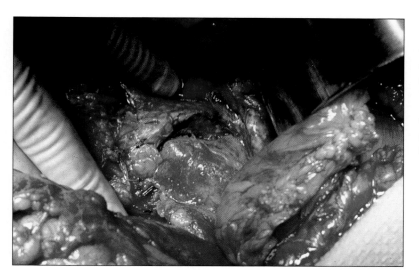

FIGURE 1-12 Traumatic transection of the pancreas with surrounding peritonitis, approximately 3 days after injury. Unfortunately, there is no evidence that prophylactic antimicrobial agents would decrease the likelihood of such infection. Indeed, the value of pancreatic resection or debridement is also uncertain. The principal infecting organisms in this situation are of enteric origin. *Escherichia coli* is the most commonly encountered organism, with enterococci, viridans streptococci, and *Klebsiella* each found in about 20% of cases. Other gram-negative rods, staphylococci, *Candida*, and anaerobes are seen less often.

WOUND INFECTION

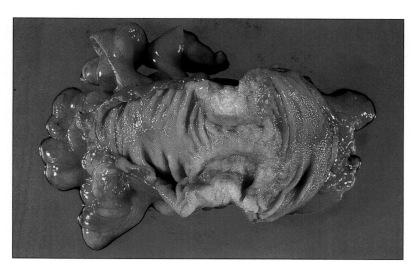

FIGURE 1-13 Resected colon with classic "apple core" carcinoma illustrating good preoperative bowel preparation with very clean mucosal surface. The two principal aspects of preoperative bowel preparation are the use of antimicrobials, such as oral neomycin plus erythromycin, and the use of mechanical cleansing by means of purgatives and enemas. Both approaches are important in order to reduce to very small numbers the huge bacterial load normally present in the colon (10^{11}–10^{12}/g of feces) and so to minimize the risk of infection.

Major aerobic pathogens in surgical wound infections

Pathogen	Infections, %
Staphylococcus aureus	17
Enterococci	13
Coagulase-negative staphylococci	12
Escherichia coli	10
Pseudomonas aeruginosa	8
Enterobacter spp	8
Proteus mirabilis	4
Klebsiella pneumoniae	3
Streptococcus spp	3
Candida albicans	2
Citrobacter spp	2
Serratia marcescens	1
Candida spp	< 1

FIGURE 1-14 Major aerobic pathogens in surgical wound infections. (*Adapted from* Kernodle and Kaiser [4].)

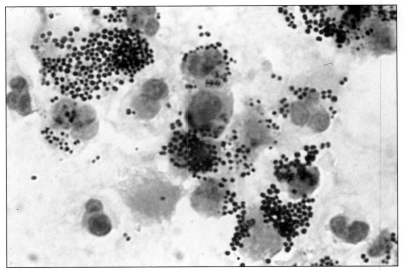

FIGURE 1-15 Gram stain of postoperative abdominal wound infection showing large numbers of intracellular gram-positive cocci in clusters (*Staphylococcus aureus*). Several organisms that may be involved in postoperative infections have distinctive morphology such that one may predict fairly accurately the identity of the organism; this is often true of the anaerobes. Accordingly, quick identification becomes a huge help to the clinician in choosing the most appropriate antimicrobial regimen early in the course of the infection and thereby minimizing the ill effects of the process. Such identification is especially important in the case of infection following bowel surgery, where there may be many different organisms, up to 10 to 20 or more, involved in the infectious process; the microbiology laboratory may need considerable time (sometimes weeks) to isolate each organism in pure culture and identify it. Although the practice is to concentrate on a smaller number of organisms (those known to be important pathogens or resistant to antimicrobial agents and those present in larger numbers), it may still take several days to identify these key organisms. The Gram stain, of course, takes only minutes to prepare and read.

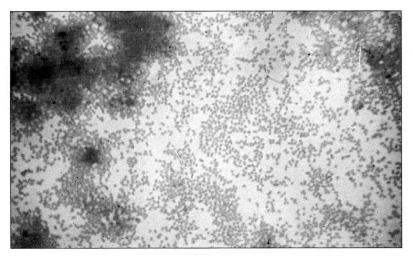

FIGURE 1-16 Microscopic examination of a pure culture of a pigmented anaerobic gram-negative rod. These organisms are coccobacillary and, in the right setting (such as respiratory tract secretions), may be confused with *Haemophilus influenzae*. These pigmenters tend to take the stain lightly, and this, coupled with their small size, may make them easy to overlook in clinical specimens where there may be many other organisms and background debris. Organisms of this type were previously known as *Bacteroides melaninogenicus*; recent taxonomic studies, however, have established that there are actually more than 15 separate species involved, and they are distributed among three different genera—*Prevotella*, *Porphyromonas*, and *Bacteroides*. The relative importance of these species remains to be established, but it appears that those now in the genus *Prevotella* are not only most important in clinical infection but more apt to be resistant to certain β-lactam antimicrobials via β-lactamase production.

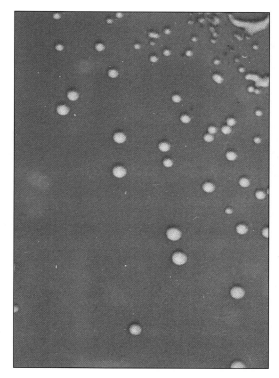

FIGURE 1-17 Pink fluorescence of colonies of pigmented, anaerobic gram-negative rods under ultraviolet light. Colonies of pigmented anaerobic gram-negative rods may be identified as such even before the colony develops its pigment (which typically takes 48 hours up to several days) by demonstrating fluorescence under ultraviolet light. The color of the fluorescence varies from orange to brick red.

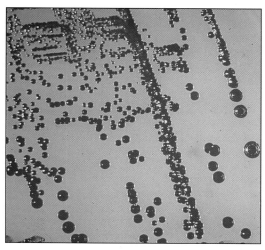

FIGURE 1-18 Colonies of pigmented, anaerobic, gram-negative rods showing characteristic brown-black color. The classic black pigment in the colonies of these anaerobic gram-negative rods was originally believed to be melanin, which led to the original designation of *Bacteroides melaninogenicus*. The pigment is now known to be hematin. The color of the pigment varies from species to species, and sometimes from strain to strain, and with the age of the colony, ranging from tan, light brown, darker brown, to black. The colony morphology is also variable. This slide shows checkerlike colonies with a central plateaulike elevation; other colonies may be perfectly smooth, mucoid, or other. Although there is a tendency for certain species to maintain distinctive colony morphology and pigmentation, as well as distinct characteristics under ultraviolet light before pigment has developed, one cannot use these attributes for accurate speciation. It is still necessary to carry out detailed biochemical tests, gas liquid chromatographic studies, and sometimes other tests for reliable identification.

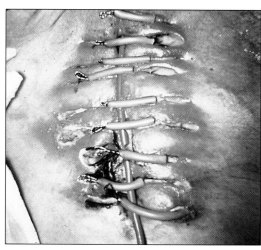

FIGURE 1-19 Wound of a patient with progressive bacterial synergistic gangrene following abdominal surgery. Often, this uncommon infection is seen in patients who have undergone thoracic or abdominal surgery, particularly if stay sutures are required (as in this case). The infection is characterized by three zones classically—a zone of necrosis centrally, a surrounding middle zone of intense purplish discoloration, and an outer zone of erythema. On occasion, this type of infection may be seen without prior surgery. The major symptom is extraordinary pain and tenderness of the lesion. The process may proceed, if not treated successfully, as a slowly advancing subcutaneous slough; on occasion, it may extend down as far as the fascia. Fever and systemic symptoms are mild. Classically, the etiology is a combination of a microaerophilic streptococcus (*Streptococcus evolutus*) and *Staphylococcus aureus*, but sometimes the streptococcus is an obligate anaerobe, and a wide variety of organisms, especially *Proteus*, may be seen instead of (or in addition to) the staphylococcus. Although reports have appeared of cures with antimicrobial therapy alone, most cases require surgical management as well.

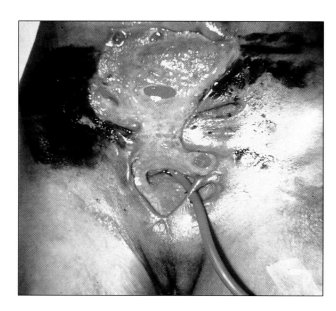

FIGURE 1-20 Progressive bacterial synergistic gangrene showing advanced stage with wound dehiscence and evisceration. The same patient as illustrated in Figure 1-19 is shown in an advanced stage of the disease with wound dehiscence and evisceration. This progression underlines the importance of recognizing the entity and treating it effectively early in the course of the process.

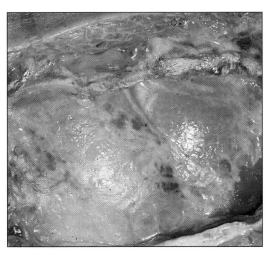

FIGURE 1-21 Necrotizing fasciitis of the abdominal wall. Pus can be seen between the fascia and abdominal wall in the upper part of the figure. The most common bacterial etiology of this entity is group A β-hemolytic streptococci. In the past, this condition was known as hemolytic streptococcal gangrene or hospital gangrene, and it was an extremely common and serious problem in US hospitals during the Civil War and in various hospitals in Europe in the 1800s. A recent upsurge in cases has occurred in the community (it is no longer a hospital problem because of modern sanitation and hospital infection-control measures) related to virulent, toxin-producing strains of *Streptococcus pyogenes* (the "flesh-eating bacteria"). Staphylococci also commonly cause this infection, and anaerobes are not uncommonly involved, particularly in the entity known as Fournier's gangrene, which typically involves the perineal area, especially in diabetics. Among the anaerobes recovered from necrotizing fasciitis are various gram-negative bacilli, including the *Bacteroides fragilis* group, various clostridia, including *Clostridium perfringens*, and anaerobic and microaerophilic streptococci. In many cases in which anaerobes are involved, facultative gram-negative rods and enterococci are also present. This entity may be a postoperative complication, as in the patient pictured, but also occurs after injury, even trivial injury.

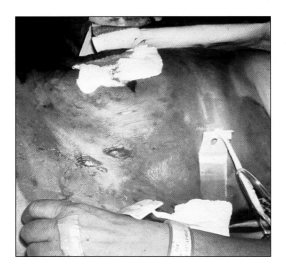

FIGURE 1-22 Clostridial myonecrosis (gas gangrene) of the abdominal wall occurring postoperatively. Note the bronzed discoloration (compare with the color of the hand and upper thigh) and the bullae. Clostridial myonecrosis is one of the most serious of the soft-tissue infections. Pain is one of the hallmarks of the process; it is typically sudden in onset and one of the first things noted by the patient. Accumulations of gas in the soft tissue, never marked in amount, may be detected in most cases, and a peculiar sweetish or mousy smell may be noted. Mental changes are not uncommon, and patients may go into shock. The most common *Clostridium* found in this process is *C. perfringens*; the other species that may be seen include *C. novyi*, *C. septicum*, *C. histolyticum*, *C. bifermentans*, and *C. fallax*.

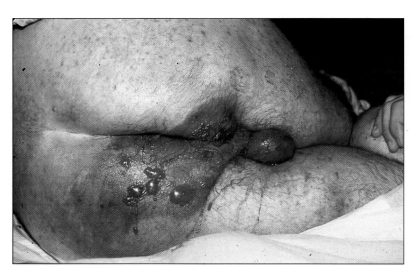

FIGURE 1-23 Clostridial myonecrosis involving the buttocks and perineum. Note the hemorrhage into the tissues and the hemorrhagic bullae. Involvement of large muscle groups is characteristic of clostridial myonecrosis. The disease may spread rapidly, if unchecked, and the mortality may be significant. Immediate debridement or amputation is crucial, and every bit of necrotic muscle must be removed to gain control. Antimicrobial therapy is also important. Penicillin G, in large doses, should be given; there is rationale for adding clindamycin or metronidazole to this regimen, because the latter drugs may shut off toxin production and also occasional strains of these clostridia may be resistant to penicillin (or clindamycin).

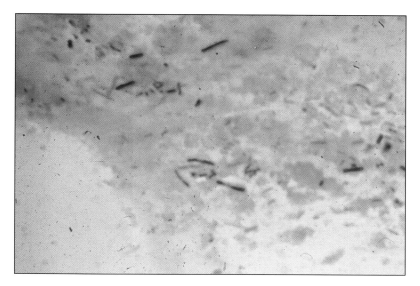

FIGURE 1-24 Tissue Gram stain from clostridial myonecrosis. A tissue specimen from the patient illustrated in Figure 1-23 shows large, boxcarlike, gram-positive rods, which are highly suggestive of *Clostridium perfringens*. There are relatively few polymorphonuclear leukocytes present, and those that are seen are badly distorted. The toxins produced by the responsible clostridia often prevent diapedesis of polymorphonuclear leukocytes into the infected area, even leading to white cell thrombi in the vessels, and may also kill or injure the leukocytes (leukocidins).

Host risk factors for wound infections following gastrointestinal surgery

Extremes of age (very old or very young)
Diabetes
Prior irradiation of the operative site
Steroids and other immunosuppressive therapy
Severe obesity
Malnutrition
Cutaneous anergy
Low expression of HLA-DR on monocytes
Remote infection at time of surgery (*eg*, urinary tract infection)
Long duration of hospitalization prior to surgery
Gastric achlorhydria (gastroduodenal surgery)
Obstruction or perforation of viscus
Preoperative ASA assessment score of 3, 4, or 5

ASA—American Society of Anesthesiologists.

FIGURE 1-25 Host risk factors for wound infection following gastrointestinal surgery. (*Adapted from* Kernodle and Kaiser [5].)

Operative risk factors for wound infection following gastrointestinal surgery

No preoperative shower or inadequate preparation of skin with antiseptics
Shaving operative site on day prior to surgery
Prolonged length of procedure
Intraoperative contamination
Homologous blood transfusion
Excessive use of electrosurgical knife
Poor hemostasis
Use of foreign material
Use of prophylactic abdominal drains
Injection of epinephrine into wound
Appendectomy-in-passing added to elective cholecystectomy
Inadequate preparation of colon (colorectal surgery)

FIGURE 1-26 Operative risk factors for wound infection following gastrointestinal surgery. (*Adapted from* Kernodle and Kaiser [5].)

Recommendations for prophylactic antibiotics in gastrointestinal surgery

Operation	Likely pathogens	Recommended drugs	Adult dosage before surgery
Gastroduodenal	Enteric gram-negative bacilli, gram-positive cocci	*High risk only:* cefazolin	1–2 g iv
Biliary tract	Enteric gram-negative bacilli, enterococci, clostridia	*High risk only:* cefazolin	1–2 g iv
Colorectal	Enteric gram-negative bacilli, anaerobes	*Oral:* neomycin + erythromycin base	1–2 g po
Appendectomy	Enteric gram-negative bacilli, anaerobes	*Parenteral:* cefoxitin or cefotetan	1–2 g iv

iv—intravenously; po—orally.

FIGURE 1-27 Recommendations for prophylactic antibiotics in gastrointestinal surgery. (*Adapted from* [6].)

PERITONITIS

Classification of peritonitis

Primary peritonitis
  Spontaneous peritonitis of childhood
  Spontaneous peritonitis of adult
  Peritonitis in CAPD
  Tuberculous peritonitis
Secondary peritonitis
  Spontaneous peritonitis (spontaneous acute)
      Gastrointestinal tract perforation
      Bowel wall necrosis
      Pelvic peritonitis
      Peritonitis after translocation of bacteria
  Postoperative peritonitis
      Anastomotic leak
      Leak at suture line
      Stump insufficiency
      Other iatrogenic leaks
  Posttraumatic peritonitis
      Blunt abdominal trauma
      Penetrating abdominal trauma
Tertiary peritonitis
      Peritonitis without pathogens
      Peritonitis with fungi
      Peritonitis with low-grade pathogenic bacteria
Intra-abdominal abscess

CAPD—continuous ambulatory peritoneal dialysis.

FIGURE 1-28 Classification of peritonitis. Peritonitis is inflammation of the serous lining of the peritoneal cavity and represents a response to various factors, including microbial agents and chemical irritants. The peritoneum covers all of the intestinal organs and abdominal wall, diaphragm, retroperitoneum, and pelvis, comprising a total area comparable to the surface area of the skin. The classification of peritonitis illustrates the various causes. Primary or spontaneous peritonitis occurs without an evident or focal gastrointestinal source (such as a perforated viscus). Secondary peritonitis, on the other hand, is associated with an antecedent gastrointestinal lesion or event and involves the gastrointestinal flora. Numerous intra-abdominal processes may give rise to peritonitis, including disease, trauma, or surgery involving any part of the gastrointestinal or genitourinary tract. Tertiary peritonitis is a new entity that encompasses patients recovering from secondary peritonitis who experience an ongoing failure of host defenses without a "true" infectious challenge. Intra-abdominal abscess may develop in all three classes of peritonitis. (*Adapted from* Condon and Wittmann [7].)

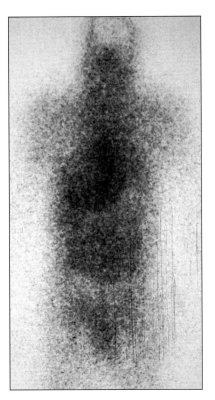

FIGURE 1-29 Technetium radionuclide scan showing diffuse peritonitis. One rarely needs to resort to this type of study to make the diagnosis.

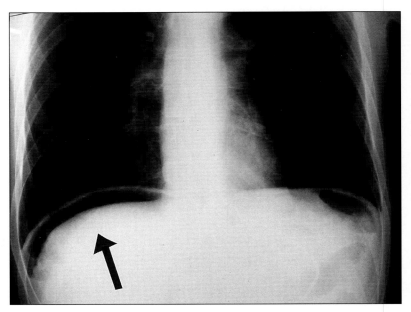

FIGURE 1-30 Abdominal radiograph showing free air under the diaphragm. The pneumoperitoneum is most easily seen under the right diaphragm (*arrow*). This picture may be seen in the immediate postoperative period as a result of exposure of the peritoneal cavity to air. In general, this finding indicates perforation of the bowel, but it may be seen occasionally in perforation of cysts in pneumatosis cystoides intestinalis or gas-producing infection in the free peritoneal cavity.

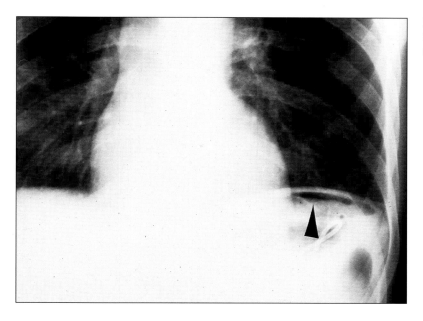

FIGURE 1-31 Abdominal radiograph showing "air" accumulation under the left diaphragm (*arrowhead*) in a patient with peritonitis secondary to perforation of a duodenal ulcer.

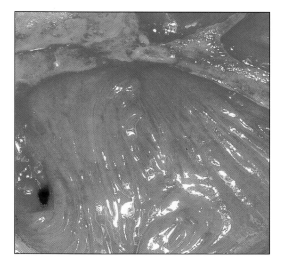

FIGURE 1-32 Small bowel fistula to the anterior abdominal wall. This type of fistula would be encountered most commonly as a complication of inflammatory bowel disease. Fistulae usually form as a result of direct extension of an ulcer, from spontaneous decompression of an abscess, or after therapeutic drainage of an abscess. Enteric or colorectal fistulae occur in 20% to 40% of patients with Crohn's disease but are rare in ulcerative colitis. Fistulae usually require surgical management supplemented by antimicrobial therapy. Occasionally, antimicrobial therapy alone may be adequate, particularly with perianal fistulae. The microbiology of fistulae has not been well studied, but clearly the luminal flora is involved, and the invasion of tissues by this flora is the rationale for antimicrobial therapy.

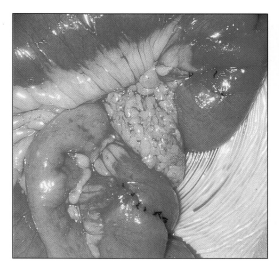

FIGURE 1-33 Small bowel obstruction secondary to an omental band. The bowel is dilated, and the serosal surface shows vascular congestion and some areas of minor hemorrhage. Without surgical decompression (relief of the obstruction), an inflammatory reaction would ultimately lead to migration of luminal organisms to the serosal surface, setting up peritonitis and perhaps intra-abdominal abscess.

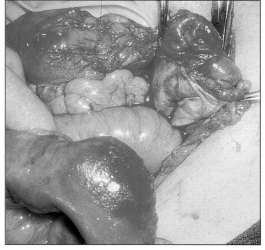

FIGURE 1-34 Segment of small bowel with one wall trapped in a Richter's hernia. This entity results when a portion of the antimesenteric wall of the bowel becomes strangulated within a hernia sac. The entrapped portion of the bowel may become gangrenous, and if the strangulation is not recognized and relieved early by appropriate surgery, abscess formation may result.

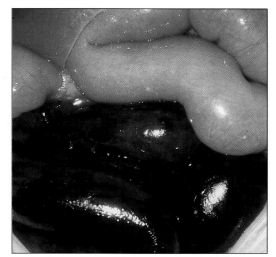

FIGURE 1-35 Strangulation obstruction leading to gangrene of the bowel secondary to volvulus, in turn related to an adhesion. Surgical management is primary and must be carried out promptly when the integrity of the bowel is compromised.

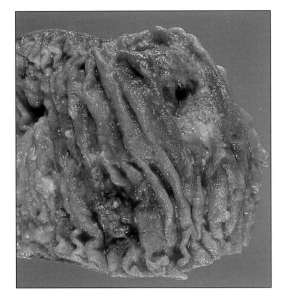

Figure 1-36 Gross specimen showing enterocolitis due to cytomegalovirus (CMV), with perforation, in an AIDS patient. This entity may also occur in transplant patients. Approximately 20% of AIDS patients develop CMV gastrointestinal disease at some time. Discrete ulcers, which may be quite large, are produced in the colon (and upper gastrointestinal tract, when that is involved). The surrounding mucosa, as in this patient, may be edematous, erythematous, granular, and friable. Localized CMV disease is more common in the right colon, but the rectosigmoid region is commonly involved in AIDS patients. Distal small bowel involvement is rare. Diagnosis requires colonoscopy, and because the changes are not specific for CMV (and the mucosa may even appear normal), biopsies should be taken. When ulcers are present, the biopsies should be from the ulcer base. The right colon is most likely to yield inclusion bodies on biopsy. Histologic examination is best for diagnosis; viral cultures may take weeks to become positive. Ganciclovir therapy is worth trying, but not all patients respond.

A. Organisms recovered in spontaneous bacterial peritonitis: Gram-negative bacteria

Gram-negative bacilli
Enterobacteriaceae
  Citrobacter amalonaticus
  Enterobacter aerogenes
  Enterobacter cloacae
  Escherichia coli
  Klebsiella pneumoniae
  Proteus
  Providencia
  Salmonella
  Serratia
  Yersinia enterocolitica

Other
  Acinetobacter
  Aeromonas hydrophila
  Aeromonas sobria
  Brucella melitensis
  Campylobacter fetus
  Flavobacterium meningosepticum
  Haemophilus
  Moraxella
  Pasteurella multocida
  Pseudomonas aeruginosa

Gram-negative cocci
  Neisseria meningitidis
  Neisseria gonorrheae

B. Organisms recovered in spontaneous bacterial peritonitis: Gram-positive bacteria

Gram-positive cocci
  Enterococcus faecium
  E. faecalis
  Streptococcus group A
  Streptococcus group B
  Streptococcus group D
    (nonenterococcal)
  Streptococcus (viridans group)
  Streptococcus, γ-hemolytic
  Streptococcus pneumoniae
  Staphylococcus aureus
  Other staphylococci

Gram-positive bacilli
  Bacillus
  Corynebacterium
  Listeria monocytogenes

C. Organisms recovered from spontaneous bacterial peritonitis: Anaerobes and other organisms

Anaerobes
  Bacteroides fragilis
  Bacteroides spp
  Clostridium perfringens
  C. cadaveris
  Lactobacillus
  Microaerophilic streptococci
  Peptostreptococcus anaerobius
  Peptostreptococcus spp
  Propionibacterium

Other
  Candida
  Chlamydia trachomatis
  Cytomegalovirus
  ECHO virus type 4
  Measles virus
  Rubella virus
  Mycobacterium tuberculosis
  Mycoplasma

ECHO—enteric cytopathogenic human orphan.

Figure 1-37 Organisms recovered in spontaneous bacterial peritonitis (SBP). **A,** Gram-negative bacteria. **B,** Gram-positive bacteria. **C,** Anaerobes and other organisms. The frequency with which bowel organisms are recovered in SBP suggests that the gut is the major source of infection, although other sources including the genitourinary tract may also contribute. Before antimicrobials were available, *Streptococcus pneumoniae* and group A streptococci were important agents of SBP in children, but these organisms are less prevalent today and have been replaced by gram-negative bacilli and, to a lesser extent, staphylococci. In adults, gram-negative bacilli also dominate, followed by streptococci and gram-positive cocci. (*Adapted from* Finegold and Johnson [8].)

Common organisms associated with CAPD-related peritonitis	
Gram-positive bacteria	60%–70%
Staphylococcus (coagulase-negative)	30%–45%
Staphylococcus aureus	10%–20%
Streptococcus	10%–15%
Enterococcus	3%–5%
Diphtheroids	1%–2%
Gram-negative bacteria	20%–30%
Enterobacteriaceae	10%–20%
Pseudomonas aeruginosa	5%–10%
Other	2%–3%
Fungi	5%–15%
Mycobacteria	0%–3%
Anaerobes, polymicrobial	0%–10%

CAPD—continuous ambulatory peritoneal dialysis.

FIGURE 1-38 Common organisms associated with continuous ambulatory peritoneal dialysis (CAPD)-related peritonitis. Peritonitis remains the most common complication of CAPD and is a primary reason for discontinuing use of this dialysis technique in patients. Overall, the average incidence of peritonitis is 1.3 to 1.4 episodes per patient per year of dialysis, although the rates vary considerably among individual patients and facilities. Peritonitis is usually caused by a single pathogen that originates from the normal flora of the skin or upper respiratory tract. (*Adapted from* Finegold and Johnson [8].)

Clinical manifestations of CAPD-associated peritonitis	
Cloudy dialysate	90%–100%
Abdominal pain	70%–80%
Fever	35%–60%
Nausea, vomiting	25%–35%
Diarrhea	< 10%
Abdominal tenderness	50%–80%
Drainage problems	15%
Peripheral leukocytes	30%–45%

CAPD—continuous ambulatory peritoneal dialysis.

FIGURE 1-39 Clinical manifestations of continuous ambulatory peritoneal dialysis (CAPD)-associated peritonitis. Criteria for the diagnosis of CAPD-associated peritonitis include: 1) signs and symptoms of peritoneal irritation; 2) cloudy dialysate effluent with a leukocyte count > 100/mm^3; and 3) positive culture of dialysate fluid. Any two of these criteria may be adequate to establish the diagnosis. Signs and symptoms of peritonitis vary from mild to severe, depending largely on the virulence of the pathogen and time course of the infection. (*Adapted from* Finegold and Johnson [8].)

INTRAPERITONEAL INFECTION

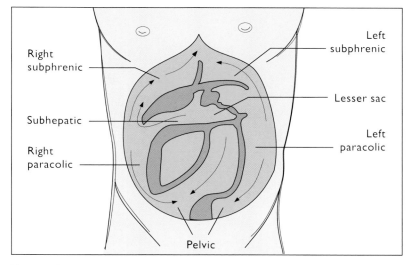

FIGURE 1-40 Diagram of the intraperitoneal spaces, showing the circulation of fluid and potential areas for abscess formation.

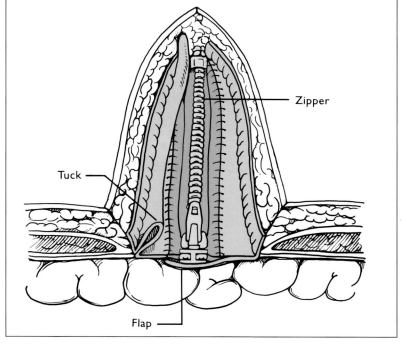

FIGURE 1-41 Zipper prosthesis for closure of abdomen in patients having planned relaparotomy approach. In severe intra-abdominal infections, reoperation for drainage may be required on multiple occasions. This "open" abdomen approach was subsequently developed so that open management and repeated drainage could be carried out. The inserted Marlex mesh with a zipper permits daily aggressive manual lavage and any needed drainage rapidly and simply. It is well tolerated [9].

Appendicitis

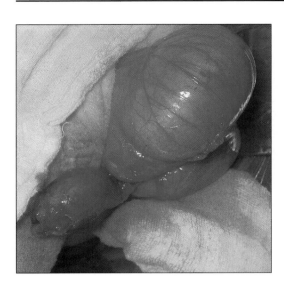

FIGURE 1-42 Intraoperative view of acute appendicitis, without gangrene or perforation. The cecum is distended. The risk of intra-abdominal or wound infection following surgery for this entity is very low; cultures of such appendices are often sterile and, when not, yield relatively low counts and often only one or two different organisms.

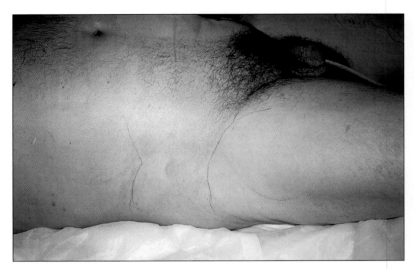

FIGURE 1-43 Right flank of a patient with appendicitis with perforation. Note the right-lower-quadrant cellulitis and edema. Appendectomy, with drainage of any intraperitoneal fluid or pus collection, and antimicrobial therapy constitute the therapy of choice. A large number of organisms is recovered from appendiceal tissue (avoiding the lumen) or intraperitoneal abscesses, and anaerobic bacteria predominate over nonanaerobes (*see* Fig. 1-45).

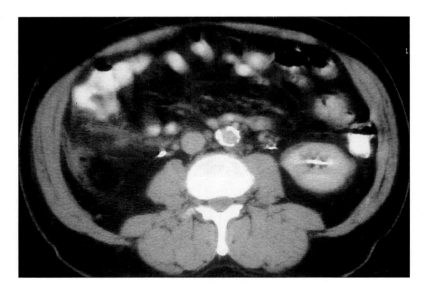

FIGURE 1-44 Computed tomography scan showing a right-lower-quadrant phlegmon and abscess secondary to perforated appendicitis. In patients with an unclear history and generalized peritonitis, such studies may reveal the underlying problem.

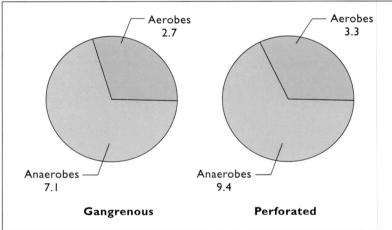

Aerobes 2.7
Anaerobes 7.1
Gangrenous

Aerobes 3.3
Anaerobes 9.4
Perforated

FIGURE 1-45 Pie chart diagram depicting the frequency of aerobic and anaerobic bacteria recovered from patients with gangrenous and perforated appendicitis. In both cases, anaerobes show a marked predominance. Mean counts of organisms recovered were 9.8 in patients with gangrenous appendicitis and 12.7 in patients with perforated appendicitis. Anaerobes predominated in both cases by almost 3:1. Among the nonaerobes, *Escherichia coli* and streptococci were the most common. Among the anaerobes, the main isolates were members of the *Bacteroides fragilis* group (*B. fragilis* and *B. thetaiotaomicron*), anaerobic cocci, and *Bilophila wadsworthia*.

A. Aerobic and anaerobic species isolated from patients with gangrenous or perforated appendicitis: Aerobic and facultative bacteria

	Gangrenous, % (*n*=27)	Perforated, % (*n*=44)	All, % (*n*=71)
Escherichia coli	70.4	77.3	74.6
Viridans streptococci	18.5	43.2	33.8
Streptococcus group D	7.4	27.3	19.7
Pseudomonas aeruginosa	11.1	18.2	15.5
Enterococcus spp	18.5	9.1	12.7
Staphylococcus spp	14.8	11.4	12.7
Pseudomonas spp	7.4	9.1	8.5
Citrobacter freundii	3.7	6.8	5.6
β-Hemolytic streptococci group F	7.4	4.5	5.6
β-Hemolytic streptococci group C	3.7	4.5	4.2
Enterobacter spp	7.4	2.3	4.2
Klebsiella spp	3.7	4.5	4.2
β-Hemolytic streptococci group G	0	4.5	2.8
Moraxella spp	3.7	2.3	2.8
Corynebacterium spp	0	2.3	1.4
Serratia marcescens	3.7	0	1.4
Eikenella corrodens	0	2.3	1.4
Hafnia alvei	3.7	0	1.4
Haemophilus influenzae	0	2.3	1.4

B. Aerobic and anaerobic species isolated from patients with gangrenous or perforated appendicitis: Anaerobic bacteria

	Gangrenous, % (*n*=27)	Perforated, % (*n*=44)	All, % (*n*=71)
Bacteroides fragilis	70.1	79.5	76.1
B. thetaiotaomicron	48.1	61.4	56.3
Bilophila wadsworthia	37.0	54.5	47.9
Peptostreptococcus micros	44.4	45.5	45.1
Eubacterium spp	40.7	29.5	33.8
B. intermedius	33.3	27.3	29.6
B. vulgatus	18.5	34.1	28.2
B. splanchnicus	25.9	27.3	26.8
Fusobacterium spp	22.2	27.3	25.4
B. ovatus	18.5	27.3	23.9
Microaerophilic streptococci	29.6	20.5	23.9
Peptostreptococcus spp	29.6	18.2	22.5
Lactobacillus spp	22.2	20.5	21.1
B. uniformis	22.2	18.2	19.7
B. distasonis	14.8	20.5	18.3
Clostridium clostridioforme	18.5	18.2	18.3
B. gracilis	11.1	15.9	14.1
Actinomyces spp	11.1	11.4	11.3
C. ramosum	11.1	9.1	9.9
Porphyromonas spp	18.5	2.3	8.5
B. buccae	3.7	6.8	5.6
B. caccae	7.4	4.5	5.6
C. innocuum	7.4	4.5	5.6
B. stercoris	7.4	4.5	5.6
C. sporogenes	3.7	6.8	5.6
Propionibacterium acnes	7.4	4.5	5.6
C. leptum	11.1	0	4.2
Desulfomonas spp	3.7	4.5	4.2
Unidentified gram-negative rod	37.0	36.4	36.6
Unidentified gram-positive rod	14.8	29.5	23.9
Unidentified pigmenting rod	18.5	18.2	18.3

FIGURE 1-46
Aerobic and anaerobic species isolated from patients with gangrenous or perforated appendicitis. **A,** Aerobic and facultative bacteria. **B,** Anaerobic bacteria [10]. (*Adapted from* Finegold and Johnson [8].)

96-195

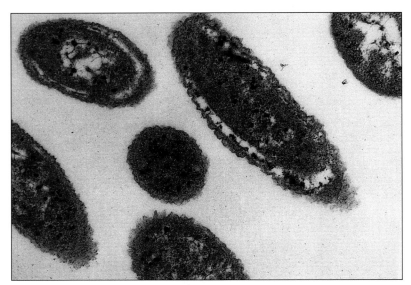

FIGURE 1-47 Transmission electron micrograph of *Bilophila wadsworthia*. This organism was the third most common anaerobic isolate from patients with gangrenous or perforated appendicitis and is found frequently in intra-abdominal infections of other types. It is an anaerobic gram-negative rod that is fairly fastidious and may take up to 1 week to grow. It is resistant to bile and therefore may be detected on *Bacteroides* bile esculin medium, which is selective for the *Bacteroides fragilis* group. Most strains are β-lactamase-positive and therefore resistant to many β-lactam antibiotics. *Bilophila* is found in the stool of most subjects studied, but only at counts of about 10^6/g. The fact that it is so prominent in infections despite relatively low counts in normal bowel flora is an indication of its virulence; the same situation occurs with *B. fragilis*. Bilophila is also found in a small percentage of saliva and vaginal fluid samples from normal individuals and occurs on occasion in a wide variety of infections throughout the body.

Diverticulitis

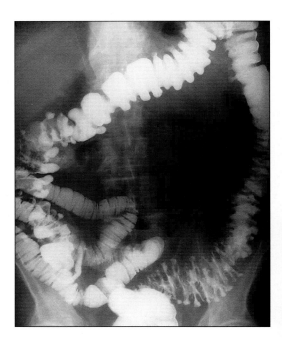

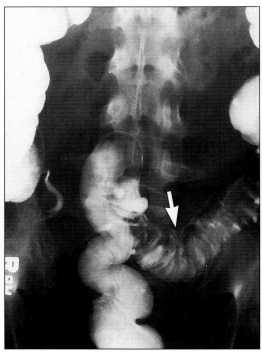

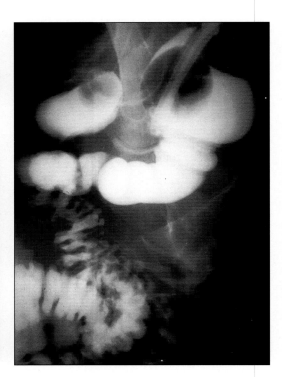

FIGURE 1-48 Barium enema showing multiple diverticula throughout the colon and sigmoid. Computed tomography (CT) scan with oral and rectal contrast material is now the procedure of first choice, because CT scans are more sensitive than radiologic examinations and better demonstrate the extent and complications of diverticular inflammation. When diverticulitis is suspected but not found, the CT scan more often shows an alternative etiology for the signs and symptoms. The value of sonography in the work-up of diverticulitis is not yet established.

FIGURE 1-49 Barium radiograph demonstrating acute diverticulitis with intramural sinus formation (*arrow*). Obstruction at the mouth of a diverticulum secondary to impaction of fecal material (fecalith) is believed to be the initiating event of diverticulitis. The obstruction leads to a compromised blood supply, and with ischemia, the risk of bacterial invasion increases. Microperforation of the colon wall leads to focal extravasation of luminal contents, in turn leading to a pericolic phlegmon. Next, necrosis occurs and a pericolic abscess is formed in the colonic mesentery.

FIGURE 1-50 Barium enema showing acute diverticulitis of the sigmoid colon.

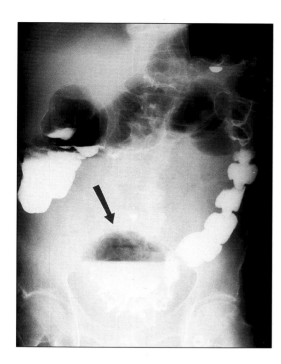

FIGURE 1-51 Pelvic abscess with large air-fluid level (*arrow*) secondary to a perforated diverticulitis. Following micro-perforation of the colon wall and necrosis, a pericolic abscess is formed in the colonic mesentery. This abscess may then enlarge and perforate to form a pelvic abscess. Rupture of the pelvic abscess would lead to generalized peritonitis and sepsis.

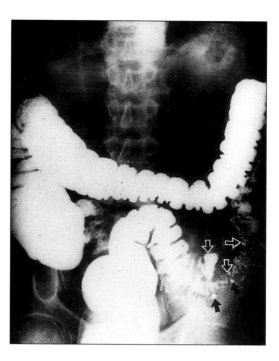

FIGURE 1-52 Barium enema of a patient with multiple diverticula, with a pericolonic abscess due to a ruptured diverticulum. The pericolonic abscess (*arrows*) is filled with barium.

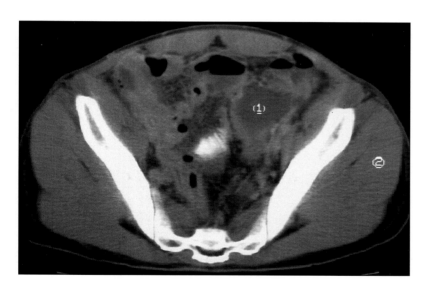

FIGURE 1-53 Pelvic computed tomography scan showing a left-lower-quadrant abscess secondary to diverticulitis (labeled *1*).

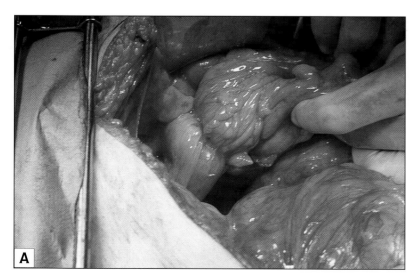

FIGURE 1-54 Colovesical fistula secondary to perforated diverticulitis. **A,** Operative view of colovesical fistula. (*continued*)

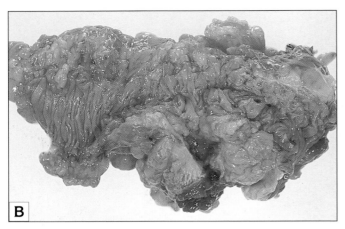

FIGURE 1-54 (*continued*) **B,** Resected specimen with colovesical fistula. In addition to pelvic abscess, complications that may be seen in diverticular disease include localized abscess, obstruction of the colon or small bowel by mass effect, and fistula formation. Therapy varies with the stage of the process. Patients with localized peritoneal irritation, abdominal pain, fever, and leukocytosis should be hospitalized and treated with bowel rest, hydration, and antimicrobial agents. More advanced disease or failure to respond to a medical regimen may require surgery, either a single or staged procedure. Staged procedures involve a first procedure with drainage, resection of the involved bowel, and a colostomy and then a second procedure for restoration of bowel continuity after approximately 3 months. Percutaneous drainage of abscesses may be feasible in certain situations.

Biliary Tract Infection

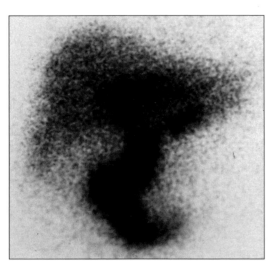

FIGURE 1-55 HIDA scan demonstrating acalculous cholecystitis. Obstruction of the common bile duct can be diagnosed by hepatobiliary scanning with the HIDA derivative. In this case, no component of the biliary system or small bowel is visualized, despite adequate hepatic uptake.

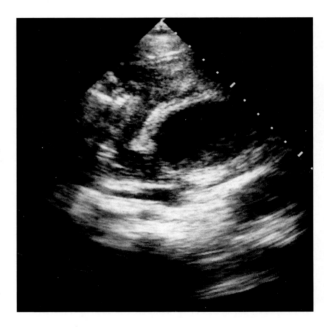

FIGURE 1-56 Ultrasound of acalculous cholecystitis showing dilated gallbladder and thickened gallbladder wall, with no stones. Ultrasound is useful for demonstrating gallbladder size, presence of stones, and degree of bile duct dilatation.

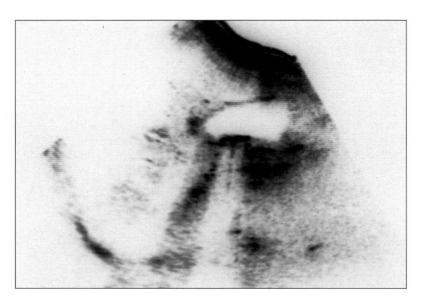

FIGURE 1-57 Ultrasound showing simple cholecystitis with gallstones and penumbra. In more than 90% of cases of acute cholecystitis, gallstones are impacted in the cystic duct. It is assumed that a sudden change in the degree of obstruction leads to a sudden increase in intraductal pressures, producing gallbladder distension and compromising blood supply and lymphatic drainage. This may proceed to necrosis of tissues and proliferation of bacteria.

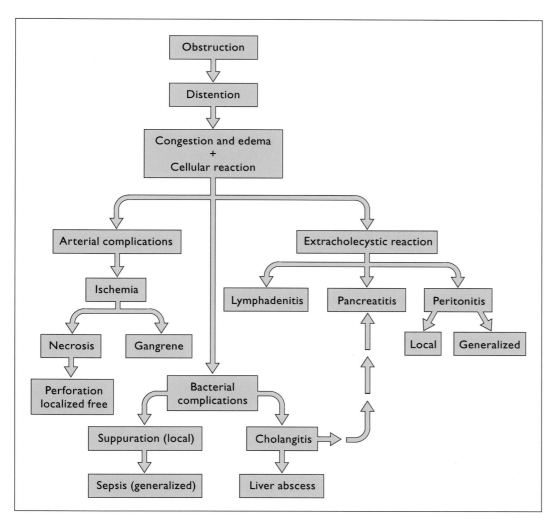

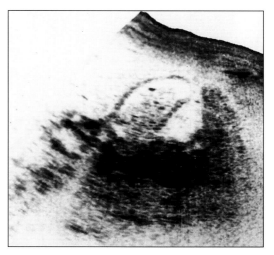

FIGURE 1-58 Pathogenesis of acute chole-cystitis. Infection develops in more than half of cases of cholecystitis. Infective complications include empyema of the gallbladder, gangrene of the gallbladder, emphysematous cholecystitis, pericholecystic abscess, cholangitis, liver abscess, peritonitis, intraperitoneal abscess, and bacteremia. (*Adapted from* Levison and Bush [11].)

Microorganisms in bile in acute cholecystitis

Aerobes–174 (87%)			
Gram-negative	132 (66%)	Gram-positive	42 (21%)
Escherichia coli	77	*Enterococcus faecalis*	30
Klebsiella	22	β-Hemolytic streptococci	4
Proteus	13	*Staphylococcus epidermidis*	4
Enterobacter	8	Viridans streptococcus	1
Pseudomonas	4		
Anaerobes–25 (13%)			
Gram-negative	2(1%)	Gram-positive	23 (12%)
Bacteroides spp	2	*Clostridium perfringens*	16
		Peptostreptococcus	7

FIGURE 1-60 Ultrasound showing cholecystitis with thickened gallbladder wall, gallstones, and an abscess adjacent to the gallbladder.

FIGURE 1-59 Microorganisms in bile in acute cholecystitis. The bacteriologic findings from one study of 199 cases are presented. The bacteria responsible for gallbladder infections reflects the normal bowel flora, particularly the duodenum. The duodenal flora in these patients is not uncommonly abnormal as a result of such factors as achlorhydria, gastric or small bowel obstruction, and small bowel diverticula or blind loops. The infecting flora of biliary tract infections usually includes *Escherichia coli, Klebsiella, Enterobacter,* and enterococci. Anaerobes are found with some frequency, particularly *Clostridium perfringens* and *Bacteroides fragilis.* Anaerobic or polymicrobic infections (involving anaerobes) are seen more often in elderly patients and those who have undergone previous biliary tract surgical procedures or manipulations. These patients usually have more severe symptoms and a higher incidence of complications. (*Adapted from* Keighley [12].)

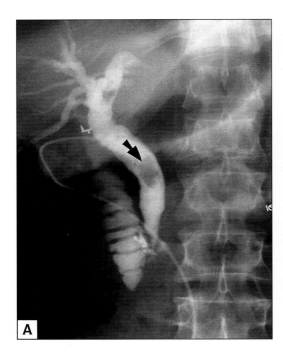

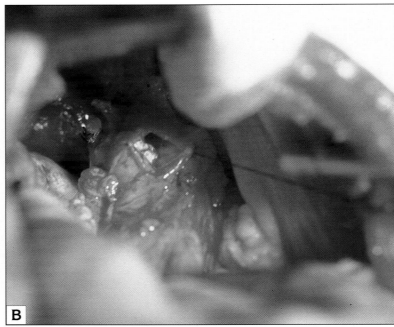

FIGURE 1-61
Acute cholecystitis.
A. Operative cholangiogram with a common bile duct stone (*arrow*). **B.** Operative view of the same patient shows the common bile duct stone and ascending cholangitis.

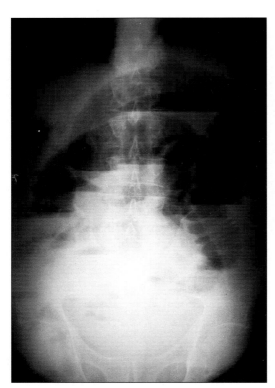

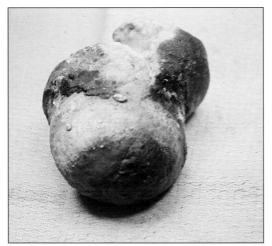

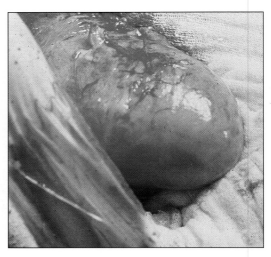

FIGURE 1-63 Large gallstone removed from a patient with gallstone ileus. The gallstone was removed from the patient shown in Figure 1-62.

FIGURE 1-64 Surgical view of empyema of the gallbladder.

FIGURE 1-62 Classic findings of "gallstone ileus" on flat plate radiograph of the abdomen. Small bowel obstruction (dilated loops of bowel with air-fluid levels) and air in the biliary tree can be seen.

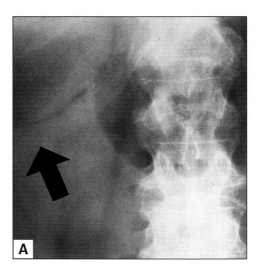

FIGURE 1-65 Emphysematous cholecystitis. **A.** The typical findings of emphysematous cholecystitis are seen on a flat plate radiograph of the abdomen. The *arrow* points to a rim of gas. (*continued*)

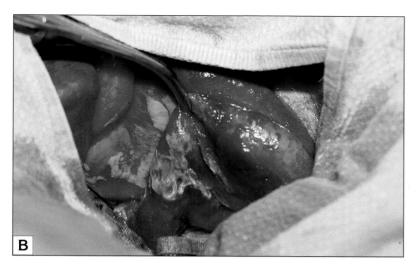

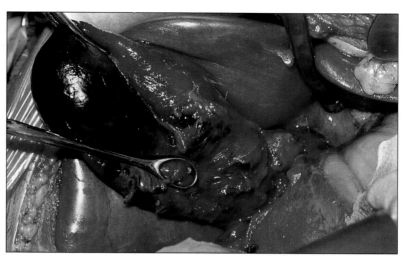

FIGURE 1-65 (*continued*) **B.** Surgery reveals empyema of the gallbladder with necrosis of the gallbladder wall.

FIGURE 1-66 Operative view of gangrenous cholecystitis (acalculous). The gallbladder is reflected upward.

Liver Abscess

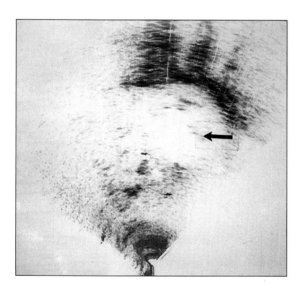

FIGURE 1-67 Abdominal ultrasound of a liver abscess. The *arrow* points to the abscess. The clinical picture of liver abscess involves fever, sometimes with chills, and aching right-upper-quadrant pain that may radiate to the right shoulder and be aggravated by inspiration. Percussion over the liver is painful, and fullness or localized edema may be noted over the lower thoracic or upper abdominal wall. Pulmonary symptoms and findings may be associated with abscesses high in the right lobe of the liver. The course is usually indolent. Laboratory abnormalities include leukocytosis with left shift, elevation of the serum alkaline phosphatase without other liver function test abnormalities. Blood cultures are positive in one third to one half of patients. Computed tomography (CT), ultrasound, and radionuclide studies are the most valuable procedures for diagnosing liver abscess. Percutaneous aspiration may be undertaken for diagnostic purposes and especially to obtain material for direct examination and culture. Most patients can be managed by percutaneous drainage under ultrasound or CT guidance plus antimicrobial therapy.

Associated conditions in liver abscess		
	Literature review	**Duke University Hospital**
	1954–1979 (*n*=885)	**1968–1982 (*n*=55)**
Biliary tract disease	33%	36%
Neoplastic disease	10%	22%
Portal system infection	12%	12%
Other infection	13%	15%
Trauma	3%	4%
Unknown	21%	15%

FIGURE 1-68 Associated conditions in liver abscess. Most cases of liver abscess are secondary to pyelophlebitis or suppurative cholangitis. Embolic abscesses are also seen. Infection may extend directly, or by way of lymphatics, following perforated gallbladder or duodenal ulcer, or from pancreatic abscess, perinephric or subphrenic abscess, or even lung abscess or thoracic empyema. Cryptogenic liver abscesses are not uncommon. (*Adapted from* Bartlett [13].)

Bacteriology of liver abcesses

	Liver isolates, *n*	Blood isolates, *n*
Anaerobes	30	14
Peptostreptococcus	6	2
Microaerophilic streptococci	7	7
Fusobacteria	5	1
Bacteroides fragilis	5	2
Other *Bacteroides* spp	5	2
Aerobes	7	6
Streptococci	4	3
Escherichia coli	2	2
Proteus	1	0

FIGURE 1-69 Bacteriology of liver abscesses. Prior to the advent of antibiotics, *Escherichia coli* and streptococci were the principal etiologic agents of liver abscess. Subsequently, other gram-negative bacilli, such as *Klebsiella, Enterobacter, Proteus,* and *Pseudomonas,* have been found with increasing frequency. The exact incidence of anaerobic infections is uncertain, but it appears that if proper collection, transport, and culture techniques were used, anaerobes would be found in at least 50% of patients, often in the absence of other flora. The most commonly encountered anaerobes are gram-negative bacilli (especially *Bacteroides fragilis, Fusobacterium,* and *Prevotella*) and anaerobic and microaerophilic streptococci.

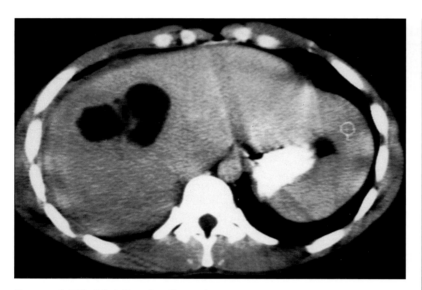

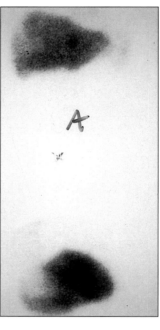

FIGURE 1-71 Liver abscess seen on technetium scan. The defect in the liver (lack of technetium uptake) indicates the space-occupying abscess.

FIGURE 1-70 Multilocular liver abscess on computed tomography scan. Multiple or multilocular liver abscesses are more common than solitary abscesses.

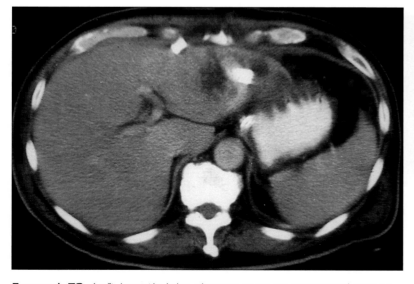

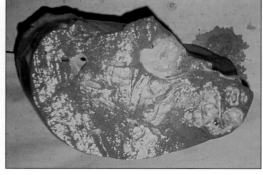

FIGURE 1-73 Autopsy specimen showing multiple pyogenic liver abscesses. The patient had *Bacteroides* bacteremia.

FIGURE 1-72 Left hepatic lobe abscess seen on computed tomography scan.

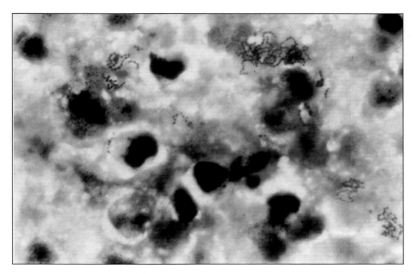

FIGURE 1-74 Direct Gram stain from liver abscess showing chains of tiny streptococci that proved to be microaerophilic streptococci.

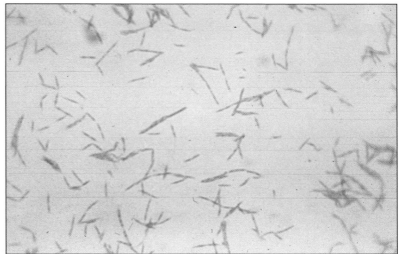

FIGURE 1-75 Microscopic appearance of *Fusobacterium nucleatum* in pure culture. Note the thin organisms with tapered ends. This organism is seen with some frequency in liver abscess.

FIGURE 1-76 Signs and symptoms of amebic liver abscess [15,16]. (*Adapted from* Reed and Ravdin [17].)

Signs and symptoms of amebic liver abscess

Presentation	Adams and MacLeod (*n*=2074)	Katzenstein *et al.* (*n*=67) Acute	Chronic
Symptom			
Fever	75	85	32
Diarrhea	14	30	30
Weight loss	NR	20	60
Cough	11	5	7
Sign			
Tender liver	80	90	90
Hepatomegaly	80	25	60
Rales/rhonchi	47	27	60

NR—not reported.

FIGURE 1-77 Complications of amebic liver abscesses [15]. (*Adapted from* Reed and Ravdin [17].)

Complications of amebic liver abscesses

Complications	Cases, *n*	Cases, %	Mortality, %
Pulmonary	146	7.8	6.2
Pleural effusion/empyema		29.0	
Hepatobronchial fistula		47.0	
Lung abscess		14.0	
Consolidation		10.0	
Abdominal rupture	38	2.0	18.4
Pericardial rupture	27	1.4	29.6

Pancreatic Infections

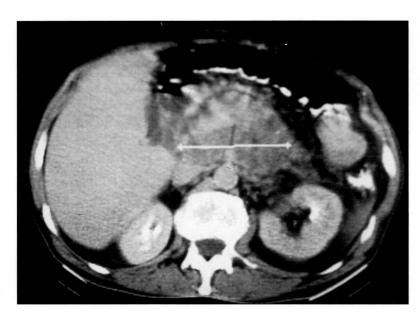

FIGURE 1-78 Computed tomography scan showing pancreatic phlegmon. Pancreatic phlegmon, or abscess, develops principally as a complication of pancreatitis of any origin (alcoholic, biliary, postoperative, or trauma-related). Infected pancreatic necrosis may also occur, less commonly, as a complication of endoscopic retrograde cholangiopancreatography, of posterior penetrating peptic ulcer, or as a secondary infection of a pseudocyst. Approximately two thirds of pancreatic abscesses are multiple; they may be solitary or multilocular.

Presenting symptoms and signs of pancreatic infections in 45 patients

Sign or symptom	No.	%
Fever	39	87
Abdominal pain	37	82
Abdominal tenderness	28	62
Palpable mass	22	50
Nausea or vomiting	21	47
Distention	12	27
Jaundice	7	16
Systemic sepsis	3	7
Pulmonary failure	2	4
Gastrointestinal bleeding	1	2

FIGURE 1-79 Presenting symptoms and signs of pancreatic infections in 45 patients. After initial improvement in a patient with pancreatitis, persistence of fever, ileus, and tenderness, or frank deterioration of the patient's condition should raise the question of abscess. Most cases manifest pain, usually epigastric in location and commonly radiating to the back or flank. Nausea and vomiting, tenderness over the area of the abscess, and guarding or rebound on examination are common. A mass or fullness may be noted. The clinical picture is nonspecific, and one cannot reliably distinguish between pancreatic abscess, sterile or infected pancreatic necrosis, and sterile or infected pancreatic pseudocyst. (*Adapted from* Klar and Warshaw [18].)

Microorganisms isolated in 45 pancreatic infections*

Escherichia	22
Enterococcus	17
Staphylococcus	16
Klebsiella	6
Proteus	4
Candida albicans	3
Pseudomonas	3
Streptococcus	2
Torulopsis glabrata	1
Haemophilus parainfluenzae	1
Diphtheroids	1
Serratia marcescens	1
Unidentified gram-positive organism	5

*> 1 organism was isolated from 20 specimens.

FIGURE 1-80 Microorganisms isolated in 45 pancreatic infections. Enteric organisms are isolated most often from pancreatic abscess, with approximately half of the cases showing a polymicrobial flora. *Escherichia coli* is the most commonly encountered organism (~35% of cases), with enterococci, viridans streptococci, and *Klebsiella* each found in approximately 20% of cases. Staphylococci and other gram-negative rods occur in < 10% of cases, with *Candida* seen only occasionally. Studies of anaerobes are not adequate to permit accurate assessment of their incidence or role in pancreatic abscess, but various studies have found them in 6% to 16% of cases, and anaerobes, including *Bacteroides fragilis*, have been found in bacteremia accompanying pancreatic abscess. The bacteriology of the infected pancreas suggests an enteric source, but animal studies have revealed that bacteria may reach the pancreas from many sources, including the colon, gallbladder, and urinary tract, as well as via the circulation, main pancreatic duct, and transperitoneally. (*Adapted from* Klar and Warshaw [18].)

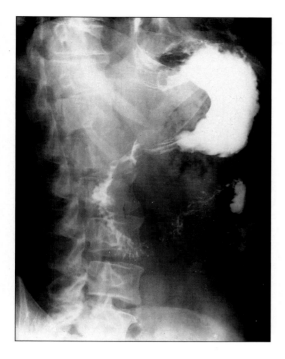

FIGURE 1-81   Abdominal radiograph showing pancreatic abscess. Note the widened duodenal loop on upper gastrointestinal study. Computed tomography (CT) scanning is the most reliable diagnostic aid, detecting pancreatic infection in 75% of cases. It also provides information on the site and size of the collection. High-dose intravenous contrast infusion in combination with CT is said to be very helpful in predicting pancreatic necrosis. Percutaneous CT-guided aspiration of material for Gram stain and culture is the most reliable way to differentiate secondary pancreatic infection from pancreatic inflammation. Blood cultures should always be done.

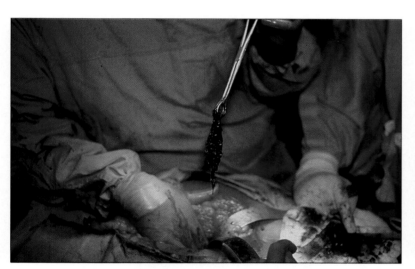

FIGURE 1-82   Operative view with necrotic retroperitoneal debris being removed from a patient with infected pancreatitis. The principal therapeutic approaches to pancreatic abscess are surgical debridement and drainage, percutaneous drainage, and antimicrobial therapy.

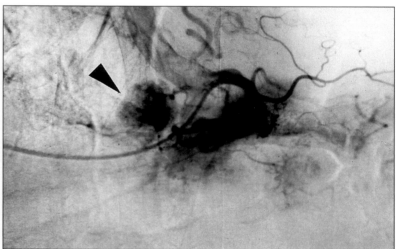

FIGURE 1-83   Arteriogram showing pseudoaneurysm (*arrowhead*) of pancreaticoduodenal arteries in pancreatitis.

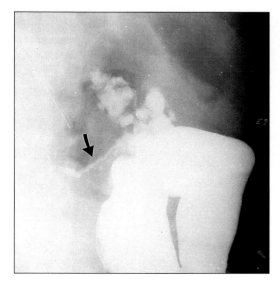

FIGURE 1-84   Barium study showing perforation of splenic flexure of the colon secondary to severe necrotizing pancreatitis. The *arrow* shows the pancreatic duct. Complications of pancreatic infection include perforation into the peritoneal cavity or into the stomach, bowel, biliary tree, or a bronchus; hemorrhage into the abscess cavity; gastrointestinal bleeding; empyema; bacteremia; and diabetes mellitus.

Intra-abdominal Abscesses

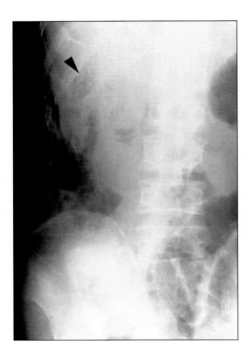

FIGURE 1-85 Abdominal radiograph showing gas in an abscess cavity (*arrowhead*) in the right upper quadrant. Intra-peritoneal abscesses are walled off from the rest of the peritoneal cavity by inflammatory adhesions, loops of bowel and their mesentery, the greater omentum, and other abdominal viscera. The principal anatomic sites of abscesses within the abdomen are the subphrenic areas (including subhepatic and right and left subdiaphragmatic abscesses), pelvis, lumbar gutters, and intermesenteric folds.

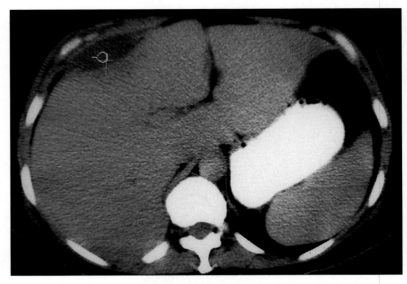

FIGURE 1-86 Right subdiaphragmatic abscess detected by computed tomography scan. Subphrenic abscess is related etiologically primarily to the stomach, duodenum, or biliary tract, with relatively few cases related to appendicitis. It may also relate to the lower bowel or female genital tract, as well as to abdominal surgery or trauma. The major routes of infection are by direct extension or via lymphatic drainage. The suprahepatic space is much more likely to be involved with abscess than the subhepatic space.

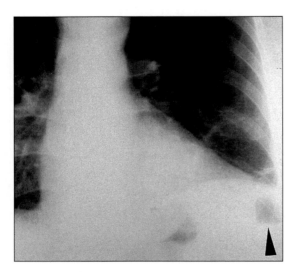

FIGURE 1-87 Chest radiograph showing elevated left diaphragm, atelectasis, left pleural effusion, and subdiaphragmatic gas (*arrowhead*) due to left subphrenic abscess. Intra-abdominal abscess presents with a variable clinical picture, ranging from an acute process with rigors, high fever, and abdominal pain and tenderness to an insidious process with few or no findings other than fever, which is almost always present. Upper abdominal abscesses may have symptoms and findings related to the chest. Pelvic abscess is characterized by pain and deep tenderness in one or both lower quadrants, fever, dysuria and urinary frequency, and diarrhea. There may be tenderness of the pelvic peritoneum and bulging of the anterior rectal wall. Complications of intra-abdominal abscess include bacteremia, fistulae, generalized peritonitis, serous pleural effusion, empyema, and mesenteric vein thrombosis.

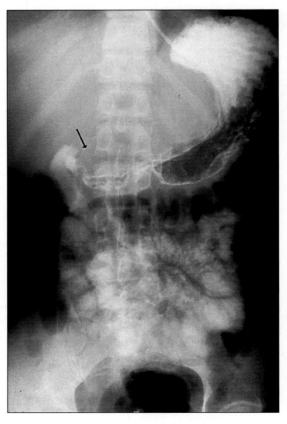

FIGURE 1-88 Barium study showing leaking anastomosis. The *arrow* points to barium that has escaped via the anastomosis. The stomach has been displaced to the left by the large abscess.

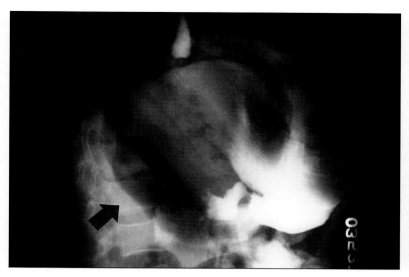

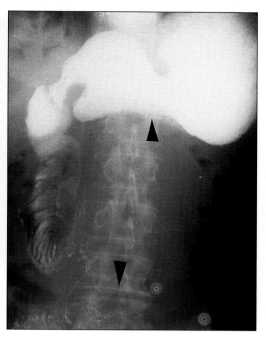

FIGURE 1-90 Radiograph demonstrating midabdominal abscess. The extent of the abscess is delineated by the *arrowheads*.

FIGURE 1-89 Upper gastrointestinal series showing large lesser sac abscess (*arrow*) secondary to posterior perforation of gastric ulcer. Lesser sac abscess is likely to originate from pancreatitis or perforations of the stomach or duodenum.

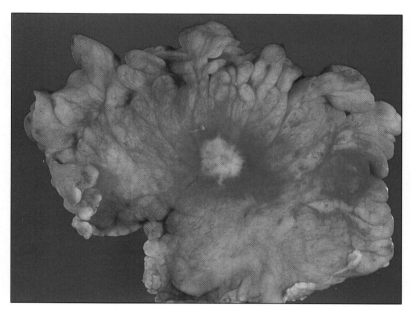

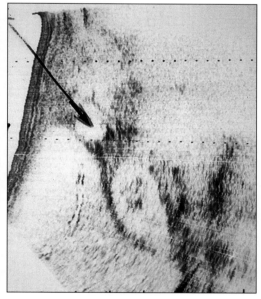

FIGURE 1-92 Ultrasound showing pericecal abscess (*arrow*). Various radiographic and other findings are useful in diagnosis. Ultrasound and computed tomography scanning are quite superior to conventional radiographic procedures. Blood cultures (both aerobic and anaerobic) should always be obtained. Laparoscopy and even laparotomy may be needed for diagnosis of difficult cases, but this is rare.

FIGURE 1-91 Resected sigmoid colon showing mesenteric abscess.

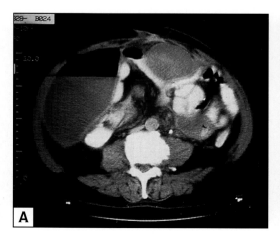

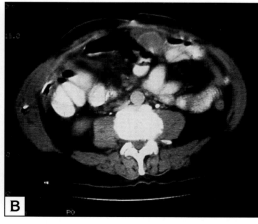

FIGURE 1-93 Retrocolic abscess. **A,** Computed tomography scan of abdomen showing large right retrocolic abscess secondary to perforation of the cecum. **B,** Marked improvement is seen following 48 hours of percutaneous drainage.

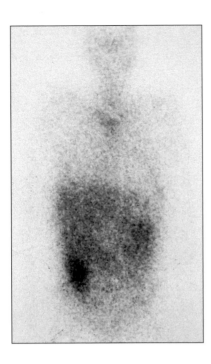

FIGURE 1-94 Gallium scan showing right-lower-quadrant abscess. The most common precursors of pelvic abscess are appendicitis (right lower quadrant), diverticulitis (left lower quadrant), or pelvic inflammatory disease. Paracolic abscess is more frequent on the right side.

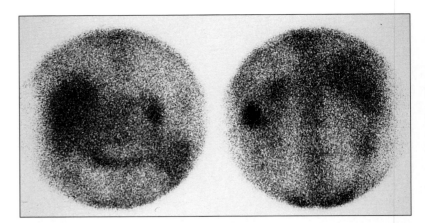

FIGURE 1-95 Technetium scan showing a splenic abscess in both anterior and posterior views. Splenic abscesses are uncommon and usually occur secondary to hematogenous dissemination of microorganisms from sources anywhere in the body. Splenic infarction is a relatively common underlying feature.

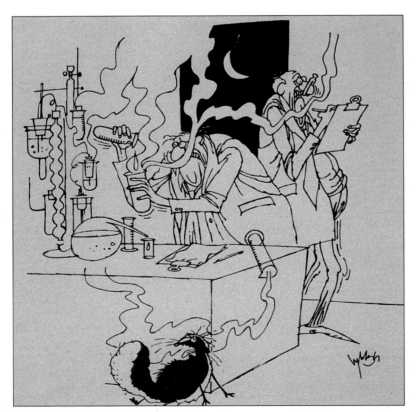

FIGURE 1-96 Cartoon depicting the foul odor that may be detected with an intra-abdominal abscess. Anaerobes are a major part of the infecting flora ordinarily found in intra-abdominal abscesses, and this odor is an important clue to their presence. However, absence of the odor does not rule out a role for anaerobes, because certain anaerobes, particularly peptostreptococci, do not produce the volatile amines and fatty acids that may account for the odor. Of course, until the abscess is exposed by surgery or spontaneous drainage to the surface of the body, the odor may not be detectable.

Comparison of common bacterial isolates from normal colonic flora and from intra-abdominal abscess

Colonic isolates		Abscess isolates	
Rank	Organism	Rank	Organism
1	*Bacteroides vulgatus*	1	*E. coli*
2	*Fusobacterium prausnitzii*	2	*B. fragilis*
3	*Bifidobacterium adolescentis*	3	*Enterococcus*
4	*Eubacterium aerofaciens*	4	Anaerobic cocci
5	*Peptostreptococcus productus* II	5	*Clostridium*
6	*Bacteroides thetaiotaomicron*	6	*Proteus*
7	*Eubacterium eligens*	7	*Fusobacterium*
8	*Peptostreptococcus productus* I	8	*Klebsiella*
9	*Eubacterium biforme*	9	*Pseudomonas*
10	*E. aerofaciens* III	10	*Staphylococcus*
11	*Bacteroides distasonis*	11	*Eubacterium*
28	*Bacteroides ovatus*		
29	*Bacteroides fragilis*		
59–75	*Enterococcus*		
76–113	*Escherichia coli, Klebsiella pneumoniae*		

FIGURE 1-97 Comparison of common bacterial isolates from normal colonic flora and from intra-abdominal abscess. The specific etiology of intra-abdominal abscesses depends on the underlying process and the flora of the gastrointestinal, biliary, or female genital tract area that gives rise to the problem. The principal pathogens encountered include various Enterobacteriaceae, other gram-negative bacilli, streptococci, *Bacteroides fragilis*, other gram-negative anaerobic rods, clostridia, and anaerobic cocci. Many other organisms, including *Salmonella*, may be involved. (*Adapted from* Rotstein and Simmons [19].)

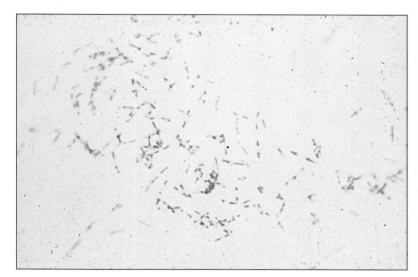

FIGURE 1-98 Gram stain of a pure culture of *Bacteroides fragilis*. The organism, like most gram-negative anaerobes, stains palely and irregularly. It is important to reduce the light in the microscopic field to detect poorly staining anaerobes. There is a moderate degree of pleomorphism also, which again is not uncommon with anaerobic bacteria. *B. fragilis* is the single most commonly encountered anaerobic organism in clinically significant infections. It is clearly a virulent organism, and the prognosis is typically poorer in a mixed anaerobic infection if this organism is present. It may be resistant to antimicrobial agents, but resistance is typically much more common in other members of the *B. fragilis* group, especially *B. thetaiotaomicron*.

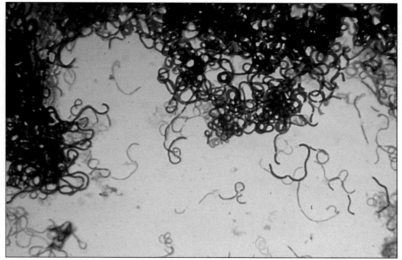

FIGURE 1-99 Gram stain of the edge of a clostridial colony. Swarming growth may be seen with a number of species of motile clostridia, and this feature may make it difficult to separate the various organisms present in a mixed infection in pure culture.

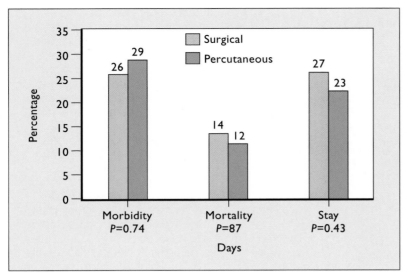

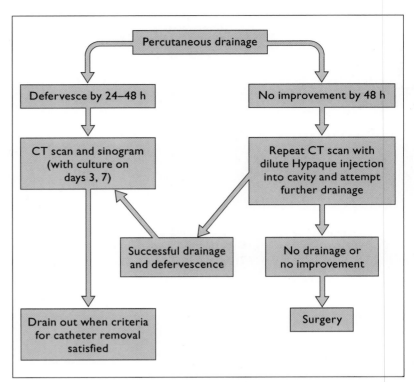

FIGURE 1-100 Percutaneous versus surgical drainage of intra-abdominal abscesses. This figure illustrates that the surgical and percutaneous drainage, done in comparable patients matched for severity of illness, produce very similar results whether one looks at mortality, morbidity, or length of hospital stay. (*Adapted from* Hemming *et al.* [20].)

FIGURE 1-101 Algorithm for the management of patients with intra-abdominal abscesses using percutaneous drainage. Antimicrobial therapy should be administered concomitantly [21]. (CT—computed tomography.) (*Adapted from* Rotstein and Simmons [19].)

Other Intra-abdominal Infections

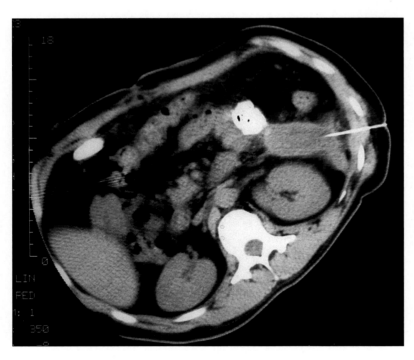

FIGURE 1-102 Left perinephric abscess being drained percutaneously under computed tomography (CT) guidance. The needle can be seen in the abscess cavity on the right of this CT scan. Perinephric abscess is an uncommon complication of urinary tract infection and usually occurs secondary to obstruction or, occasionally, bacteremia. Diabetes mellitus is an important predisposing factor. Although patients may have a dramatic clinical picture with fever, unilateral abdominal and flank pain, and symptoms of lower urinary tract infection, the picture may be quite insidious and difficult to diagnose. CT scan and, to a lesser extent, renal ultrasound have improved our capability of early diagnosis considerably. The most common CT findings are thickening of Gerota's fascia, renal enlargement, and fluid and/or gas surrounding the kidney. In addition to antimicrobial therapy, drainage is important. In most cases, patients do well with percutaneous drainage; if this fails, surgery is necessary.

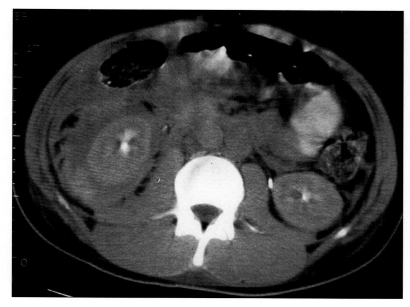

FIGURE 1-103 Computed tomography scan showing right per-inephric abscess, with intra-abdominal gas. The infecting organisms are most often gram-negative enteric bacilli, but occasionally gram-positive cocci may be involved when the infection is of hematogenous origin. Multiple organisms can be recovered in approximately one fourth of cases. On occasion, anaerobes or fungi, especially *Candida*, may be isolated.

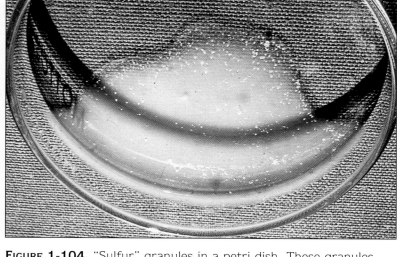

FIGURE 1-104 "Sulfur" granules in a petri dish. These granules resemble grains of elemental sulfur and hence, the name. They are, in fact, colonies of various species of *Actinomyces* or related organisms. Demonstration of such granules in abscess contents or purulent drainage is very important, because it essentially makes the diagnosis of actinomycosis, although there may be a number of accompanying organisms (especially *Actinobacillus actinomycetemcomitans* and pigmented anaerobic gram-negative bacilli). Recovery of these granules is also important in that one can recover pure cultures of the offending actinomyces from washed granules, and culture of the material without washing allows recovery of accompanying organisms. Knowledge of the presence of *Actinomyces* permits the laboratory to use special media and prolonged cultivation to recover these fastidious organisms.

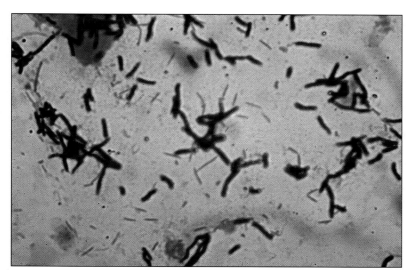

FIGURE 1-105 Gram stain of "sulfur" granule (unwashed) from a patient with actinomycosis. Note the larger, branching rods that are gram-positive (*Actinomyces*) and the smaller, thinner, fusiform-shaped rods that are gram-negative (*Fusobacterium*). The very distinctive microscopic morphology of these organisms (and many other anaerobes, as well as some nonanaerobes) permits their immediate presumptive identification with a high degree of accuracy. This tentative identification permits tailored antimicrobial therapy to be instigated early, whereas culture of such material may take several days or longer for isolation and identification of the various bacteria.

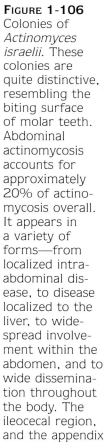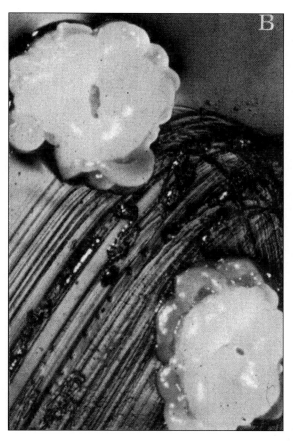

FIGURE 1-106 Colonies of *Actinomyces israelii*. These colonies are quite distinctive, resembling the biting surface of molar teeth. Abdominal actinomycosis accounts for approximately 20% of actinomycosis overall. It appears in a variety of forms—from localized intra-abdominal disease, to disease localized to the liver, to widespread involvement within the abdomen, and to wide dissemination throughout the body. The ileocecal region, and the appendix in particular, is the site most commonly involved in abdominal actinomycosis, but there are reports of involvement of all other areas of the intestinal tract, gallbladder, pancreas, abdominal wall, and pelvis, in addition to the liver. The disease is usually restricted to a single organ; disseminated infection is rare.

REFERENCES

1. Draser BS, Hill MJ: *Human Intestinal Flora.* London: Academic Press; 1974.

2. Finegold SM, Baron EJ, Wexler HM: *A Clinical Guide to Anaerobic Infections.* Princeton Scientific Publishing/Star Publishing Co.; 1992.

3. Jones RC: Surgical infections in trauma. *In* Gorbach SL, Bartlett JG, Blacklow NR (eds.): *Infectious Diseases.* Philadelphia: W.B. Saunders; 1992:773–778.

4. Kernodle DS, Kaiser AB: Postoperative infections and antimicrobial prophylaxis. *In* Mandell GL, Bennett JE, Dolin R (eds.): *Principles and Practice of Infectious Diseases,* 4th ed. New York: Churchill Livingstone; 1995:2742.

5. Kernodle DS, Kaiser AB: Prophylaxis for gastrointestinal surgery. *In* Blaser MJ, Smith PD, Ravdin JI, *et al.* (eds.): *Infections of the Gastrointestinal Tract.* New York: Raven Press; 1995:1329–1344.

6. Antimicrobial prophylaxis in surgery. *Med Lett* 1995, 37:79–82.

7. Condon RE, Wittmann DH: Approach to the patient with intraabdominal infection. *In* Gorbach SL, Bartlett JG, Blackow NR (eds.): *Infectious Diseases.* Philadelphia: W.B. Saunders; 1992:654–660.

8. Finegold SM, Johnson CC: Peritonitis and intraabdominal infections. *In* Blaser MJ, Smith PD, Ravdin JI, *et al.* (eds.): *Infections of the Gastrointestinal Tract.* New York: Raven Press; 1995:369–403.

9. Hedderich GS, *et al.*: The septic abdomen: Open management with Marlex mesh with a zipper. *Surgery* 1986, 99:399.

10. Bennion RS, Thompson JE, Baron EJ, Finegold SM: Gangrenous and perforated appendicitis with peritonitis—treatment and bacteriology. *Clin Ther* 1990, 12:31–44.

11. Levison ME, Bush LM: Peritonitis and other intra-abdominal infections. *In* Mandell GL, Bennett JE, Dolin R (eds.): *Principles and Practice of Infectious Diseases,* 4th ed. New York: Churchill Livingstone; 1995:705–740.

12. Keighley MR: Micro-organisms in bile: A preventable cause of sepsis after biliary surgery. *Ann R Coll Surg Engl* 1997, 59:328.

13. Bartlett JG: Pyogenic liver abscess. *In* Gorbach SL, Bartlett JG, Blacklow NR (eds.): *Infectious Diseases.* Philadelphia: W.B. Saunders; 1992:726–732.

14. Sabbaj J, Sutter VL, Finegold SM: Anaerobic pyogenic liver abscesses. *Ann Intern Med* 1972, 77:627–638.

15. Adams EB, MacLeod IN: Invasive amebiasis: II. Amebic liver abscess and its complications. *Medicine (Balt)* 1977, 56:325–334.

16. Katzenstein D, Rickerson V, Braude A: New concepts of amebic liver abscess derived from hepatic imaging, serodiagnosis, and hepatic enzymes in 67 consecutive cases in San Diego. *Medicine (Balt)* 1982, 61:237–246.

17. Reed SL, Ravdin JI: Amebiasis. *In* Blaser MJ, Smith PD, Ravdin JI, *et al.* (eds.): *Infections of the Gastrointestinal Tract.* New York: Raven Press; 1995:1065–1080.

18. Klar E, Warshaw AL: Infection after acute peritonitis. *In* Gorbach SL, Bartlett JG, Blacklow NR (eds.): *Infectious Diseases.* Philadelphia: W.B. Saunders; 1992:743–750.

19. Rotstein OD, Simmons RL: Intraabdominal abscesses. *In* Gorbach SL, Bartlett JG, Blacklow NR (eds.): *Infectious Diseases.* Philadelphia: W.B. Saunders; 1992:668.

20. Hemming A, Davis NL, Robins RE: Surgical versus percutaneous drainage of intra-abdominal abscess. *Am J Surg* 1991, 161:593–595.

21. Rotstein OD: Peritonitis and intra-abdominal abscesses. *In* Wilmore DW (ed.): *Care of the Surgical Patient,* vol 2, sect IX, ch 8. New York: Scientific American, Inc.; 1989:3–24.

SELECTED BIBLIOGRAPHY

Bennion RS, Baron EJ, Thompson JE Jr, *et al.*: The bacteriology of gangrenous and perforated appendicitis—revisited. *Ann Surg* 1990, 211:165–171.

Finegold SM, Johnson CC: Peritonitis and intraabdominal abscess. *In* Blaser ML, Smith PD, Ravdin JI, *et al.* (eds.): *Infections of the Gastrointestinal Tract.* New York: Raven Press; 1995:369–403.

Finegold SM, Sutter VL, Mathisen GE: Normal indigenous intestinal flora. *In* Hentges DJ (ed.): *Human Intestinal Microflora in Health and Disease.* New York: Academic Press; 1983:355–446.

Levison ME, Bush LM: Peritonitis and other intra-abdominal infections. *In* Mandell GL, Bennett JE, Dolin R (eds.): *Principles and Practice of Infectious Diseases,* 4th ed. New York: Churchill Livingstone; 1995:705–740.

Wilson SE, Finegold SM, Williams RA (eds.): *Intra-abdominal Infection.* New York: McGraw-Hill; 1982.

CHAPTER 2

Hepatitis

Lionel Rabin

HEPATITIS DUE TO THE HEPATOTROPIC VIRUSES

Overview of the six hepatotropic viruses

Virus	Nucleic acid	Mode of transmission	Chronicity	Treatment available?
Hepatitis A	RNA	Fecal-oral	No	No
Hepatitis B	DNA	Blood, semen, saliva	Yes	Yes
Hepatitis C	RNA	Blood, sexual(?)	Yes	Yes
Hepatitis D	RNA	Blood, semen	Yes	Yes
Hepatitis E	RNA	Fecal-oral	No	No
Hepatitis G	RNA	Blood	?	?

FIGURE 2-1 Overview of the six hepatotropic viruses. Acute viral hepatitis can be caused by at least six different viral agents. Although the clinical syndrome of acute hepatitis is very similar with each of these agents, each virus is entirely distinct and unrelated. Accurate diagnosis depends on correct use and interpretation of serologic tests.

FIGURE 2-2 Comparative morphology of the hepatitis viruses A, B, C, D, and E. (ds—double-stranded; ss—single-stranded; +—positive sense; -—negative sense.)

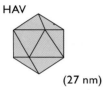

HAV

27–28 nm
Icosahedral, nonenveloped
7.5-kb RNA, linear, ss, +
Heparnavirus (Picornaviridae)

(27 nm)

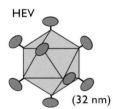

HEV

32–34 nm
Nonenveloped, icosahedral
7.6-kb RNA, linear, ss, +
Alphavirus-like

(32 nm)

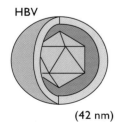

HBV

42 nm
Double-shelled virion, with
  nucleocapsid core
3.2-kb DNA, circular, ss/ds
Hepadnavirus

(42 nm)

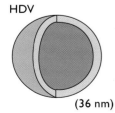

HDV

35–37 nm
Hybrid particle with HBsAg coat
  + HDV core
1.7-kb RNA, linear, ss, −
?

(36 nm)

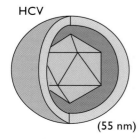

HCV

30–60 nm (?)
Enveloped
9.4-kb RNA, linear, ss, +
Flavivirus-like

(55 nm)

Hepatitis A Virus

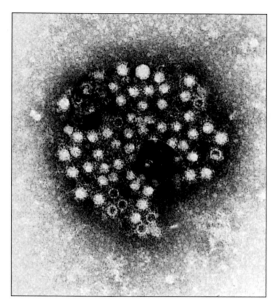

FIGURE 2-3 Electron micrograph of the hepatitis A virus. The micrograph discloses virus particles, 27 to 28 nm in diameter, aggregated by antibody. (*From* Battegay *et al.* [1]; with permission.)

Clinical and epidemiologic features of viral hepatitis A	
Incubation (days)	15–45, mean 25
Onset	Acute
Age preference	Children, young adults
Transmission	
Fecal-oral	+++
Percutaneous	Unusual
Perinatal	–
Sexual	±
Clinical	
Severity	Mild
Fulminant	0.1%
Chronicity	0%
Carrier	None
Cancer	None
Mortality	0.2%
Prophylaxis	Immunoglobulin
	Inactivated vaccine
Therapy	None

FIGURE 2-4 Clinical and epidemiologic features of hepatitis A. Note the very low mortality rate, absence of chronicity or carrier state, and no known risk for hepatocellular carcinoma.

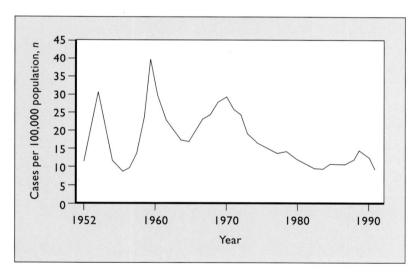

FIGURE 2-5 Reported incidence of hepatitis A in the United States between 1952 and 1991. The low incidence in developed countries is most probably related to safe water supplies and the appropriate handling and treatment of human wastes. Approximately 32% of cases of sporadic viral hepatitis in the United States are due to hepatitis A virus. (*Courtesy of* C.N. Shapiro, MD.)

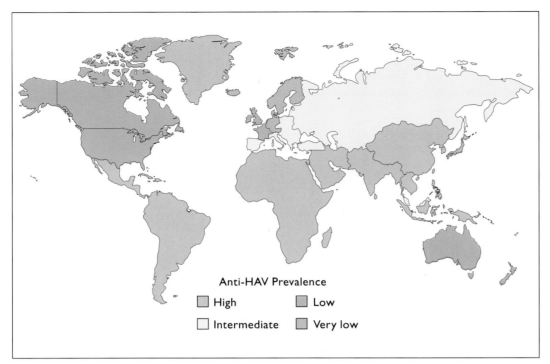

FIGURE 2-6 Worldwide prevalence of hepatitis A virus (HAV). (*Courtesy of* E.E. Mast, MD, MPH.)

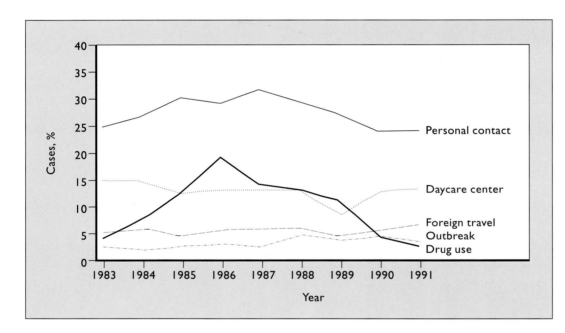

FIGURE 2-7 Risk factors associated with reported cases of hepatitis A in the United States between 1983 and 1991. For institutions (including elderly and extended-care facilities) and daycare centers that fail to maintain high or acceptable standards of hygiene, risk of hepatitis A infection is high among patients and staff. (*Courtesy of* C.N. Shapiro, MD.)

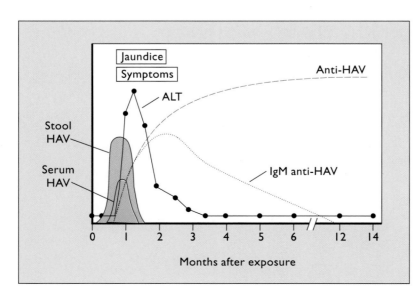

FIGURE 2-8 Typical time course of hepatitis A with emphasis on serologic manifestations. Demonstration of IgM anti–hepatitis A virus (HAV) is diagnostic of hepatitis A infection. IgM anti–HAV occurs at the time of onset of symptoms and may persist for months. (ALT—alanine aminotransferase.)

Recommendations for immunoglobulin prophylaxis for hepatitis A

Preexposure prophylaxis

Susceptible travelers to developing countries, especially when living in rural areas, eating or drinking in settings of poor or uncertain sanitation, or having close contact with local persons. Persons who plan to reside in developing areas for long periods should receive IG regularly every 5 months. For persons who require repeated IG, screening of immune status is useful to avoid unnecessary doses of IG.

Postexposure prophylaxis

Serologic screening of contacts for anti–hepatitis A virus before giving IG is not recommended (costs and time delay).

Close personal contact. All household and sexual contacts of persons with hepatitis A.

Daycare center. All staff and attendees of daycare centers with children in diapers if ≥ one child or employee is diagnosed as having hepatitis A, or cases are diagnosed in ≥ two households of center attendees.

Schools. Routine administration not indicated for pupils or teachers in contact with a patient. During classroom-centered outbreak, IG may be given.

Hospitals. Routine IG prophylaxis for hospital personnel is not indicated. In outbreaks, prophylaxis of persons exposed to feces from infected patients may be indicated.

Offices and factories. Routine administration not indicated for persons having casual contact with infected person.

Common-source exposure. IG might be effective in preventing food-borne or water-borne hepatitis A if exposure is recognized in time. If a food handler is diagnosed, IG should be administered to other food handlers but is usually not recommended to patrons. IG for patrons may be considered if all of the following conditions exist:

1. Infected person is directly involved in handling foods, without gloves, that are not cooked before being eaten.
2. Hygienic practices of food handler are deficient or the food handler has had diarrhea.
3. Patrons can be identified and treated within 2 weeks of exposure.

IG—immunoglobulin.

FIGURE 2-9 Recommendations for immunoglobulin prophylaxis for hepatitis A. (*Adapted from* Centers for Disease Control and Prevention [2].)

Hepatitis B Virus

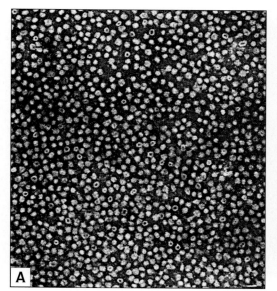
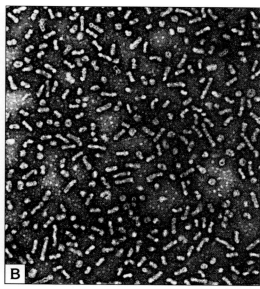
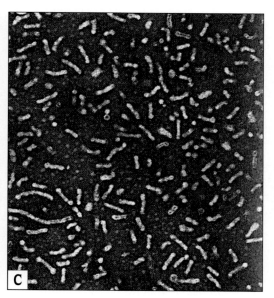

FIGURE 2-10 Electron micrograph of hepatitis B viral forms in blood of an infected patient showing sucrose density gradient fractions after rate-zonal sedimentation of particles. The concentration of incomplete forms in blood usually greatly exceeds the concentration of complete virions or Dane particles. (*continued*)

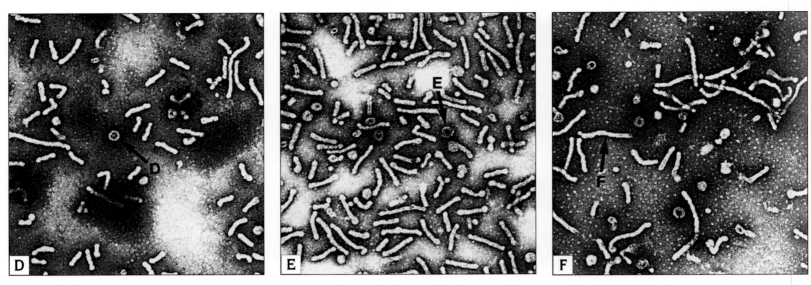

FIGURE 2-10 (*continued*) *D,* Virion (*arrow*) with an electron-dense core; *E,* empty virion (*arrow*); *F,* filamentous form (*arrow*). (*Courtesy of* J.L. Gerin, MD; *from* Robinson [3]; with permission.)

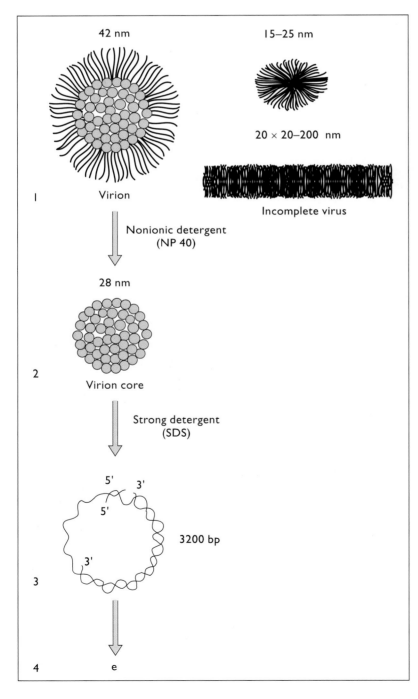

FIGURE 2-11 Diagrammatic representation of hepatitis B viral forms found in blood of infected patients. *1,* Hepatitis B surface antigen (HBsAg) (*a, d/y, w/r*) bearing particles in blood. *2,* Virion core with hepatitis B core antigen (HBcAg) on its surface and containing DNA, and DNA polymerase and protein kinase activities. *3,* Viral DNA is a circular, double-stranded molecule with a single-stranded gap up to 50% of the circle length. DNA polymerase repairs the single-stranded gap, making 3200 base-pair (bp) molecules. The 5' end of the long strand has covalently attached protein. *4,* Hepatitis B e antigen (HBeAg) is released from the virion core by detergent (SDS) treatment and found as soluble antigen in serum. (*Adapted from* Robinson [3].)

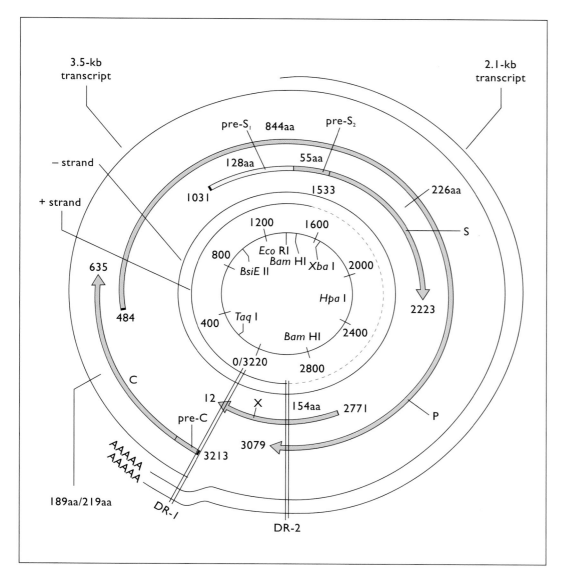

FIGURE 2-12 Organization of the hepatitis B virus (HBV) genome. Hepatitis B virus consists of a small, circular, partially double-stranded DNA genome. The genome has four genes: S, C, P, and X. The S gene produces hepatitis B surface antigen (HBsAg); the C gene produces hepatitis B core antigen (HBcAg) and hepatitis B e antigen (HBeAg); the P gene produces polymerase for viral replication; and the X gene is a transactivating factor. (*Adapted from* Robinson [3].)

Clinical and epidemiologic features of hepatitis B

Incubation (days)	30–150, mean 75
Onset	Insidious or acute
Age preference	Young adults (sexual and percutaneous),
Transmission	babies, toddlers
Fecal-oral	–
Percutaneous	+++
Perinatal	+++
Sexual	++
Clinical	Occasionally severe
Severity	0.1%–1%
Fulminant	5%
Chronicity	0.1%–30%
Carrier	+ (neonatal infection)
Cancer	0.5%–2%
Mortality	Hepatitis B immunoglobulin
Prophylaxis	Recombinant vaccine
Therapy	Interferon 40% effective

FIGURE 2-13 Clinical and epidemiologic features of hepatitis B. The development of the carrier state varies widely among geographic locations and among subpopulations within some countries. Risks for chronicity, cirrhosis, and hepatocellular carcinoma are also increased with hepatitis B virus infections.

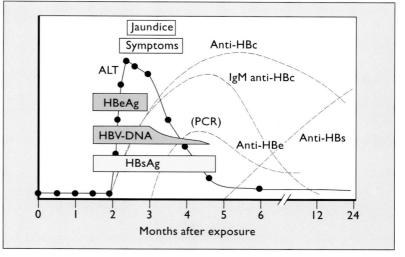

FIGURE 2-14 Typical clinical, serologic, and virologic time course of hepatitis B. (ALT—alanine aminotransferase; HBc—hepatitis B core; HBeAg—hepatitis B e antigen; HBsAg—hepatitis B surface antigen; HBV—hepatitis B virus; PCR—polymerase chain reaction.) (*From* Hsu *et al.* [4].)

Hepatitis B virus serologic markers in different stages of infection and convalescence

HBsAG	Anti-HBs	Anti-HBc IgG	Anti-HBc IgM	HBeAg	Anti-HBe	Diagnostic interpretation
+	−	−	−	+ or −	−	Late incubation period of hepatitis B
+	−	+	+	+	−	Acute hepatitis B
−	−	+	−	−	−	HBsAg-negative acute hepatitis B
+	−	+++	+ or −	−	+	Healthy HBsAg carrier
+	−	+++	+ or −	+	−	Chronic hepatitis B
−	++	++	+ or −	−	+	HBV infection in recent past
−	+ or −	+ or −	−	−	−	HBV infection in distant past
−	++	−	−	−	−	Recent HBV vaccination

HBc—hepatitis B core; HBeAg—hepatitis B e antigen; HBsAg—hepatitis B surface antigen; HBV—hepatitis B virus.

FIGURE 2-15 Variations in hepatitis B virus serologic markers in different stages of hepatitis B infection, convalescence, and recovery. The potential for diagnostic confusion requires careful evaluation of clinical and serologic findings. The figure does not include all possible variations. Approximately 5% to 10% of patients with hepatitis B infection become hepatitis B surface antigen carriers. (*Adapted from* Robinson [3].)

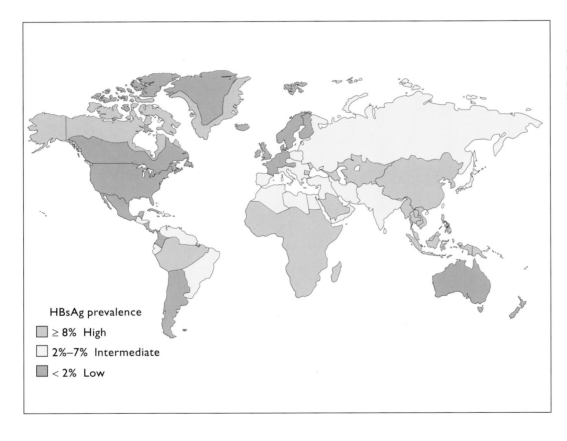

HBsAg prevalence

▢ ≥ 8% High

▢ 2%–7% Intermediate

▢ < 2% Low

FIGURE 2-16 Worldwide prevalence of hepatitis B. High prevalence zones where the carrier rate approaches or occasionally exceeds 20% include sub-Saharan Africa and Southeast Asia. (HBsAg—hepatitis B surface antigen.) (*Courtesy of* E.E. Mast, MD, MPH.)

Groups with increased risk of hepatitis B virus infection

Medical, dental, and laboratory workers and others with exposure to human blood
Homosexual men
Heterosexuals with multiple sex partners or with sexually transmitted diseases
Highly hepatitis B virus–endemic populations, *eg*, Alaskan natives
Household contacts of HBsAg-positive individuals
Parenteral drug users who share needles
Hemophilia patients
Hemodialysis patients
Patients for whom multiple blood or blood product infusions are anticipated
Prison inmates and staff
Staff and patients of institutions for mentally disabled
Travelers to highly hepatitis B virus–endemic areas with anticipated exposure to human blood, sexual contacts with locals, or prolonged living in households with locals
Newborn infants of serum HBsAg-positive mothers

HBsAg—hepatitis B surface antigen.

FIGURE 2-17 Groups with increased risk for hepatitis B virus infection. Individuals in any of these risk groups are recommended to receive the hepatitis B vaccine. (*From* Robinson [3].)

Hepatitis B vaccines and doses licensed for use in the United States

Vaccination group	Hepatavax-B		Recombivax HB		Engenix-B	
	µg	mL	µg	mL	µg	mL
Infants of HBsAg-positive mothers	10	0.5	5	0.5	10	0.5
Others < 10 yrs of age	10	0.5	2.5	0.25	10	0.5
Ages 10–19 yrs	20	1.0	5	0.5	20	1.0
Ages > 19 yrs	20	1.0	10	1.0	20	1.0
Immunologically impaired including dialysis patients	40	2.0	40	1.0	40	2.0

HBsAg—hepatits B surface antigen.

FIGURE 2-18 Hepatitis B vaccines licensed for use in the United States. Doses are given three times, at 0, 1, and 6 months. For Hepatavax-B, the plasma vaccine is no longer manufactured in the United States. For immunocompromised persons, including dialysis patients, Recombivax HB is given in concentrated form, and doses of Engenix-B are given at 0, 1, 2, and 6 months rather than 0, 1, and 6 months. (*Adapted from* Advisory Committee on Immunization Practices [5].)

Anti–hepatitis B surface antigen seroconversion rates after hepatitis B vaccination

Neonates	>95%
Age (yrs)	
2–19	~99%
20–29	~95%
30–39	~90%
40–49	~85%
50–59	~70%
>59	~50%
Renal failure, HIV infection, other immunosuppression	50%–70%
Liver disease	60%–70%

FIGURE 2-19 Anti–hepatitis B virus seroconversion rates after hepatitis B vaccination. There is an increased rate of failure to seroconvert in patients with renal failure, HIV infection, immunosuppression, hepatic disease, and age > 59 years. (*From* Robinson [3].)

Hepatitis D Virus

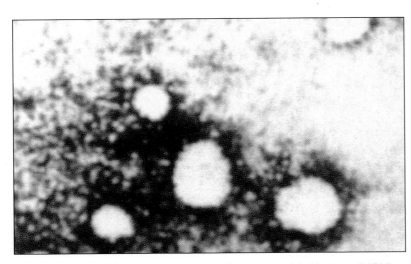

FIGURE 2-20 Electron micrograph of the hepatitis D virus (HDV). HDV is a unique RNA virus resembling plant satellite viruses or viroids. It is a defective or incomplete virus that requires the "helper" function of hepatitis B virus. Patients who develop delta infection are hepatitis B surface antigen–positive. Delta occurs as a coinfection, with up to 5% of patients having simultaneous acute delta infection and acute hepatitis B. (*Courtesy of* Abbott Laboratories; *from* Kuhns [6]; with permission.)

Clinical and epidemiologic features of hepatitis D	
Incubation (days)	15–150, mean 30
Onset	Insidious or acute
Age preference	Any age (similar to HBV)
Transmission	
Fecal-oral	–
Percutaneous	+++
Perinatal	+
Sexual	++
Clinical	
Severity	Occasionally severe
Fulminant	5%–20%
Chronicity	5%–70%
Carrier	Variable
Cancer	±
Mortality	2%–20%
Prophylaxis	HBV vaccine (none for HBV carriers)
Therapy	Unknown

HBV–hepatitis B virus.

FIGURE 2-21 Clinical and epidemiologic features of hepatitis D. In acute hepatitis B virus/hepatitis D virus coinfection, the frequency of chronicity is essentially the same as that for hepatitis B virus; however, in hepatitis D virus superinfection, chronicity ranges from 5% to 70%. Delta hepatitis, whether acute or chronic, tends to be more severe than either typical or chronic hepatitis B by itself.

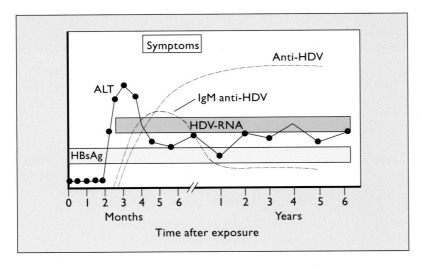

FIGURE 2-22 Clinical, virologic, and serologic courses of a typical case of acute hepatitis D superinfection in a patient with chronic hepatitis B, leading to chronic hepatitis D virus (HDV) infection. (ALT—alanine aminotransferase; HBsAg—hepatitis B surface antigen.) (*From* Hsu *et al.* [4].)

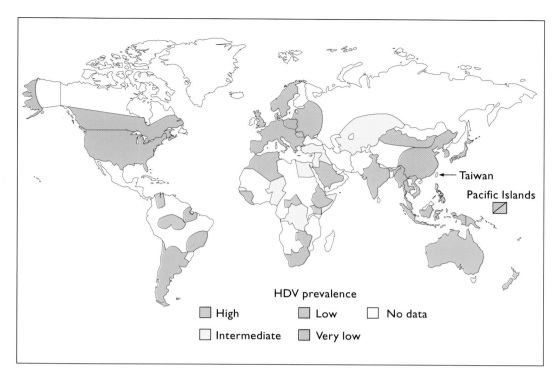

FIGURE 2-23 Worldwide distribution of hepatitis D virus (HDV) infection. (*Courtesy of* E.E. Mast, MD, MPH.)

Taiwan

Pacific Islands

HDV prevalence

☐ High ☐ Low ☐ No data

☐ Intermediate ☐ Very low

Hepatitis C Virus

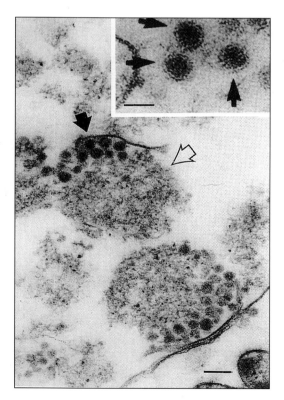

FIGURE 2-24
Electron micrographic evidence of the hepatitis C virus. Standard thin section electron micrography shows an HPBALL cell harvested on day 25 of culture. Cytoplasmic vesicles containing viruslike particles (*arrow*) approximately 50 nm in diameter associated with amorphous material (*open arrow*). Inset, A higher magnification of the viruslike particles (*arrows*). (Bar=100 nm.) (*From* Shimizu *et al.* [7]; with permission.)

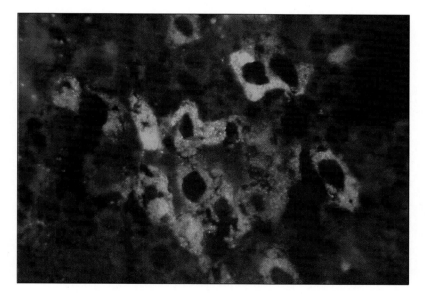

FIGURE 2-25 Hepatitis C virus antigen (HCVAg) in cytoplasm of hepatocytes, identified by fluorescein isothiocyanate–labeled polyclonal IgG anti-HCVAg. Liver biopsy specimen from a hepatitis C virus–infected patient shows very prominent deposits of HCVAg, with a distinct granular pattern in the hepatocyte located in the center of the field. (*Courtesy of* K. Krawczynski, MD, PhD.)

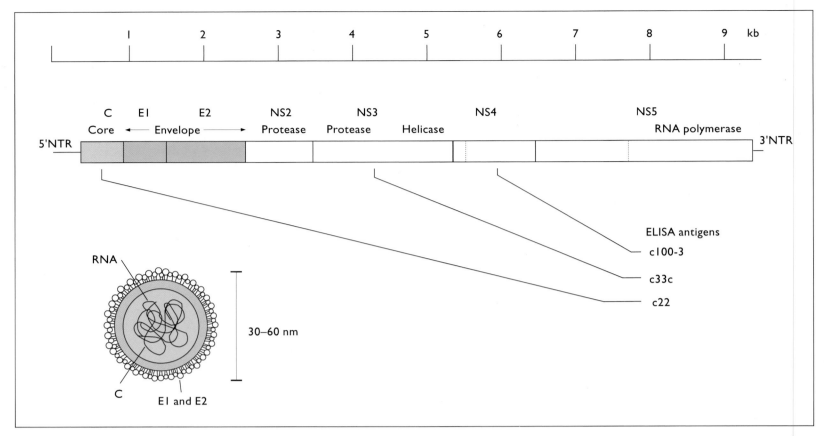

FIGURE 2-26 Organization of the hepatitis C virus genome. Hepatitis C is due to a small flavivirus-like RNA virus with a linear, single-stranded genome of approximately 10 kb.

(ELISA—enzyme-linked immunosorbent assay; NTR—nontranslated region.) (*From* Lemon and Brown [8].)

Clinical and epidemiologic features of hepatitis C	
Incubation (days)	15–120, mean 50
Onset	Insidious
Age preference	Any age, but more common in adults
Transmission	
Fecal-oral	–
Percutaneous	+++
Perinatal	±?
Sexual	±?
Clinical	
Severity	Moderate
Fulminant	0.1%
Chronicity	85%
Carrier	0.5%–1.0%
Cancer	+
Mortality	0.2%
Prophylaxis	None
Therapy	Interferon 50% effective

FIGURE 2-27 Clinical and epidemiologic features of hepatitis C. Fulminant cases due to hepatitis C are rare. Many patients are asymptomatic, and severity in symptomatic cases usually ranges from mild to moderate. Progression to chronicity is common, however.

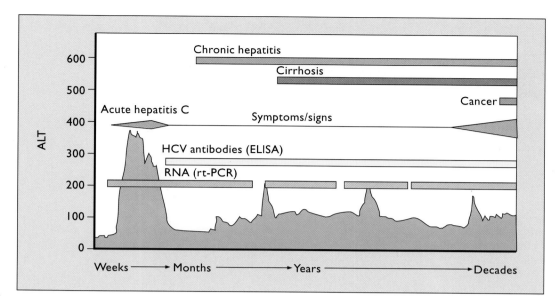

FIGURE 2-28 Natural history of hepatitis C. Chronicity may develop over months, years, or decades and may lead to cirrhosis and an increased risk for hepatocellular carcinoma. (ALT—alanine aminotransferase; ELISA—enzyme-linked immunoassay; HCV—hepatitis C virus; rt-PCR—reverse transcriptase polymerase chain reaction.) (*From* Lemon and Brown [8].)

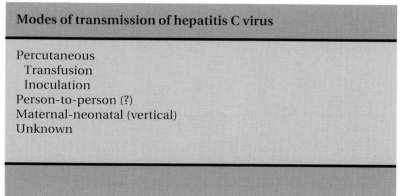

Modes of transmission of hepatitis C virus

Percutaneous
  Transfusion
  Inoculation
Person-to-person (?)
Maternal-neonatal (vertical)
Unknown

FIGURE 2-29 Modes of transmission of hepatitis C virus.

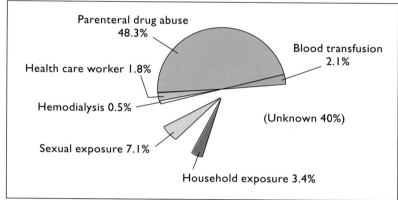

FIGURE 2-30 Risk factors associated with non-A, non-B hepatitis in young adults (aged 15–44 years) in the United States. Almost 40% of patients with hepatitis C virus infection have no known risk factor or history of illicit drug abuse. The incidence of anti–hepatitis C virus antibody is approximately 70% among parenteral drug abusers, 70% among hemophiliacs, 20% to 30% among oncology and renal dialysis patients, and 2% to 6% among health care workers. (*Adapted from* Alter *et al.* [9].)

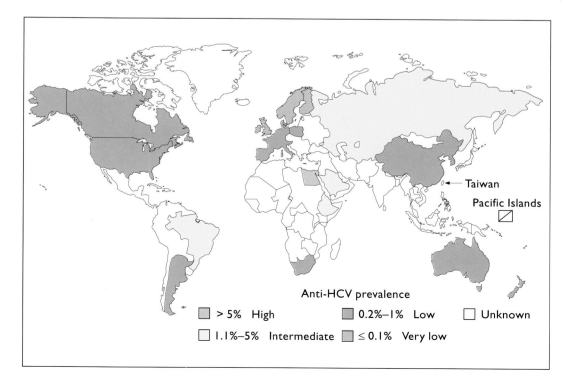

FIGURE 2-31 Worldwide prevalence of hepatitis C. Prevalence of anti–hepatitis C virus (HCV) is determined by EIA-1 or EIA-2 with supplemental testing. (*Courtesy of* E.E. Mast, MD, MPH.)

Tests for hepatitis C virus

Enzyme-linked immunoassay
Recombinant immunoblot assay
Polymerase chain reaction
Binding DNA
Genotyping

FIGURE 2-32 Tests for hepatitis C. Current (second-generation) sensitive enzyme-linked immunoassays detect several polypeptides from different regions of the hepatitis C virus genome: from the core (c22), NS3 (c33c), and NS4 (c100 and 5-1-1 regions). Antibody to hepatitis C virus is detected in approximately 95% of chronic cases but in only 50% to 60% of acute cases at the onset of illness. Antibody may arise as late as 4 to 6 weeks after onset or may not be detected in patients with self-limited disease. Determining whether a result is a false-positive may require a confirmatory test, such as a recombinant immunoblot assay, which has a high degree of specificity, or the polymerase chain reaction amplification for detection of viral RNA in serum and/or tissue.

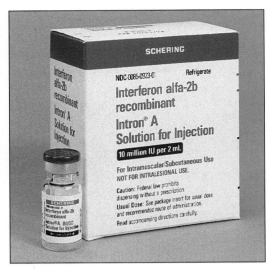

FIGURE 2-33 Interferon alfa-2b treatment of hepatitis C. No specific anti–hepatitis C virus therapy has been recommended, but interferon alfa-2b, the only Food and Drug Administration–approved treatment for chronic hepatitis C, has been shown to be effective in approximately 50% of cases. (*Courtesy of* Schering-Plough, Kenilworth, NJ.)

Hepatitis E Virus

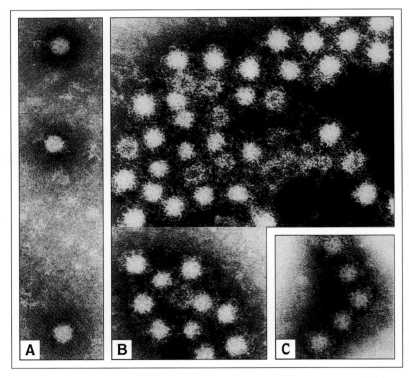

FIGURE 2-34 Electron micrograph of the hepatitis E virus (HEV) particles. Virus particles were present in bile collected 30 days after inoculation of a cynomologus monkey with HEV. **A,** Immune electron microscopy (IEM) carried out with anti-HEV–negative serum demonstrated three particles without associated antibody. **B** and **C,** IEM carried out with anti-HEV–positive serum from a convalescent patient demonstrated complexes of virus particles with associated immunoglobulin molecules. (Bar=100 nm.) (*From* Ticehurst *et al.* [10]; with permission.)

Clinical and epidemiologic features of hepatitis E

Incubation (days)	15–60, mean 30
Onset	Acute
Age preference	Young adults (20–40 yrs)
Transmission	
Fecal-oral	+++
Percutaneous	–
Perinatal	–
Sexual	–
Clinical	
Severity	Mild
Fulminant	1%–2%
Chronicity	0%
Carrier	None
Cancer	None
Mortality	0.2%
Prophylaxis	Unknown
Therapy	None

FIGURE 2-35 Clinical and epidemiologic features of hepatitis E. Hepatitis E virus is a nonenveloped virus like hepatitis A virus (HAV) and shares several key features with HAV, such as fecal-oral transmission and apparent lack of chronicity, but unlike HAV, it has a tendency to cause fatal fulminant hepatitis in pregnant women (up to 20% of cases occur in the last trimester of pregnancy).

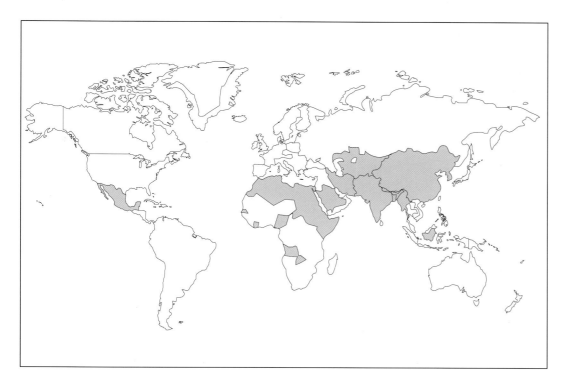

FIGURE 2-36 Worldwide distribution of endemic and sporadic cases of hepatitis E. Most cases occur in Asia, Africa, and Mexico. (*Courtesy of* E.E. Mast, MD, MPH.)

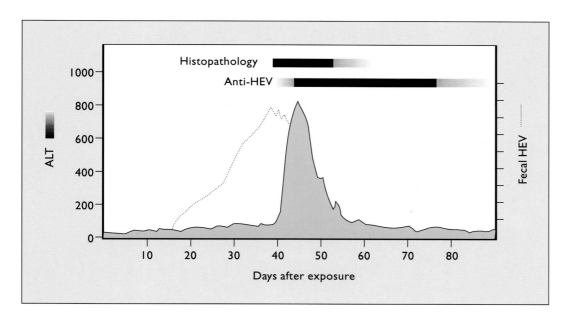

FIGURE 2-37 Course of events during a self-limited case of hepatitis E. (ALT—alanine aminotransferase; HEV—hepatitis E virus.) (*From* Lemon [11].)

Hepatitis G Virus

Hepatitis G virus: A newly discovered hepatitis virus

9.5-kb RNA virus, ss, positive sense; similar to flaviviruses and HCV

Transmission via transfusion (and other percutaneous routes?)

Accounts for 0.4% of all community-acquired viral hepatitis, 1.4% of community-acquired non-A, non-B hepatitis

Causes persistent infection with slow progression, generally mild to chronic hepatitis

Coinfection with HCV possible, and occasionally hepatitis B virus

Data suggest prevalence of hepatitis G virus in blood donors exceeds HCV and is not related to alanine transaminase status

HCV—hepatitis C virus; SS—single-stranded.

FIGURE 2-38 Features of the hepatitis G virus (HGV). A newly discovered virus, HGV appears to be a novel flavivirus-like agent. It can be transmitted experimentally to nonhuman primates. HGV infection may explain the occurrence of non-A, non-B, non-C posttransfusion hepatitis [12,13].

Clinical and epidemiologic features of hepatitis G

Age preference	Young adults (similar to hepatitis C virus)
Transmission	Transfusion, possibly intravenous drug use, high-risk sexual activity
Clinical	
Severity	Generally mild
Fulminant	Reported
Chronicity	Yes
Cancer	Undetermined
Mortality	Reported

FIGURE 2-39 Clinical and epidemiologic features of hepatitis G. Hepatitis G virus (HGV) disease is generally mild, causing low-level alanine transaminase elevations. HGV and hepatitis C virus infection can be simultaneously transmitted and result in persistent coinfection. HGV infection alone may be persistent and accompanied by chronic hepatitis. Coinfection with hepatitis B virus has also been encountered. One report from Japan of six cases of fulminant hepatitis of unknown etiology, disclosed that three patients showed positive signals for HGV on semi-nested polymerase chain reaction [12–14].

CLINICAL COURSE AND DIAGNOSIS

Symptoms associated with hepatitis A, B, and non-A, non-B in adults

Finding	Prevalence of symptoms		
	Hepatitis A, % (18 patients)	Hepatitis B, % (214 patients)	Hepatitis non-A, non-B, % (68 patients)
Jaundice	88	83	82
Dark urine	68	79	89
Fatigue	63	74	77
Light-colored stools	58	48	37
Loss of appetite	42	56	62
Distaste for cigarettes (in smokers only)	45	57	63
Nausea or vomiting	26	46	56
Abdominal pain	37	51	51
Fever or chills	32	25	25
Headache	26	26	25
Muscle pain	26	21	17
Diarrhea	16	30	15
Constipation	16	17	19
Joint pain	11	30	21
Sore throat	0	12	14

FIGURE 2-40 Comparison of symptoms associated with hepatitis A, B, and non-A, non-B. Findings were obtained from US Army personnel hospitalized with serologic confirmation of hepatitis virus infection. (*From* Lemon and Day [15].)

Serologic Diagnosis

A. Serologic tests for identification of hepatitis viruses

Serologic test	Comment
IgM anti-HAV	Acute hepatitis A
IgG anti-HAV	Previous resolved infection with HAV
HBsAg	Acute or chronic hepatitis B
Anti-HBs	Indicates protective immunity
Anti-HBc	Antibody directed against internal HBcAg
HBeAg	Indicates presence of complete (infectious) hepatitis B virus
Anti-HBe	Indicates loss of complete virus and decreased likelihood of transmission
Anti-HCV	Probable presence of HCV
Anti-HDV	Presence of HDV

HAV—hepatitis A virus; HBcAg— hepatitis B core antigen; HBeAg—hepatitis B e antigen; HBsAg—hepatitis B surface antigen; HCV—hepatitis C virus; HDV—hepatitis D virus.

FIGURE 2-41 Serologic markers for viral hepatitis. **A,** Serologic tests for identification of hepatitis viruses A to D. **B,** Serologic markers in different stages and etiologies of viral hepatitis (A, B, C, D, and E.) (Panel 41A *adapted from* Maddrey [16]; panel 41B *from* Kuhns [6].)

B. Viral hepatitis diagnostic markers

Stage of infection	HAV	HBV	HCV	HDV	HEV
Acute disease	IgM anti-HAV	IgM anti-HBc	Anti-HCV	HDAg	Anti-HEV
Chronic disease	—	HBsAg	Anti-HCV	Anti-HD	—
Infectivity	HAV RNA	HBeAg, HBsAg, HBV DNA	Anti-HCV, HCV RNA	Anti-HD, HDV RNA	HEV RNA
Recovery	None	Anti-HBe, Anti-HBs	None	None	None
Carrier state	—	HBsAg	None	Anti-HD, HDAg	—
Screen for immunity	Total anti-HAV	Anti-HBs, total anti-HBc	None	None	Anti-HEV

HAV—hepatitis A virus; HBV—hepatitis B virus; HBc—hepatitis B core; HBeAg—hepatitis B e antigen; HBsAg—hepatitis B surface antigen; HCV—hepatitis C virus; HDV—hepatitis D virus; HDAg—hepatitis D antigen; HEV—hepatitis E virus.

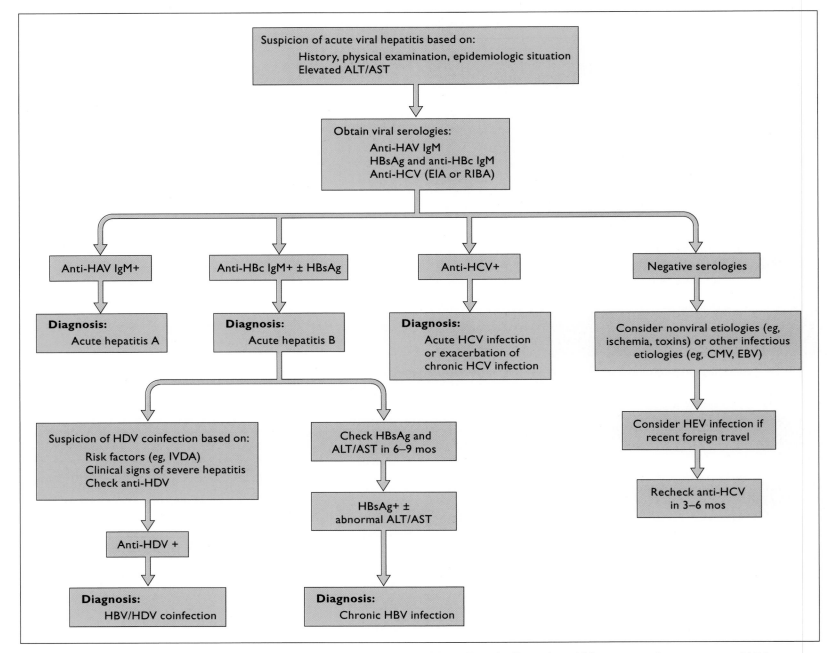

FIGURE 2-42 Algorithm for diagnostic investigation of suspected viral hepatitis. The rate of possible coinfection, superinfection, or drug-induced etiologies must also be considered in cases with confusing or atypical clinical and serologic findings. (ALT—alanine aminotransferase; AST—aspartate aminotransferase; CMV—cytomegalovirus; EBV—Epstein-Barr virus; EIA—enzyme immunoassay; HAV—hepatitis A virus; HBc—hepatitis B core; HBsAg—hepatitis B surface antigen; HBV—hepatitis B virus; HCV—hepatitis C virus; HEV—hepatitis E virus; HDV—hepatitis D virus; IVDA—intravenous drug abusers; RIBA—recombinant immunoblot assay.) (*From* Hsu [4].)

Histologic Diagnosis

Normal liver histology

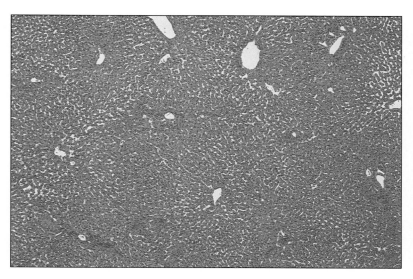

FIGURE 2-43 Normal lobular (acinar) architecture of liver. Hematoxylin-eosin–stained section of liver displays normal lobular (acinar) architecture: central veins (terminal hepatic venules), portal areas, and liver cell plates.

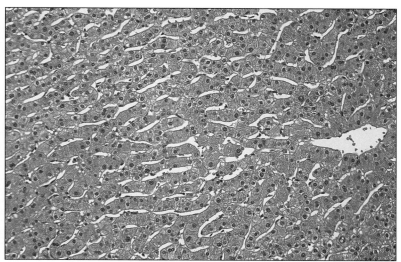

FIGURE 2-44 Histologic section of normal liver with central vein and liver cell plates. At this magnification, sinusoids and several Kupffer's cells are recognized.

Acute viral hepatitis

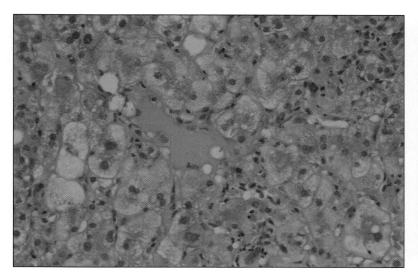

FIGURE 2-45 Liver section showing acute viral hepatitis with marked hepatocellular unrest (anisocytosis and anisonucleosis). Many hepatocytes are ballooned. An occasional focus of necrosis with inflammatory response is also present. Cell membranes of many swollen or ballooned hepatocytes are indistinct or lysed. (Hematoxylin-eosin stain; original magnification, × 80.)

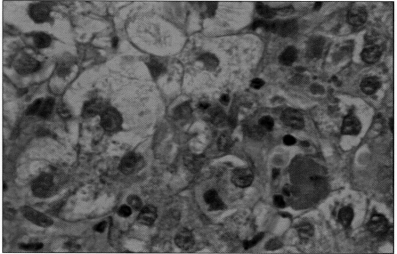

FIGURE 2-46 Liver histology in acute viral hepatitis, with marked ballooning degeneration of hepatocytes and acidophilic (apoptotic) body formation. Ballooned cells (whether singly, in groups, or diffusely) may undergo necrosis by rupture or lysis. Acidophilic/apoptotic body formation is preceded by acidophilic degeneration characterized by cell shrinkage, increased eosinophilia, increased angularity and loss of attachment to neighboring cells, nuclear pyknosis, karyorrhexis or karyolysis. Portions of a degenerating or dying hepatocyte may break off, forming apoptotic bodies. Acidophilic/apoptotic bodies extruded into sinusoids are eventually phagocytosed by Kupffer cells [17]. (Hematoxylin-eosin stain; original magnification, × 175.)

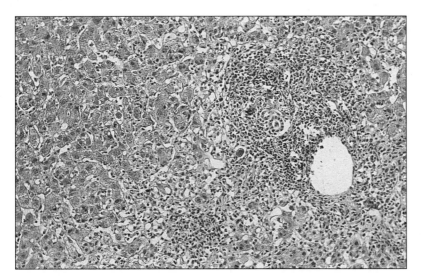

FIGURE 2-47 Liver histology in acute viral hepatitis, showing lobular disarray with prominent portal, mainly chronic, inflammation. In many cases, intrahepatic cholestasis is absent or slight, except in the cholestatic variant.

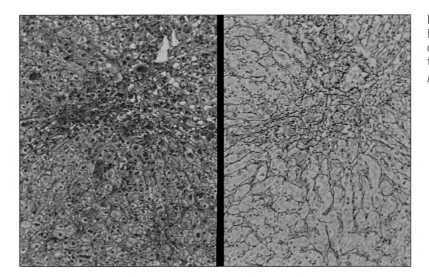

FIGURE 2-48 Liver histology during subsiding phase of acute viral hepatitis. Lobular disarray is much less intense. Regenerative changes become more apparent with increasing numbers of bi- or trinucleate hepatocytes. (*Left panel*, hematoxylin-eosin stain; *right panel*, reticulin; original magnification, × 25.)

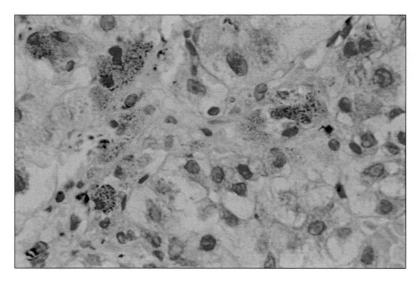

FIGURE 2-49 High power view of subsiding phase of acute viral hepatitis. In foci of parenchymal necrosis, hypertrophied Kupffer cells contain varying admixtures of lipofuscin and hemosiderin. Hemosiderin is not seen in early necroinflammatory injury (Mallory's iron method; original magnification, × 125.)

Chronic hepatitis

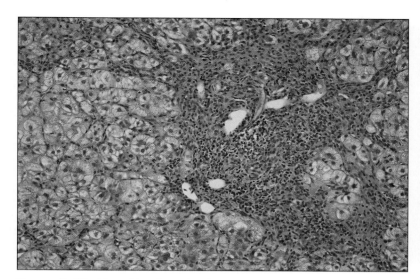

FIGURE 2-50 Liver histology in chronic hepatitis. An expanded portal area contains a heavy infiltrate of chronic inflammatory cells, focal entrapment of small groups, or individual hepatocytes giving rise to limiting plate irregularity (Hematoxylin-eosin stain; original magnification, × 45.)

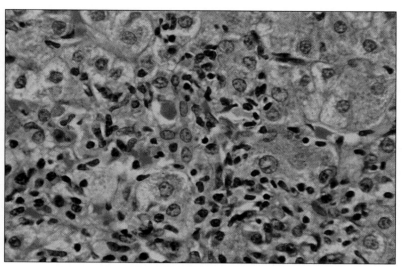

FIGURE 2-51 Higher power view in chronic hepatitis showing junction of the portal area and adjacent parenchyma infiltrated by chronic inflammatory (mainly plasma) cells. A free acidophilic body, hepatocellular entrapment, and disruption of limiting plate can be seen. (Hematoxylin-eosin stain; original magnification, × 100.)

Fulminant hepatitis

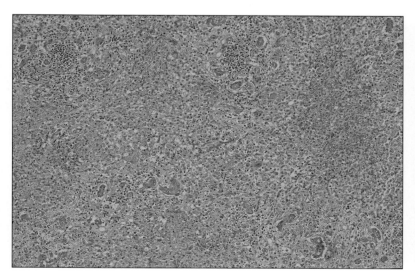

FIGURE 2-52 Liver histology in fatal fulminant hepatitis. The figure displays acute viral hepatitis with massive necrosis and marked hepatocellular loss. Relatively few remaining islands of liver cells are seen. Reactive ductal (cholangiolar) proliferation is seen in zone 1 (periportal areas). (Hematoxylin-eosin stain; original magnification, × 25.)

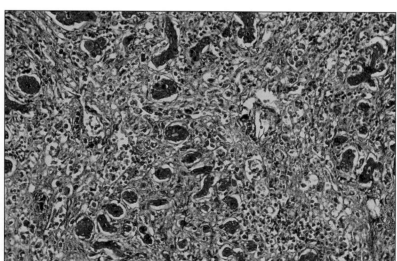

FIGURE 2-53 Fatal fulminant viral hepatitis with virtual total loss of hepatocytes. Reactive ductal proliferation is distributed in zone 1. (Masson-trichrome stain; original magnification, × 30.)

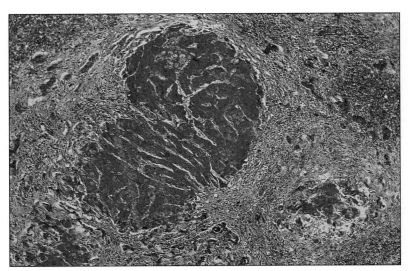

FIGURE 2-54 Subacute fatal hepatitis. Submassive, bridging necrosis is seen with an island of hepatic nodular regeneration. Scattered reactive ductal proliferation and occasional residual hepatocytes are seen in necrotic areas. (Masson-trichrome stain; original magnification, × 16.)

Differential diagnosis of chronic hepatitis

Viral hepatitis	Drug-induced
Hepatitis B	Isoniazid
Hepatitis D	Methyldopa
Hepatitis C	Diclofenac
Hepatitis G	Oxyphenisatin
	Glafenine
Inherited metabolic disease	nitrofurantoin
Wilson's disease	Pemoline
α_1-Antitrypsin deficiency	Dantrolene
Autoimmune	
Cryptogenic	

FIGURE 2-55 Differential diagnosis of chronic hepatitis. Agents other than the hepatotropic viruses should be considered.

Sequelae

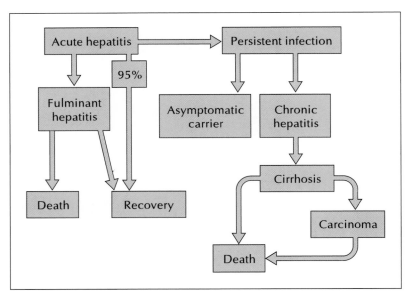

FIGURE 2-56 Clinical sequelae of chronic hepatitis. Chronicity does not develop in hepatitis A or E. The asymptomatic carrier state involves hepatitis B only.

Consequences of viral hepatitis infection

	Hepatitis				Hepatocellular
Agent	Acute	Fulminant	Chronic	Cirrhosis	carcinoma
A	+	+	0	0	0
B	+	+	5%–10%	+	+
C	+	?	~50%	+	+
D	+	+	Coinfection, < 5%	+	+
			Superinfection, ~50%		
E	+	+	0	0	0

FIGURE 2-57 Possible outcomes of infection with the five major hepatitis viruses (A, B, C, D, and E). The rates of chronicity with hepatitis B vary by age, with 20% to 50% of infected infants and children developing chronicity. In hepatitis D virus infection, under 5% of patients with coinfection develop chronicity, but approximately 50% of those with superinfection do. Data on hepatitis G are incomplete, although chronicity has been described as well as fulminant hepatitis in one report [12–14]. (*From* Krawitt [18].)

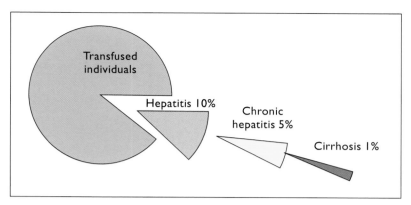

FIGURE 2-58 Progression of posttransfusion non-A, non-B hepatitis. The incidence of acute disease is approximately 10%. Approximately half of these cases (*ie*, 5% of the total number transfused) develop chronic hepatitis, and approximately 20% of the chronic hepatitis group develop cirrhosis. With the availability of donor screening for anti-hepatitis C virus antibody and techniques of greater sensitivity and specificity, the incidence of acute posttransfusion hepatitis may now have been reduced to approximately 2%. (*Adapted from* Clinical Teaching Project, American Gastroenterologic Association.)

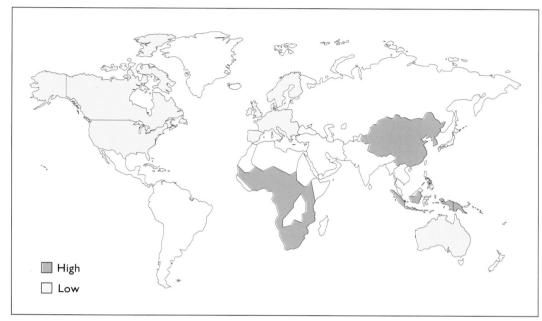

FIGURE 2-59 Worldwide variations in the incidence of primary hepatocellular carcinoma. There is a high incidence in sub-Saharan Africa and Far East Asia. This map is similar to the one for hepatitis B infection (*see* Fig. 2-16). (*Adapted from* Clinical Teaching Project, American Gastroenterological Association.)

ETIOLOGIES OF HEPATIC INJURY
Common Hepatotropic Viruses

A. Histopathologic findings in acute viral hepatitis

1. Lobular disarray
2. Hepatocellular ballooning degeneration
3. Acidophilic (eosinophilic) degeneration
4. Acidophilic/apoptotic body formation
5. Hepatocellular necrosis (lysis), focal or bridging
6. Steatosis, variable (mild to moderate severity)
7. Mononuclear cell infiltration of parenchyma and portal tracts
8. Kupffer cell hypertrophy, laden with lipofuscin; in subsiding phase (~ 7–10 days), hemosiderin accumulates
9. Variable degrees of cholestasis

B. Histopathologic findings in chronic hepatitis

Portal area changes
 1. Chronic inflammation ± lymphoid aggregates or follicles
 2. Bile duct degeneration
Periportal changes
 1. Piecemeal necrosis
 2. Ductular (cholangiolar) proliferation (variable) ± acute cholangiolitis
 3. Fibrosis ± bridging
Parenchymal (intra-acinar) change
 1. Hepatocellular degeneration (necrosis or apoptosis, focal, zonal, or multiacinar)
 2. Kupffer cell hypertrophy
 3. Ground-glass cells (in hepatitis B surface antigen carriers)
Cirrhosis (end stage)

FIGURE 2-60 Typical histopathologic findings in acute viral and chronic hepatitis. **A,** Acute viral hepatitis. **B,** Chronic hepatitis. The morphologic changes in hepatitis of viral etiology are often similar or overlap whether the hepatitis is type A, B, C, D, E, or autoimmune. In addition, many drug-induced hepatitides also mimic viral hepatitis. Certain patterns of injury and/or recognition of morphologic etiologic markers may help define the type of hepatitis with greater certainty. Ground-glass change, due to proliferation of smooth endoplasmic reticulum, is a characteristic change in chronic hepatitis B virus infection but may also be the result of drug-induced etiology. Morphologic findings must always be correlated with appropriate clinical/laboratory data.

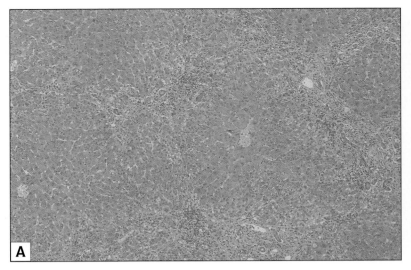

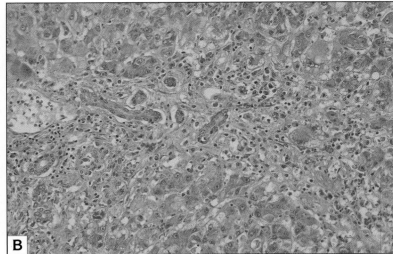

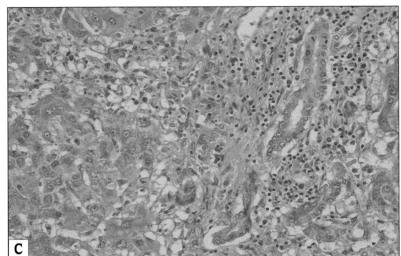

FIGURE 2-61 Acute necroinflammatory injury in hepatitis A. Three liver sections, of increasing magnification, show that the brunt of injury is in periportal (zone 1) areas in this patient with IgM anti–hepatitis A virus antibody. (Hematoxylin-eosin stain. **A,** Original magnification, × 16; **B,** × 50; **C,** × 66.)

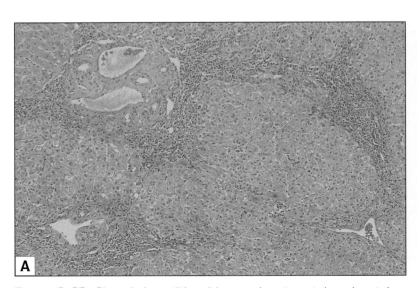

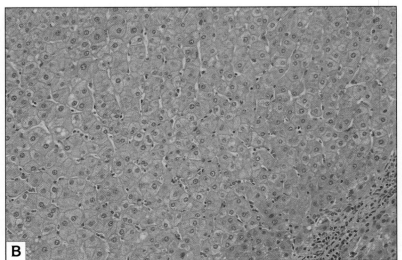

FIGURE 2-62 Chronic hepatitis with prominent portal-periportal chronic inflammation and limiting plate irregularity (piecemeal necrosis) due to hepatitis B. **A,** On low power, an occasional focus of parenchymal necrosis can be seen. (Hematoxylin-eosin stain; original magnification, × 25.) **B,** On higher power examination, an area of parenchyma contains an occasional hepatocyte with highly suggestive ground-glass change. (Hematoxylin-eosin stain; original magnification, × 50.)

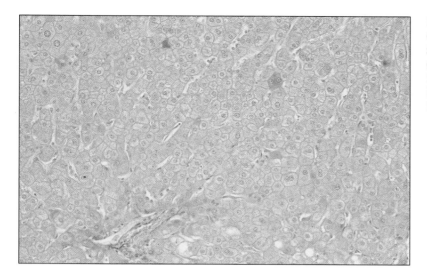

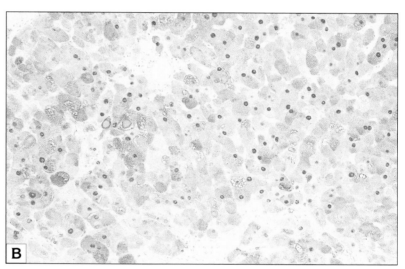

FIGURE 2-63 Victoria blue staining of ground-glass change in chronic hepatitis B. In the same case as shown in Figure 2-62, several hepatocytes show Victoria blue-positive cytoplasmic ground-glass change. As with the aldehyde fuchsin or orcein staining methods, the ground-glass material is consistent with hepatitis B surface antigen. The staining is negative in acute hepatitis B. (Original magnification, × 50.)

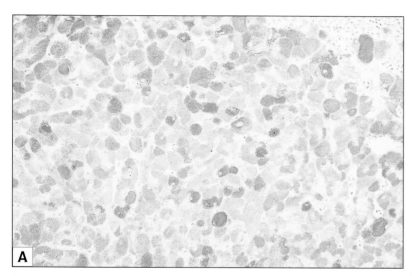

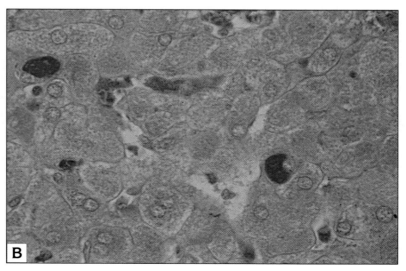

FIGURE 2-64 Immunoperoxidase stains in chronic hepatitis B. **A,** Immunoperoxidase staining for hepatitis B surface antigen (HBsAg). The immunoperoxidase technique is far more sensitive than Skikata staining methods (Victoria blue, orcein, or aldehyde fuchsin). The figure shows diffuse immunoreactivity for HBsAg, with strongly reactive hepatocytes as well as areas of weak

immunoreactivity. Note that nuclei do not contain HBsAg. In some hepatocytes, the staining is membranous. **B,** Immunoperoxidase staining for hepatitis B core antigen (HBcAg). There is strong immunoreactivity for HBcAg in the nuclei of affected hepatocytes and prominent spillover into the cytoplasm (*Both panels*, original magnification, × 50.)

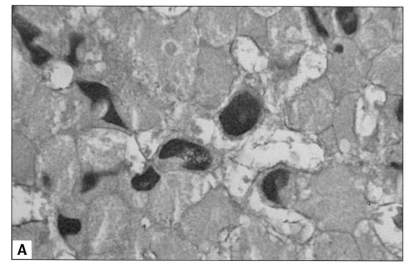

FIGURE 2-65 Skikata staining methods in ground-glass change. **A,** Aldehyde fuchsin-positive ground-glass cells in a patient with cirrhosis and serologic evidence of hepatitis B infection.

B, Orcein-positive ground-glass cells in a patient with documented hepatitis B. (*Both panels*, original magnification, × 110.)

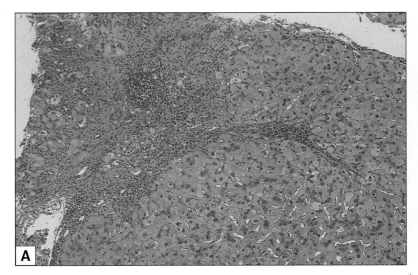

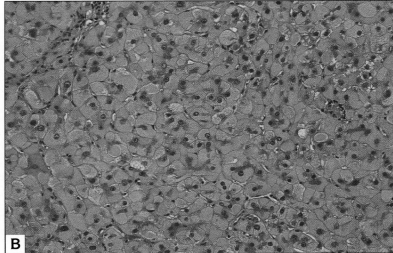

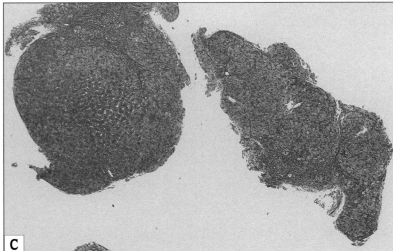

FIGURE 2-66 Cirrhotic liver with evidence of chronic necroinflammatory disease in chronic hepatitis B virus infection. **A,** On hematoxylin-eosin staining, the cytoplasm of many hepatocytes appears pale. (Original magnification, × 25.) **B,** Higher magnification displays striking, diffuse ground-glass change of hepatocytes. In several hepatocytes, nuclei are pushed toward the cell membrane. (Original magnification, × 50.) **C,** Masson-trichrome staining shows fragmentation and nodularity of the biopsy specimen. (Original magnification, × 10.)

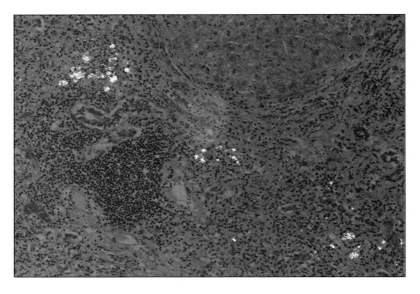

FIGURE 2-67 Polarized light microscopy in cirrhosis secondary to hepatitis B infection. Under polarized light, many portal-septal macrophages contain birefringent crystalline or granular material consistent with talc. Talc is often mixed as a filler material with drugs, and its finding correlates with past parenteral drug abuse. (Original magnification, × 40.)

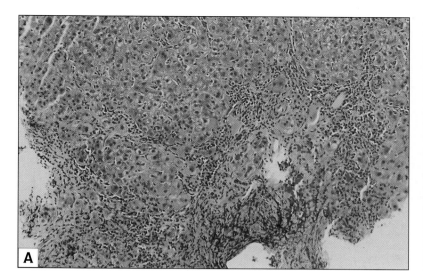

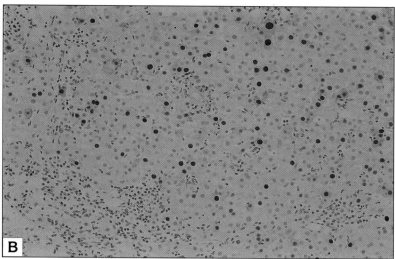

FIGURE 2-68 Liver biopsy in chronic hepatitis B with delta infection. **A,** No ground-glass hepatocytes are present on hematoxylin-eosin staining, but the patient was seropositive for hepatitis B surface antigen (HBsAg). Immunoperoxidase staining disclosed reactivity for HBsAg but none for hepatitic B core antigen. (Original magnification, × 40.) **B,** Immunoperoxidase staining confirms delta antigen in many hepatic nuclei. Some delta antigen is present in the cytoplasm.

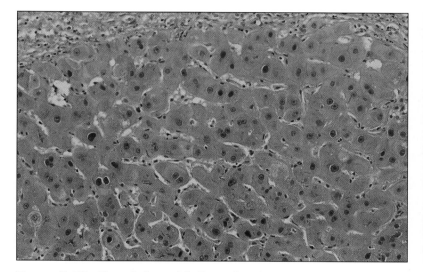

FIGURE 2-69 Chronic hepatitis B carrier. Liver biopsy specimen shows liver cell dysplasia characterized by nuclear hyperchromatism, increased nuclear size, and increased cell size. There is insufficient evidence that liver cell dysplasia is premalignant. (Hematoxylin-eosin stain; original magnification, × 50.)

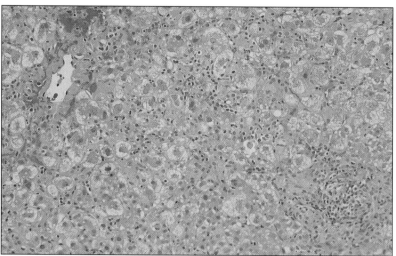

FIGURE 2-70 Liver histology in acute hepatitis C. The patient is seropositive for hepatitis C antibody.

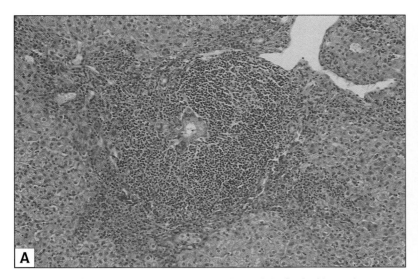

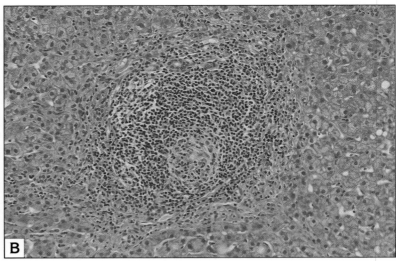

FIGURE 2-71 Liver biopsy in chronic hepatitis C. **A,** Note the prominent portal inflammation and occasional peripheral piece-meal necrosis. This section also exhibits a striking chronic nonsuppurative ductal injury (so-called Poulsen lesion), which resembles primary biliary cirrhosis [19]. **B,** Section displaying one of many portal-containing lymphoid aggregates with germinal center formation. Portal lymphoid infiltrates with germinal center formation, although not pathognomonic, occur with relatively increased frequency in chronic hepatitis C. (*Both panels,* hematoxylin-eosin stain. Original magnification; *panel 71A,* × 33; *panel 71B,* × 50.)

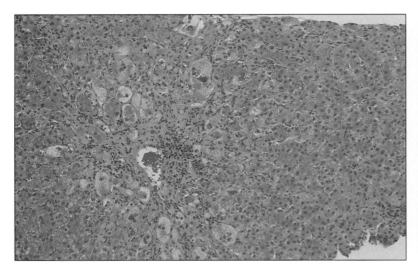

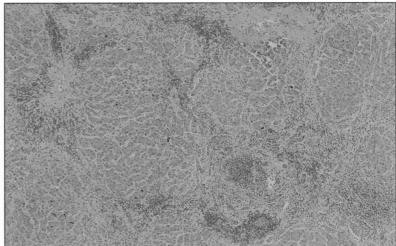

FIGURE 2-72 Liver biopsy showing postinfantile giant cell hepatitis. A liver biopsy from an adult patient seropositive for hepatitis C virus displays necroinflammatory injury with striking zone 3 (centrilobular) giant cell transformation. Postinfantile giant cell hepatitis has been described in patients with hepatitis B and C and autoimmune chronic hepatitis. In our experience, the presence of postinfantile giant cell hepatitis suggests autoimmune chronic hepatitis with somewhat greater frequency than either hepatitis B or C. (Hematoxylin-eosin stain; original magnification, × 50.)

FIGURE 2-73 Fatal acute hepatitis E clinically resembling infectious hepatitis A in a pregnant patient. Serologic tests for hepatitis A virus, hepatitis B virus, and hepatitis C virus in this patient were all negative. The clinical and geographic setting suggested hepatitis E. The injury due to hepatitis E virus is morphologically similar to acute hepatitis A with prominent periportal (zone 1) injury. (Hematoxylin-eosin stain; original magnification, × 13.2.)

Nonhepatotropic Viruses

Hepatitis from nonhepatotropic viruses	
Herpesviruses	Arboviruses
Herpes simplex virus I and II	Yellow fever
Varicella-zoster	Crimean-Congo fever
Cytomegalovirus	Rift Valley fever
Epstein-Barr virus	Dengue fever
Adenovirus	Kyasanur Forest disease
Enteric viruses	Korean hemorrhagic fever
Coxsackievirus B	Arenaviruses
Echovirus	Lassa fever
Paramyxovirus	Argentinian/Bolivian hemor-
Rubeola	rhagic fever
Togavirus	Filoviruses
Rubella	Marburg virus
	Ebola virus

FIGURE 2-74 Hepatitis due to nonhepatotropic viruses. A large number and variety of nonhepatotropic viruses may also infect and damage the liver, in addition to their more typical systemic or tissue/organ effects. Epidemiologic, geographic, and occupational information and a high index of clinical suspicion are required to determine whether the hepatitis in a given patient is due to one of these viruses or to one of the hepatotropic viruses (A, B, C, D, E, or G.)

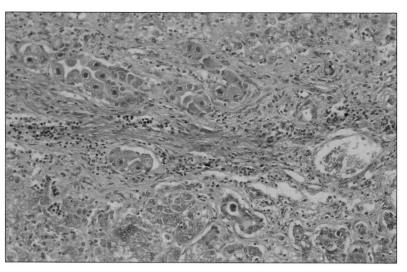

FIGURE 2-75 Neonatal cytomegalovirus hepatitis. Many biliary epithelial cells contain cytomegalovirus inclusions. (Hematoxylin-eosin stain; original magnification, × 50.)

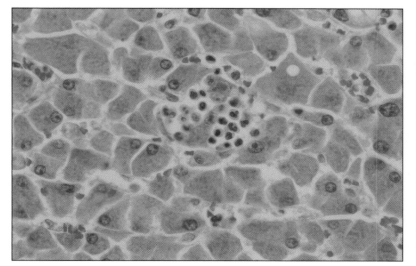

FIGURE 2-76 Liver biopsy with a focus of acute necrosis due to cytomegalovirus (CMV) hepatitis. One hepatocyte contains a CMV inclusion. In immunosuppressed patients, foci of acute necrosis with polymorphonuclear cell response, even in the absence of detectable inclusions, should suggest CMV disease. (Hematoxylin-eosin stain; original magnification, × 132.)

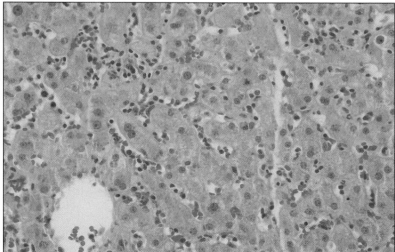

FIGURE 2-77 Liver biopsy showing a mononucleosis-like pattern in proven cytomegalovirus infection. The biopsy shows a chronic inflammatory cell infiltrate in sinusoids, granuloma-like focus, and a rare free acidophilic/apoptotic body. (Hematoxylin-eosin stain; original magnification, × 80.)

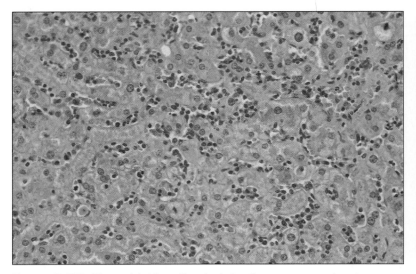

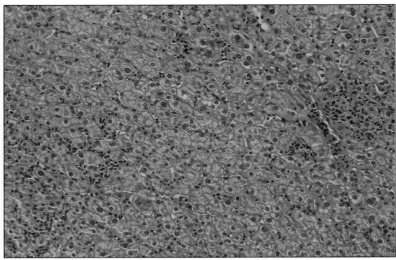

FIGURE 2-78 Sinusoidal beading in infectious mononucleosis. An extensive hepatic sinusoidal chronic inflammatory cell infiltrate, an occasional mitotic figure, and a rare free acidophilic/apoptotic body can be seen. The sinusoidal "beading," or "Indian file" appearance, is characteristic for infectious mononucleosis. The diagnosis was confirmed serologically. (Hematoxylin stain; original magnification, × 50.)

FIGURE 2-79 Serologically confirmed case of infectious mononucleosis showing sinusoidal beading and a solitary noncaseating granuloma. (Hematoxylin-eosin stain. Original magnification, × 80.)

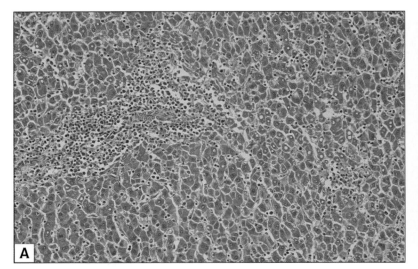

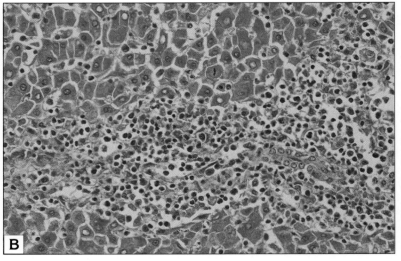

FIGURE 2-80 Fatal infectious mononucleosis. The patient suffered a ruptured spleen. **A,** Note the prominent portal-periportal chronic inflammation, spotty sinusoidal chronic inflammatory cell infiltration, a rare focus of necrosis, and dissociation of liver cell plates.

B, A higher-power field demonstrates prominent portal-periportal chronic inflammation. Note the hepatic mitotic figure in the upper half of the field near the limiting plate. (Hematoxylin-eosin stain. Original magnification: *panel 80A,* × 40; *panel 80B,* × 80.)

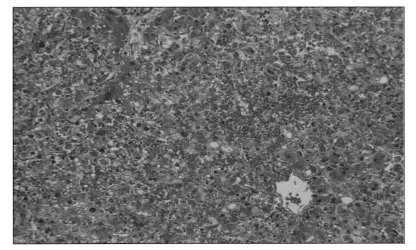

FIGURE 2-81 Liver necrosis and congestion in yellow fever. The liver specimen exhibits extensive coagulative necrosis and congestion with sparing of a rim of periportal (zone 1) and pericentral (zone 3) hepatocytes. These changes are consistent with yellow fever.

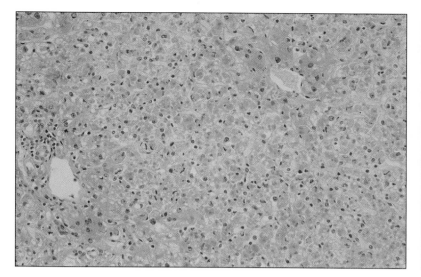

FIGURE 2-82 Fatal case of yellow fever. Midzonal (zone 2) coagulative necrosis is seen with several acidophilic cells (Councilman bodies) and fine lipid vacuolation (*see* Fig. 2-83). A ring of viable hepatocytes surround terminal hepatic vein (central veins) and periportal areas. (Hematoxylin-eosin stain; original magnification, × 50.)

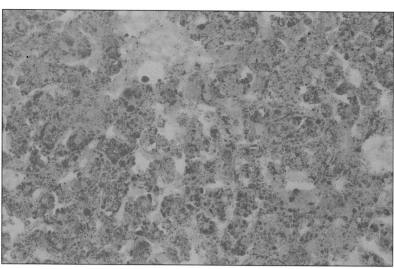

FIGURE 2-83 Frozen oil-red-O section of liver displaying diffuse fine lipid vacuolation in yellow fever. (Original magnification, × 80.)

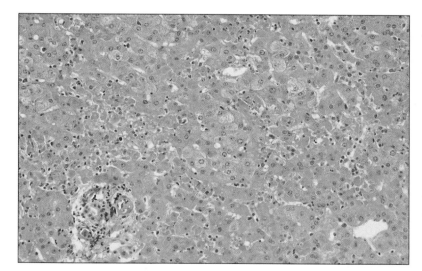

FIGURE 2-84 Lassa fever. Note the prominent focal coagulative necrosis and many apoptotic (Councilman-like) bodies. Some cases may resemble yellow fever. Lassa fever is caused by an arenavirus, and viral particles may be readily detected by electron microscopy. (Hematoxylin-eosin stain; original magnification, × 50.)

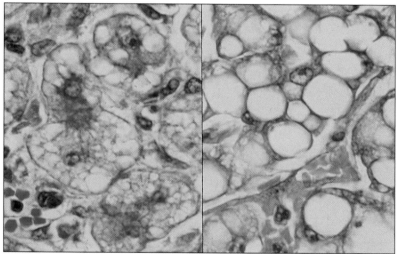

FIGURE 2-85 Reye's syndrome (postviral infection). In early childhood to adolescence, patients appearing to recover from a viral infection (*eg*, chickenpox, influenza) who are treated with aspirin may develop a type of fatty change. *Left*, Swollen hepatocytes with microvesicular steatosis. Microvesicular steatosis, however, also occurs in various other conditions, such as acute fatty metamorphosis of pregnancy, tetracycline or valproate hepatotoxicity, Jamaican vomiting sickness, defects in ureagenesis, and alcoholic foamy degeneration. *Right*, Nonspecific large vacuolar steatosis. This type of fatty change may occur in obesity, alcoholism, diabetes mellitus, or corticosteroid therapy. (Hematoxylin-eosin stain. Original magnification; *left panel*, × 40; *right panel*, × 140.)

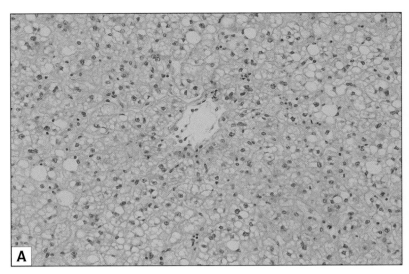 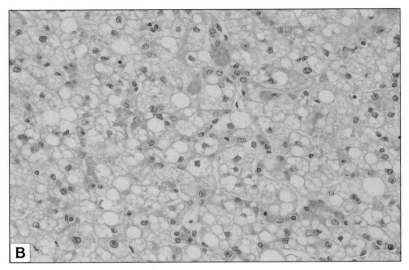

FIGURE 2-86 Reye's syndrome. **A** and **B**, Note the marked predominance of microvesicular steatosis. (Hematoxylin-eosin stain. Original magnification; *panel 86A,* × 50; *panel 86B,* × 66.)

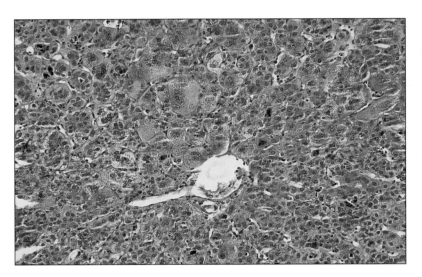

FIGURE 2-87 Liver section showing neonatal hepatitis with partial giant cell transformation due to rubella. Neonatal giant cell hepatitis is associated with many conditions, ranging from hepatitis of viral etiology, biliary atresia, α_1-antitrypsin deficiency, Alagille syndrome, rubella, etc. (Hematoxylin-eosin; original magnification, × 45.)

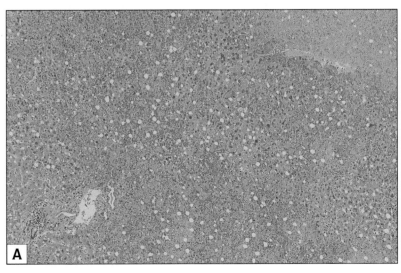 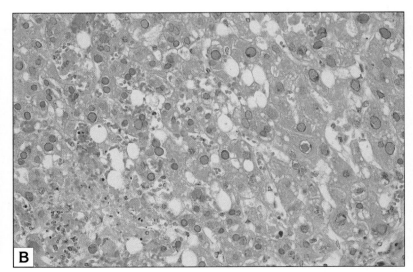

FIGURE 2-88 Disseminated herpes simplex. **A,** Liver section obtained at autopsy from an adult shows extensive coagulative necrosis and congestion as well as a nonspecific scattered steatosis. There is no specific pattern to the necrosis. No etiologic marker is discernible at this magnification. **B,** At the junction of the coagulative necrosis and adjacent viable hepatic parenchyma, many hepatic nuclei in the viable liver contain Cowdry A type inclusions. In some nuclei, the inclusion material is surrounded by a halo, due to shrinkage artifact. Many inclusions fill the nuclei, pushing the chromatin to the nuclear membrane and producing a finely beaded appearance along the nuclear membrane. (*Both panels,* hematoxylin-eosin stain. Original magnification; *panel 88A,* × 16; *panel 88B,* × 66.)

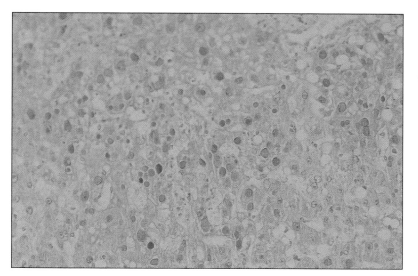

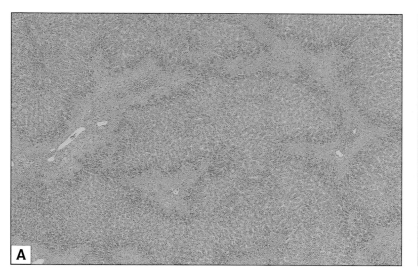

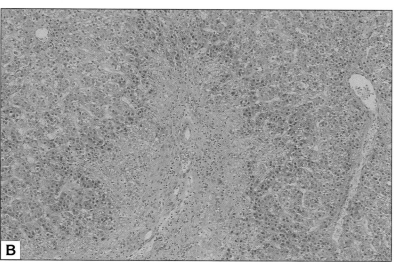

FIGURE 2-89 Confirmation of herpes simplex infection by immunoperoxidase staining. Available immunoperoxidase staining for herpes simplex virus does not distinguish between types I or II. Neonatal herpes infection may also cause severe hepatic necrosis with fatal consequences. Neonatal herpes is mostly acquired during vaginal delivery from mothers infected with genital herpes. Maternal genital herpes is an indication for cesarean delivery. (Original magnification, × 50.)

FIGURE 2-90 Adenovirus hepatitis. **A,** Liver obtained at autopsy shows extensive zone 1 (periportal) bridging necrosis. The inflammatory cell response is minimal. Hepatocytes adjacent to the necrosis are hypereosinophilic with hyperchromatic nuclei.

B, Periportal necrosis with adjacent hypereosinophilic hepatocytes and prominent nuclei. (Hematoxylin-eosin stain. Original magnification; *panel 90A,* × 10; *panel 90B,* × 25.)

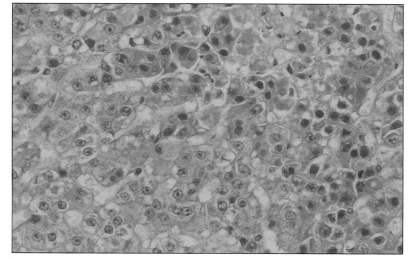

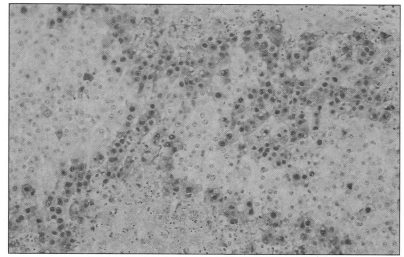

FIGURE 2-91 Liver section in adenovirus hepatitis showing hypereosinophilic hepatocytes adjacent to an area of necrosis. The nuclei in many viable hepatocytes contain inclusion material similar to herpes inclusions. (Hematoxylin-eosin stain; original magnification, × 100.)

FIGURE 2-92 Immunoperoxidase stain showing strong immunoreactivity for adenovirus in affected hepatic nuclei with spillover into the cytoplasm. (Original magnification, × 50.)

Bacterial Infection With Possible Hepatic Involvement

Bacteria causing infections with possible hepatic involvement	
Actinomyces	*Mycobacterium*
Bacteroides	*Nocardia*
Bartonella	*Proteus*
Brucella	*Pseudomonas*
Chlamydia	Rickettsia
Clostridium	*Salmonella*
Coxiella (Q fever)	Spirochetes
Escherichia coli	*Staphylococcus*
Francisella (tularemia)	*Streptococcus*
Klebsiella	*Yersinia*
Listeria	

FIGURE 2-93 Bacteria causing infections with possible hepatic involvement. Up to 50% of pyogenic liver abscesses are bacteriologically negative on culture. Abscesses may be caused by aerobic, anaerobic, or microaerophilic gram-positive or gram-negative organisms. The most frequent organism cultured is *Escherichia coli.*

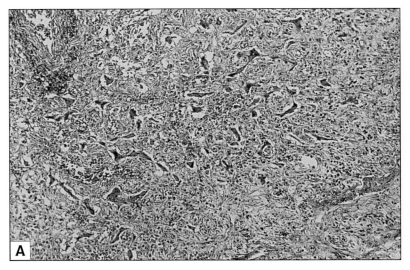

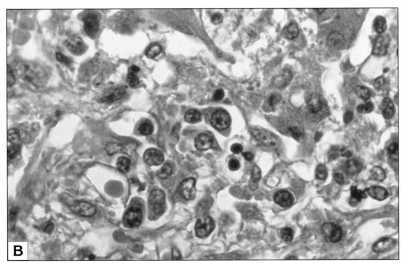

FIGURE 2-94 Congenital syphilis. **A,** Liver section shows widespread hepatocellular dropout, residual distorted hepatic plates, and slight stromal collagnation. (Masson-trichrome stain; original magnification, × 70.) **B,** A necrotic focus of parenchyma with chronic inflammatory cells and macrophages. A few distorted hepatocytes also are present. (Hematoxylin-eosin stain, original magnification, × 175.)

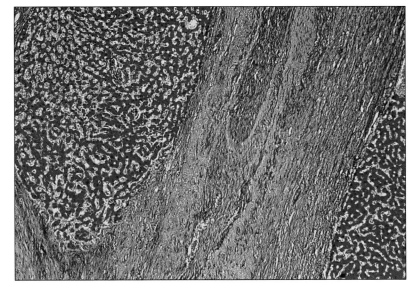

FIGURE 2-95 Hepar lobatum in syphilis. Distorted hepatic architecture results from a broad band of fibrosis separating multiacinar (multilobular) areas of parenchyma. (Masson-trichrome stain; original magnification, × 35.)

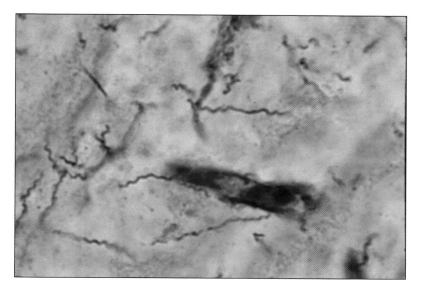

FIGURE 2-96 High magnification of an area of hepatic necrosis reveals spirochetes of *Treponema pallidum.* (Warthin-Starry stain; original magnification, × 465.)

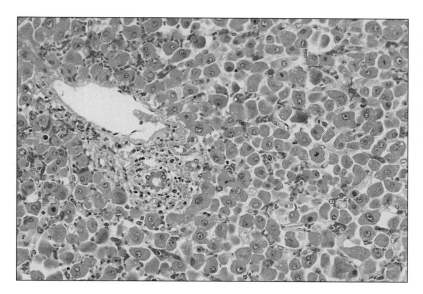

FIGURE 2-97 Leptospirosis. Sections of liver obtained at autopsy exhibit moderate to marked hepatocellular unrest, including many mitoses, dissociation of liver cell plates (loss of cohesion between cells), and spotty mild portal chronic inflammation. A clinical diagnosis of leptospirosis was confirmed. Although spirochetes are found in affected livers in approximately 25% to 30% of leptospirosis cases, the unequivocal presence of a spirochete in the liver of this patient was not demonstrated. (Hematoxylin-eosin stain; original magnification, × 66.)

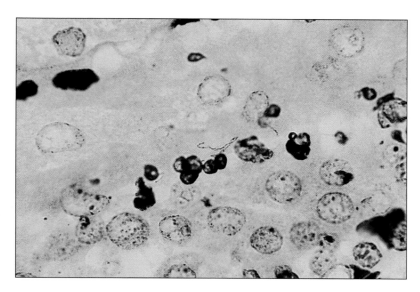

FIGURE 2-98 Leptospirosis in kidney tubule. Although spirochetes could not be found in the liver of this patient with documented leptospirosis (*see* Fig. 2-95), a few spirochetes were identified in the kidney. This section shows several spirochetes in a kidney tubule. (Warthin-Starry stain; original magnification, × 330.)

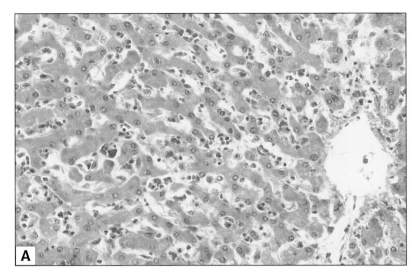

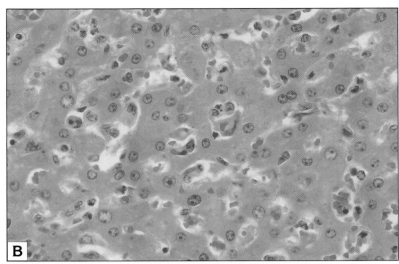

FIGURE 2-99 Relapsing fever. **A,** Liver section exhibits sinusoidal congestion, focal Kupffer cell hyperplasia, and increased numbers of inflammatory cells. **B,** On higher power, note the focal Kupffer cell hyperplasia with erythrophagocytosis. (*Both,* hematoxylin-eosin stain. Original magnification; *panel 99A,* × 80; *panel 99B,* × 132.)

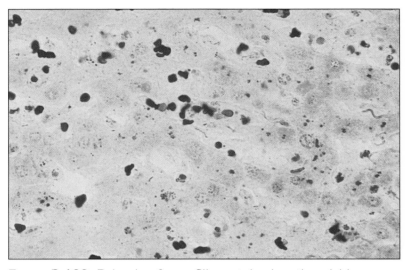

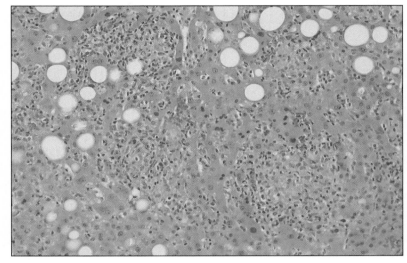

FIGURE 2-100 Relapsing fever. Silver-stained section yields a spirochete (*Borrelia* spp) lying free in sinusoid in the center of the field. (Warthin-Starry stain; original magnification, × 160.)

FIGURE 2-101 Liver biopsy specimen containing poorly formed noncaseating granulomas secondary to Q fever (*Coxiella burnettii*). (Hematoxylin-eosin stain.)

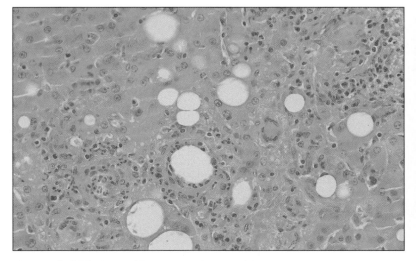

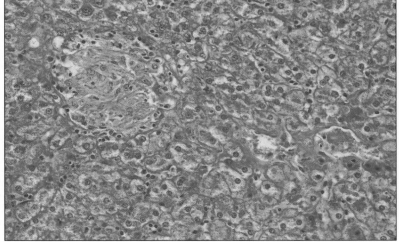

FIGURE 2-102 Liver biopsy specimen with noncaseating granulomata due to Q fever. In the lower center of the field is a dough-nut-shaped granuloma with inflammatory cells and a fibrin ring. Although not pathognomonic, fibrin-ring granulomas may be associated with Q fever. (Hematoxylin-eosin stain; original magnification, × 80.)

FIGURE 2-103 Liver biopsy with solitary noncaseating granuloma due to *Brucella abortus*. Clinical and serologic studies confirmed the diagnosis of *B. abortus* infection. (Hematoxylin-eosin stain; original magnification, × 80.)

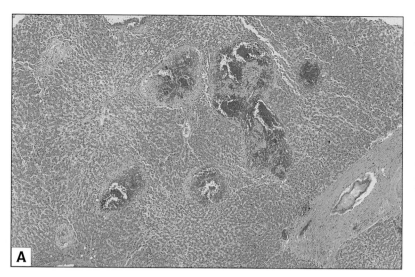

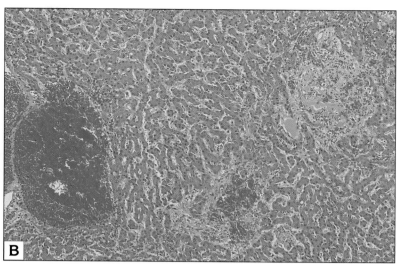

FIGURE 2-104 Bacillary necropeliosis. **A,** Liver obtained at autopsy shows "punched out" hemorrhagic areas. The patient was HIV-positive. **B,** Foci demonstrate fully formed "blood lakes" as well as degenerating granuloma-like areas with slight or spotty hemorrhage. (*Both panels,* hematoxylin-eosin stain. Original magnification; *panel 104A,* × 10; *panel 104B,* × 25.)

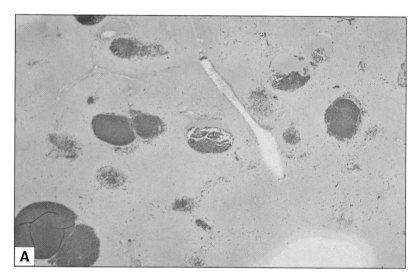

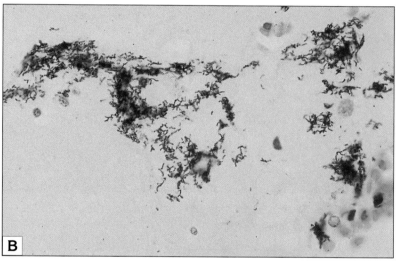

FIGURE 2-105 Warthin-Starry preparation of liver showing hemorrhagic or peliotic areas. **A,** On low-power magnification, clusters of black material can be seen in several peliotic areas. **B,** High-power magnification of one of these peliotic areas discloses clusters of entangled bacilli consisting of *Bartonella* species. (Original magnification, × 198.)

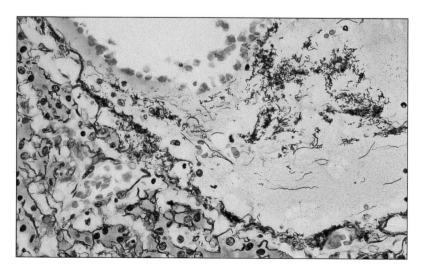

FIGURE 2-106 Necropeliotic area infiltrated by bacilli. A modification of Manuel's reticulum stain discloses clusters of entangled bacilli at the periphery of a peliotic lesion. In one area, organisms are beginning to infiltrate an adjacent sinusoid. (Wenger-Angritt reticulin method; original magnification, × 100.)

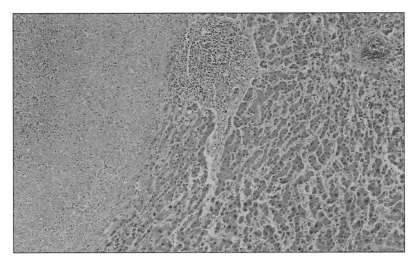

FIGURE 2-107 Listeriosis in an adult. Listeriosis is a worldwide infectious disease caused by *Listeria monocytogenes*, a gram-positive bacillus. Liver lesions may include focal necrosis, microabscesses, and abscess formation. In neonatal listeriosis, lesions may appear granulomatoid or granulomatous. In this figure, a liver section shows a large area of necrosis and portal inflammation from a fatal case of listeriosis in an adult. (Hematoxylin-eosin stain; original magnification, × 25.)

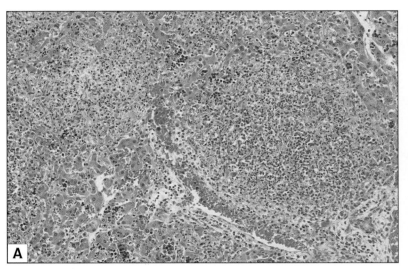

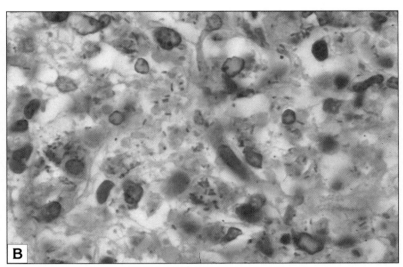

FIGURE 2-108 Listeriosis in a newborn (granulomatosis infantiseptica). **A,** Liver section displays haphazard microabscess formation with neutrophils and some macrophages. There is a suggestion of poorly formed granulomatous reaction. (Hematoxylin-eosin stain; original magnification, × 40.) **B,** Brown-Hopps stain displays numerous gram-positive intracellular bacilli in an area of necrosis. (Original magnification, × 400.)

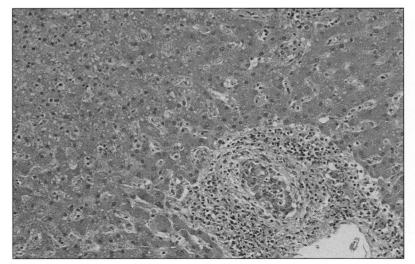

FIGURE 2-109 Toxic shock syndrome. A liver section shows acute cholangitis and finely vacuolated hepatocytes, combined with microvesicular steatosis, in a patient with fatal toxic shock syndrome. (Hematoxylin-eosin stain; original magnification, × 50.)

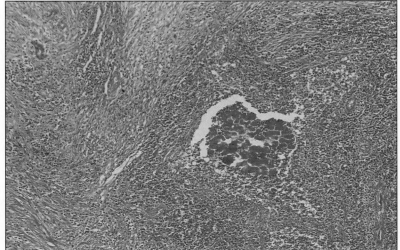

FIGURE 2-110 Botryomycosis. Liver section displays abscess formation that contains granules consisting of bacterial microcolonies. The colonies are surrounded by polymorphonuclear leukocytes. These changes are consistent with botryomycosis. Botryomycotic lesions are similar to lesions of mycetoma and actinomycosis on hematoxylin-eosin–stained sections. (Original magnification, × 25.)

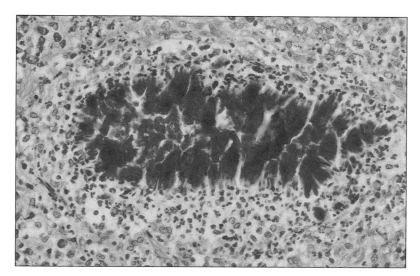

FIGURE 2-111 Botryomycosis with the Splendore-Hoeppli phenomenon. Densely packed microorganisms are surrounded at the periphery by radiating eosinophilic deposits. In thick sections, deposits appear as rings. In this section, gram-negative rods are difficult to identify in the center of the granule. (Humberstone, original magnification, × 100.)

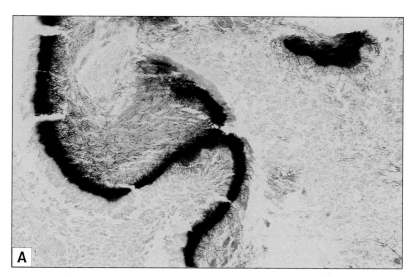

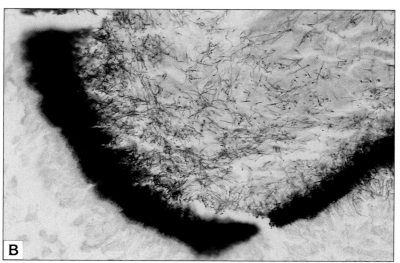

FIGURE 2-112 Disseminated actinomycosis. **A,** Filaments of actinomycosis are recognizable on medium-power magnification by the Gomori methenamine silver staining method. **B,** On high-power magnification, the filaments of actinomycosis are more readily recognized. Peripheral clubbing of "sulfur" granule is suggested. The center of granules may contain structures mimicking gram-positive cocci or even gram-negative bacilli. (Original magnification: *panel 112A,* × 50; *panel 112B,* × 132.)

Mycobacterial Infections

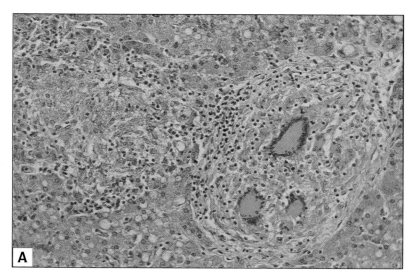

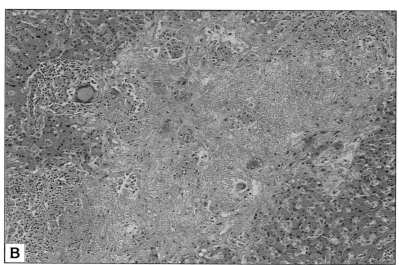

FIGURE 2-113 Miliary tuberculosis. **A,** Liver biopsy specimen shows a noncaseating granuloma containing Langhan's giant cells. Further studies confirmed miliary tuberculosis. **B,** Liver biopsy specimen showing confluent caseating ("necrotizing") granulomas in a patient with miliary tuberculosis. (Hematoxylin-eosin stain; original magnification, × 35.)

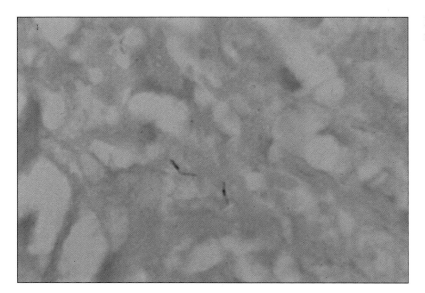

FIGURE 2-114 Acid-fast bacilli detected in liver tissue in a case of miliary tuberculosis. (Original magnification, × 260.)

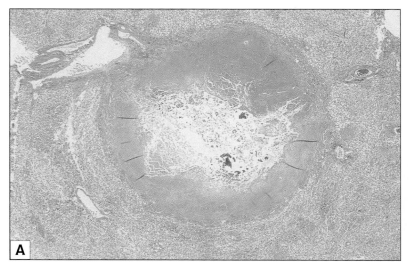

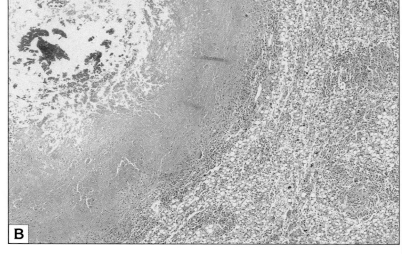

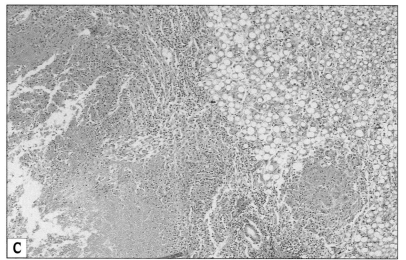

FIGURE 2-115 Tuberculous cholangitis. **A,** Caseous necrosis involves most of the wall of the interlobular bile duct. Bile is present in the lumen. **B,** Higher magnification shows that in the liver parenchyma adjacent to the interlobular bile duct, there are poorly formed granulomas. **C,** Caseous necrosis of the interlobular bile duct wall and a granuloma in adjacent parenchyma (*lower right*) are seen. Nonspecific hepatocellular steatosis also is present. (*All panels,* hematoxylin-eosin stain. Original magnification; *panel 115A,* × 5; *panel 115B,* × 16; *panel 115C,* × 25.)

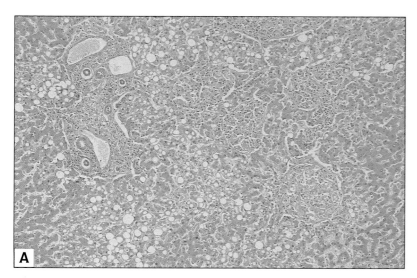

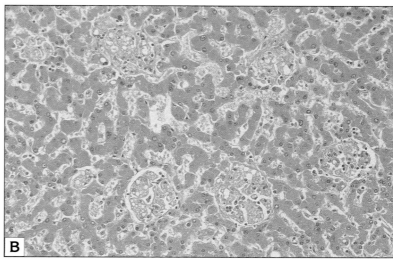

FIGURE 2-116 Lepromatous leprosy. **A,** Liver section shows portal and parenchymal collections of macrophages displaying lipid vacuolization or xanthoma-like foci. Such collections of macrophages characterize lepromatous leprosy. In tuberculid leprosy, granulomatous lesions resembling those of sarcoidosis occur. **B,** Magnified view of parenchymal foci of lepromatous leprosy. (Hematoxylin-eosin stain. Original magnification; *panel 116A*, × 25; *panel 116B*, × 50.)

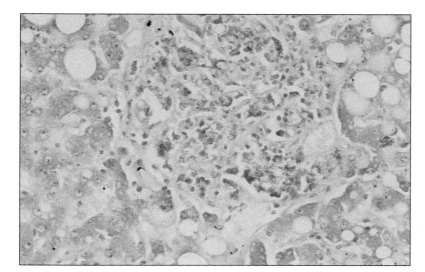

FIGURE 2-117 Lepromatous leprosy. Small acid-fast bacilli are seen in vacuolated macrophages and individual Kupffer cells from a case of lepromatous leprosy. (Fite-Faraco stain; original magnification, × 150.)

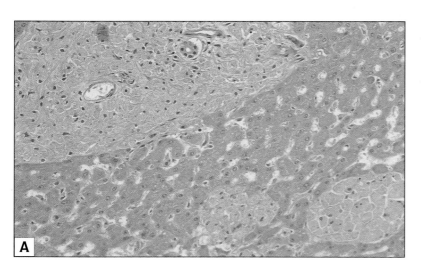

FIGURE 2-118 Disseminated *Mycobacterium avium* complex infection. **A,** Liver section from an HIV-positive patient displays a striking accumulation of finely granular, foamy-looking portal macrophages as well as granuloma-like clusters of Kupffer cells throughout the liver parenchyma. (Hematoxylin-eosin stain.) (*continued*)

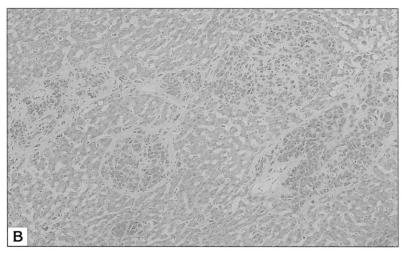

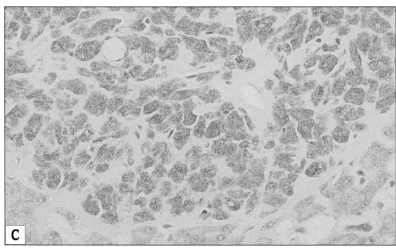

FIGURE 2-118 (*continued*) **B** and **C.** On Ziehl-Neelsen staining, the macrophage system cells are filled with an abundance of acid-fast bacilli consistent with *Mycobacterium avium intracellulare.* The bacilli are also periodic acid–Schiff positive. (Original magnification: *panel 118B,* × 25; *panel 118C,* × 100.)

Parasitic Infections With Possible Liver Involvement

A. Protozoal and helminthic infections with possible hepatic involvement: Protozoa
Amebiasis Cryptosporidiosis Malaria Pneumocystosis Toxoplasmosis Visceral leishmaniasis (kala-azar)

B. Protozoal and helminthic infections with possible hepatic involvement: Helminths	

Cestodes
  Echinococcosis
Nematodes
  Ascariasis
  Capillariasis
  Strongyloidiasis
	Trematodes
	  Clonorchiasis
	  Fascioliasis
	  Opisthorchiasis
	  Paragonimiasis
	  Schistosomiasis
	Pentastomids
	  Pentastomiasis

FIGURE 2-119 Protozoal and helminthic infections with possible hepatic involvement. **A,** Protozoa. **B,** Helminths.

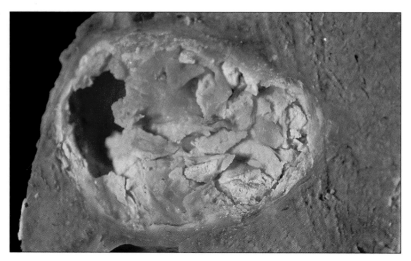

FIGURE 2-120 Gross cross-section of liver with a hydatid (echinococcal) cyst. The cyst consists of a large unilocular cyst with daughter cysts.

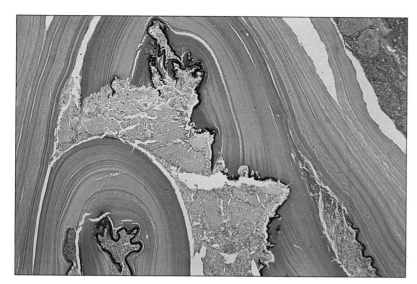

FIGURE 2-121 Section of a hydatid (echinococcal) cyst wall displaying a laminated membrane and germinal layer. (Masson-trichrome stain; original magnification, × 18.)

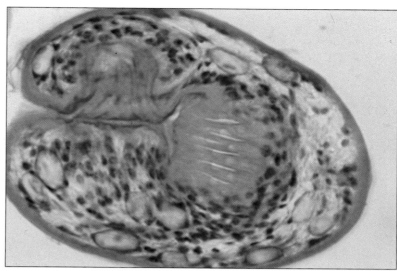

FIGURE 2-122 Scolex of *Echinococcus granulosus*. The scolex is invaginated and has a double row of hooklets. (Hematoxylin-eosin stain; original magnification, × 175.)

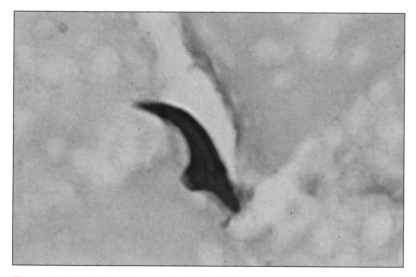

FIGURE 2-123 Hooklet or "scimitar" from *Echinococcus granulosus* showing acid-fast positivity. (Original magnification, × 345.)

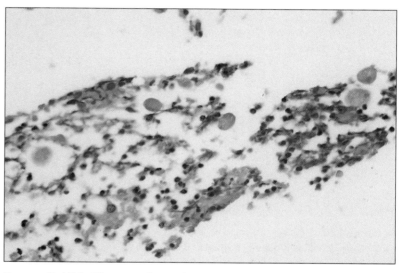

FIGURE 2-124 Fine-needle aspirate of liver containing several trophozoites of *Entamoeba histolytica*. (Hematoxylin-eosin stain; original magnification, × 115.)

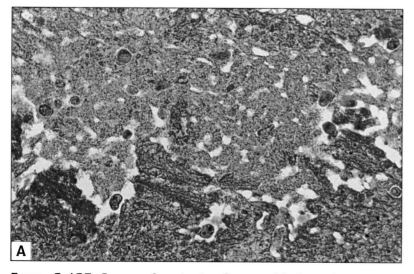

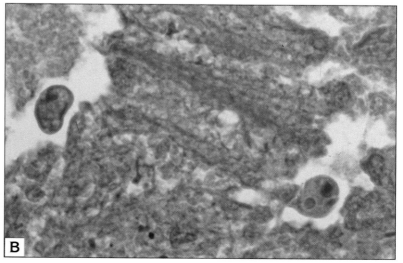

FIGURE 2-125 Smear of contents of an amebic liver abscess. **A,** Abscess contents, described as "anchovy paste," shows several scattered trophozoites in amorphous, necrotic tissue. No inflammatory response is seen. (Periodic acid–Schiff stain; original magnification, × 55.) **B,** High magnification shows trophozoites of *Entamoeba histolytica* containing round nuclei and central karyosomes. (Hematoxylin-eosin stain; original magnification, × 165.)

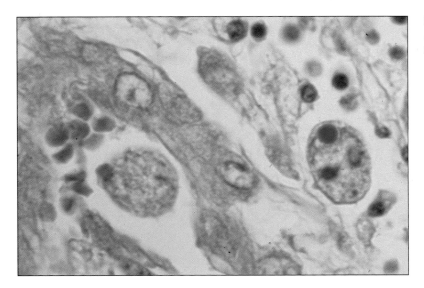

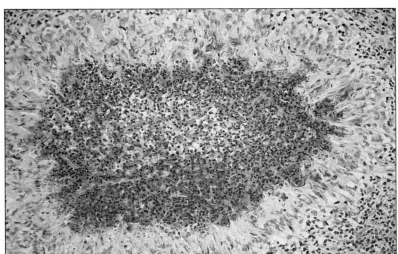

FIGURE 2-126 Gridley ameba stain shows a trophozoite of *Entamoeba histolytica* containing red blood cells. (Original magnification, × 230.)

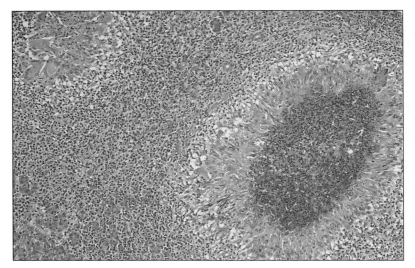

FIGURE 2-127 Necrotizing eosinophilic granulomatous inflammation secondary to visceral larva migrans (*Toxocara canis*). Note palisading at the periphery of the lesion. The central necrotic portion has an abundance of eosinophils and many scattered crystalline structures. The surrounding inflammatory response is also rich in eosinophils. No parasite is identified, but the patient was found to have visceral larva migrans. (Hematoxylin-eosin stain, × 28.)

FIGURE 2-128 Visceral larva migrans. Biebrich scarlet staining demonstrates the many eosinophils and Charcot-Leyden crystals. (Original magnification, × 45.)

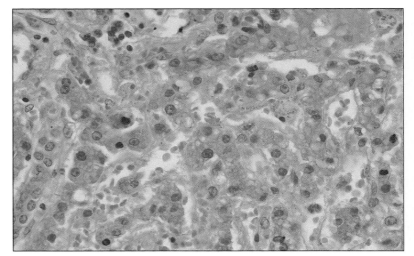

FIGURE 2-129 Kala-azar (visceral leishmaniasis). The liver section shows several hypertrophied or swollen Kupffer cells containing many small ovoid leishmania. (Hematoxylin-eosin stain; original magnification, × 132.)

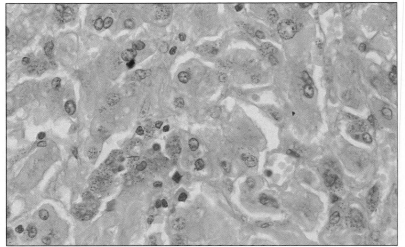

FIGURE 2-130 Kala-azar (visceral leishmaniasis). The liver displays occasional swollen Kupffer cells containing many periodic acid–Schiff-positive diastase-resistant leishmania. (Periodic acid–Schiff with diastase predigestion. Original magnification, × 160.)

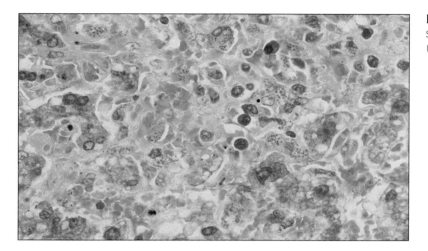

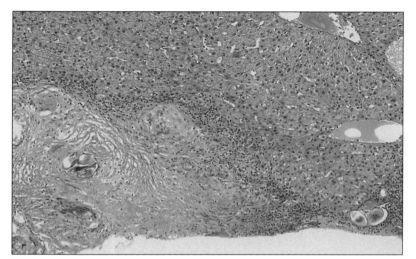

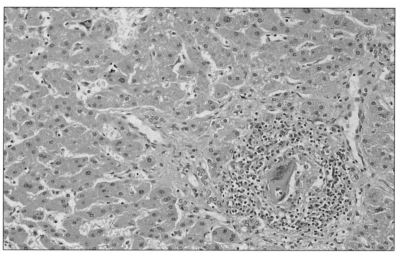

FIGURE 2-131 Kala-azar. Giemsa-stained section exhibits scattered swollen Kupffer cells containing many phagocytosed leishmania. (Original magnification, × 160.)

FIGURE 2-132 Schistosomiasis. The ova of *Schistosoma mansoni* are seen in the portal-periportal area with a foreign-body type reaction. Eggs can also be seen in the lower right corner of the section, and there is increased fibrous tissue in the portal area. Of the five species of *Schistosoma* (trematode, blood flukes) that infect humans, two species—*S. mansoni* and *S. japonicum*—account for most cases of hepatobiliary involvement. Tissue damage is essentially a consequence of the deposition of the schistosomal eggs, especially in the smaller intrahepatic portal vessels. (Hematoxylin-eosin stain; original magnification, × 33.)

FIGURE 2-133 Eggs of *Schistosoma mansoni* with a granulomatous response and eosinophilia. Schistosome eggs evoke a granulomatous reaction. Advanced schistosomiasis results in portal and septal fibrosis, eventually giving rise to Symmers' portal fibrosis. Note also the accumulation of brown-black pigment ("schistosomal pigment") in portal macrophages and scattered Kupffer cells. Schistosomal pigment is indistinguishable from malarial pigment and is a breakdown product of hemoglobin. Schistosomal pigment may be seen even in the absence of ova. (Hematoxylin-eosin stain; original magnification, × 50.)

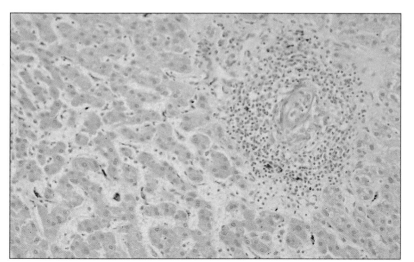

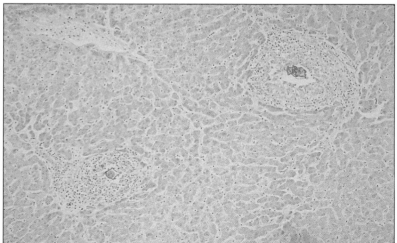

FIGURE 2-134 Schistosomal pigment stains negative for iron. (Mallory's iron stain; original magnification, × 50.)

FIGURE 2-135 Two portal areas, each containing a degenerating egg, displaying the acid-fast staining of the chitinous walls of *Schistosoma mansoni* ova. The chitinous walls of both *S. mansoni* and *S. japonicum* are acid-fast. (Acid-fast stain; original magnification, × 25.)

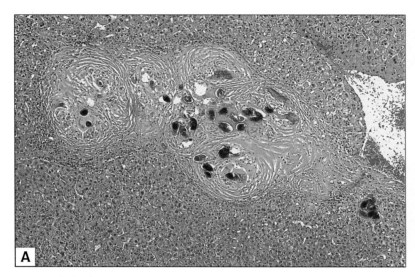

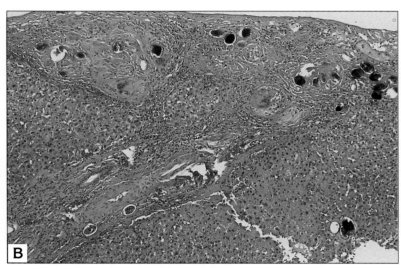

FIGURE 2-136 Liver sections revealing ova of *Schistosoma japonicum*. **A,** Marked infestation by ova of *S. japonicum* with a prominent granulomatous response and fibrous expansion of portal areas. Whereas the eggs of *S. mansoni* usually measure 114 to 175 µm × 45 to 68 µm and have a prominent lateral spine, the eggs of *S. japonicum* are smaller, ranging from 70 to 100 µm × 50 to 65 µm, with a minute spine on one side. **B,** In another section, *Schistosoma japonicum,* note the prominent subcapsular as well as portal involvement. (*Both panels,* hematoxylin-eosin stain; original magnification, × 20.)

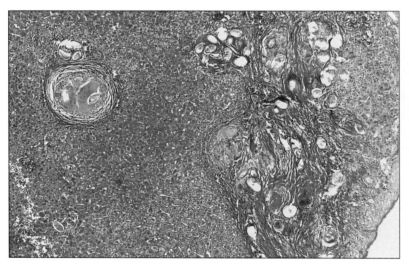

FIGURE 2-137 Marked fibrosis evoked by the many ova of *Schistosoma japonicum*. Fibrous tissue (collagen) appears blue. (Masson-trichrome stain; original magnification, × 20.)

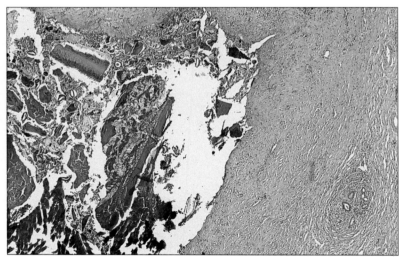

FIGURE 2-138 Ascariasis. Bile duct containing bile, debris, and *Ascaris* eggs. Note the marked fibrous thickening of the bile duct. The lining epithelium has been denuded. Peribiliary glands can be seen in the lower right field. Approximately 25% of the world's population is infected with *Ascaris lumbricoides*. (Hematoxylin-eosin stain; original magnification, × 13.2.)

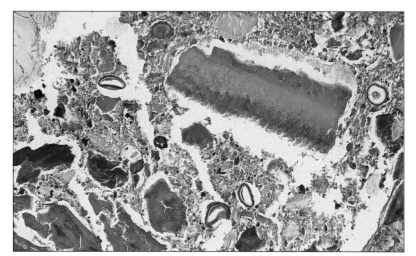

FIGURE 2-139 Ascariasis. Contents of bile duct with bile, debris, and several *Ascaris* ova. Fertilized eggs measure 45 to 75 µm × 35 to 50 µm, are round or oval-shaped, and are thick-shelled. They may be mamillated or smooth. Shells are negative on acid-fast staining. Nonfertilized eggs range from 88 to 94 µm × 44µm, are thin-shelled, and are either smooth or mamillated. (Hematoxylin-eosin stain; original magnification, × 40.)

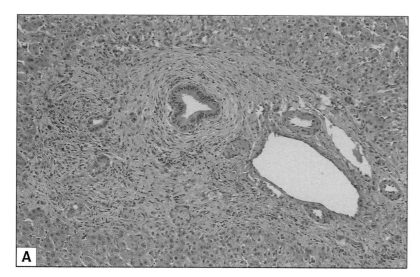

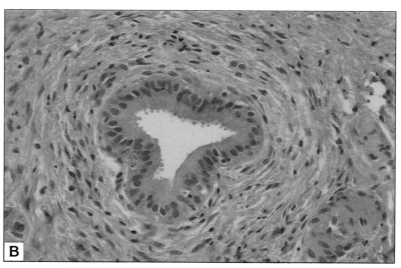

FIGURE 2-140 Cryptosporidiosis. **A,** Liver biopsy from an HIV-positive patient shows a portal area with periductal "onion-skin" fibrosis. Within the lumen of the duct are many small microorganisms attached to the lining epithelium. **B,** Higher magnification shows the many small organisms attached to the bile duct epithelium, which are consistent with *Cryptosporidium.* (Hematoxylin-eosin stain. Original magnification: *panel 140A,* × 33; *panel 140B,* × 100.)

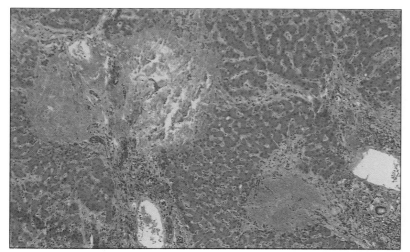

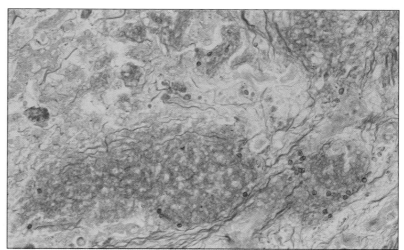

FIGURE 2-141 Disseminated *Pneumocystis carinii* infection. A liver section obtained at autopsy shows amorphous necrotic foci without any significant inflammatory cell response. The patient was HIV-positive. (Hematoxylin-eosin stain; original magnification, × 25.)

FIGURE 2-142 Silver stain of organisms in disseminated pneumocystosis. In the same patient as in Fig. 2-141, Gomori's methenamine silver preparation discloses the presence of several organisms consistent with *Pneumocystis carinii.* The cause of death in this patient was attributed to widespread *P. carinii* infection. Methenamine silver stains readily demonstrate cyst walls. Trophozoites of *P. carinii* are best demonstrated with the Giemsa staining method, and Gram stain tissue methods are also useful to detect cysts and trophozoites.

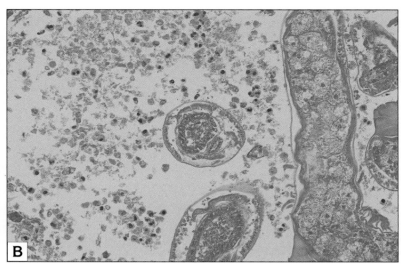

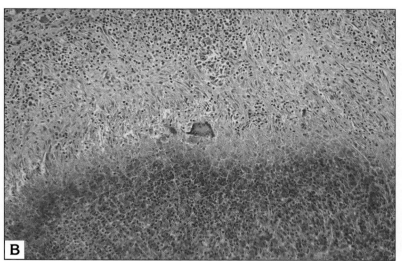

FIGURE 2-143 Capillariasis. Lesions in the liver result from deposition of eggs, adult worms, or their degenerating remnants. Areas of necrosis with peripheral granulomatous inflammation resembling lesions of visceral larva migrans (VLM) may be encountered. Unlike VLM, in which larvae are rarely found, the necrotic abscesslike areas in capillariasis may contain the adult worms or their parts. **A,** Low-power photomicrograph shows a large, irregular-abscesslike necrotic area containing parts of the adult worm, *Capillaria hepatica.* **B,** Parts of the adult male worm. (Hematoxylin-eosin stain. Original magnification: *panel 143A,* × 5; *panel 143B,* × 80.)

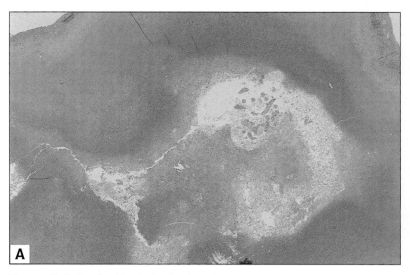

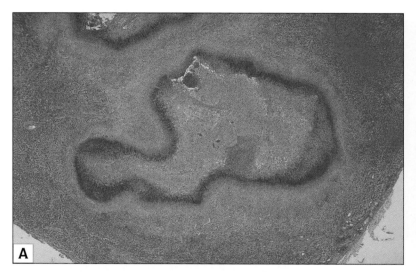

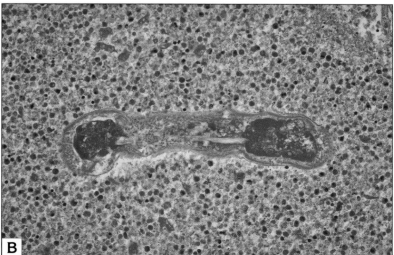

FIGURE 2-144 Capillariasis. **A,** Extensive areas of necrosis with peripheral granulomatous chronic inflammation due to *Capillaria hepatica.* Note the similarity to the lesion of visceral larva migrans. Parts of a worm are present in the necrotic area. Eggs of *Capillaria hepatica,* if present, resemble those of *Trichuris trichiura.* The inflammatory response often exhibits a marked number of eosinophils. Humans become infected by ingesting the livers of infected animals (usually rodents). **B,** Higher magnification of the periphery of a necrotic area displays the granulomatous reaction. **C,** Portion of an adult worm in a necrotic area. (Hematoxylin-eosin stain.)

Fungal Infections With Possible Hepatic Involvement

Mycotic infections with possible hepatic involvement
Candidiasis
Aspergillosis
Histoplasmosis
Coccidioidomycosis
North American blastomycosis
Cryptococcosis
Mucormycosis
African histoplasmosis
Paracoccidioidomycosis

FIGURE 2-145 Mycotic infections with possible hepatic involvement.

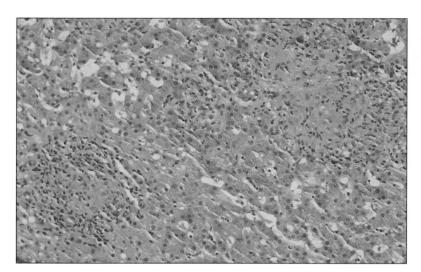

FIGURE 2-146 Disseminated histoplasmosis. A liver biopsy specimen contains noncaseating granulomatous inflammation. No specific etiologic agent is identified in this figure. (Hematoxylin-eosin stain; original magnification, × 50.)

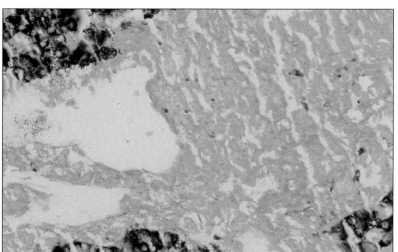

FIGURE 2-147 Disseminated histoplasmosis. Gomori methenamine silver preparation discloses a few small yeastlike organisms consistent with *Histoplasma.* In nonfatal cases of histoplasmosis, granulomas may become hyalinized and/or focally calcified. In old, hyalinized granulomas, organisms may be found on rare occasions. (Original magnification, × 100.)

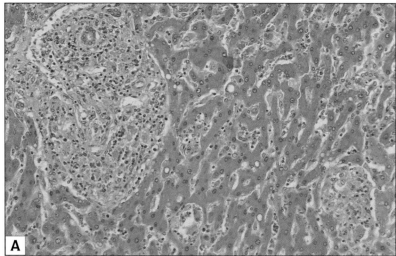

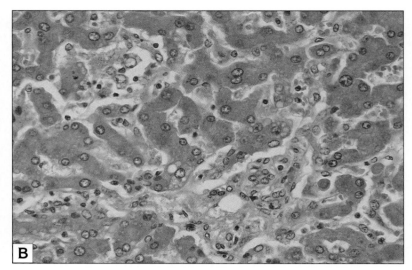

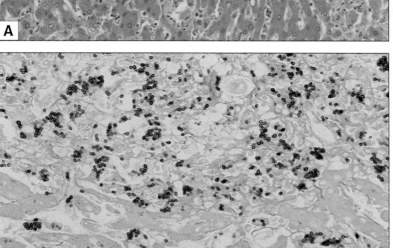

FIGURE 2-148 Disseminated histoplasmosis. **A,** Section of liver shows prominent hypertrophy of portal macrophages as well as groups and individual Kupffer cells. (Hematoxylin-eosin stain; original magnification, × 50.) **B,** On higher magnification, the swollen portal macrophages and Kupffer cells contain small organisms with nuclei surrounded by an artifactual clear zone (due to fixation). These organisms are *Histoplasma capsulatum*. (Hematoxylin-eosin stain; original magnification, × 100.) **C,** The yeast-like organisms of *H. capsulatum* are readily demonstrated with the Gomori methenamine silver stain. This section exhibits the marked involvement of portal macrophages and many Kupffer cells. The patient died of disseminated histoplasmosis.

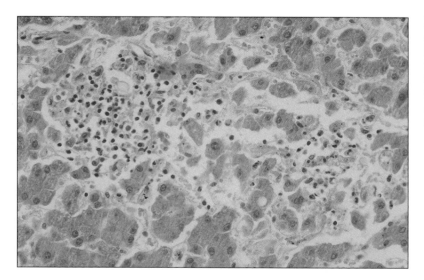

FIGURE 2-149 Cryptococcosis. Liver involvement in disseminated cryptococcosis may evoke a variety of alterations, ranging from little or no inflammatory response to polymorphonuclear exudation and/or granuloma formation. In this section, there is an area of necrosis containing small and large forms of pale bluish-gray organisms. In some cases, small forms may resemble those of *Histoplasma*, and large forms without capsules, *Blastomyces*. (Hematoxylin-eosin stain; original magnification, × 80.)

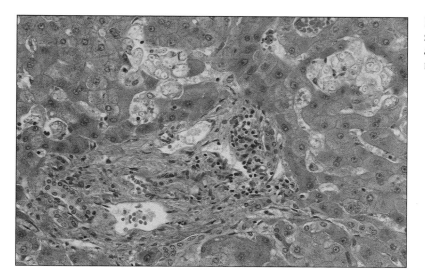

FIGURE 2-150 Liver in disseminated cryptococcosis, showing occasional clusters of *Cryptococcus neoformans*. Note the absence of an inflammatory cell response. (Hematoxylin-eosin stain; original magnification, × 40.)

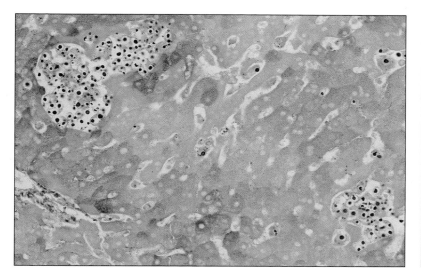

FIGURE 2-151 Gomori-methenamine-silver staining in disseminated cryptococcosis. Clusters and single fungal organisms consistent with *Cryptococcus neoformans* can be seen. (Original magnification, × 66.)

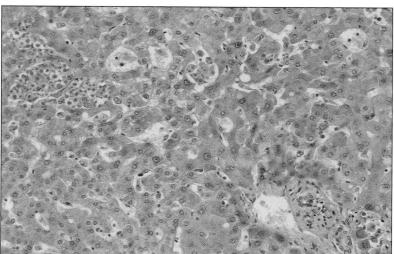

FIGURE 2-152 Mucinous capsule of cryptococcosis demonstrated with the mucicarmine staining method. Nonencapsulated forms may also be seen. (Original magnification, × 50.)

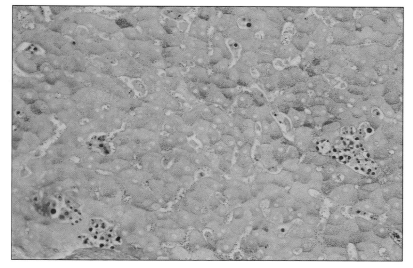

FIGURE 2-153 Mucinous capsule of cryptococcosis also stains blue with the Alcian blue–periodic acid–Schiff staining method. (Original magnification, × 66.)

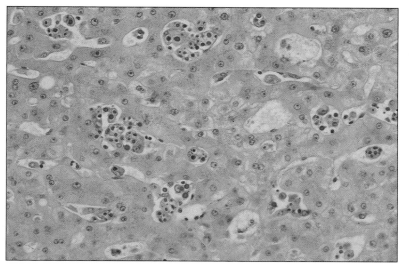

FIGURE 2-154 Cryptococcosis demonstrated with periodic acid–Schiff stain with diastase predigestion. (Original magnification, × 66.)

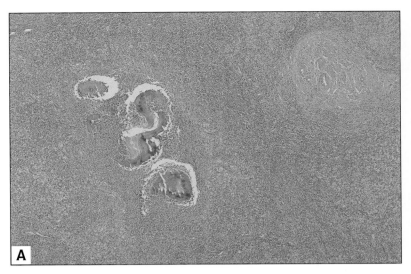

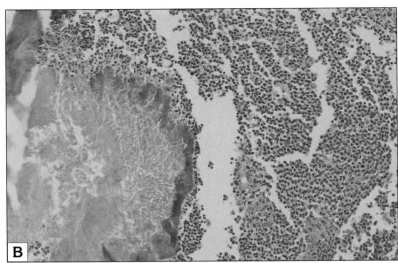

FIGURE 2-155 Liver section with extensive involvement by actinomycosis. **A,** Note the so-called "sulfur" granules in the abscessed area. **B,** On higher magnification, the sulfur granule is surrounded by pus cells. Peripheral clubbing of the granule is not apparent. (Hematoxylin-eosin stain. Original magnification; *panel 155A,* × 10; *panel 155B,* × 50.)

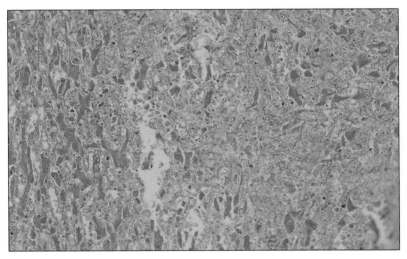

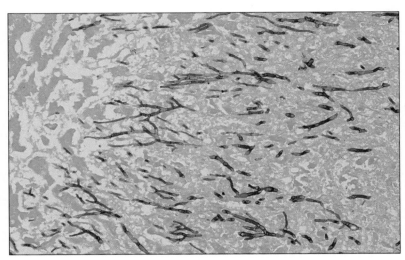

FIGURE 2-156 Aspergillosis. Section of liver obtained at autopsy contains a large necrotic area with little or no inflammatory cell response. In the necrotic area, there are a few barely perceptible fungal structures. (Hematoxylin-eosin stain; original magnification, × 66.)

FIGURE 2-157 Gomori methenamine silver stain shows many dichotomous branching septate hyphae in aspergillosis. The branches appear to follow a similar direction. These features are characteristic for aspergillosis.

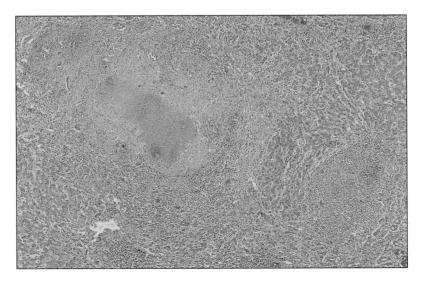

FIGURE 2-158 Coccidioidomycosis, showing granulomata including one with central necrosis. Structures consistent with fungal spores are present. Coccidioidomycosis is caused by *Coccidioides immitis.* (Hematoxylin-eosin stain; original magnification, × 13.2.)

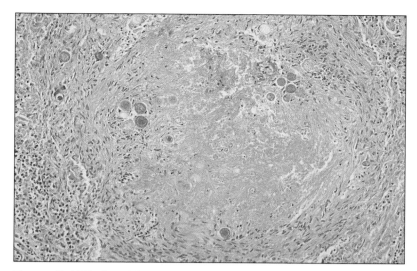

FIGURE 2-159 Coccidioidal sporangia and sporangiospores. Note the thick walls of the fungal spores. Mature sporangia range from 30 to 60 μm in diameter. Sporangiospores vary from 1 to 5 μm in diameter. (Hematoxylin-eosin stain; original magnification, × 40.)

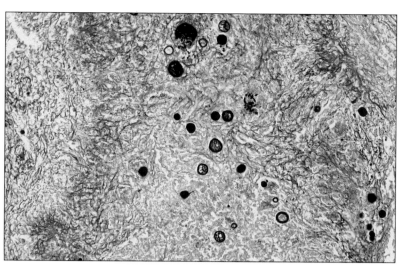

FIGURE 2-160 Coccidioidal sporangia and sporangiospores (endospores) demonstrated by Gomori methenamine silver staining. Note the release of sporangiospores from a ruptured sporangium (*top center*). (Original magnification, × 50.)

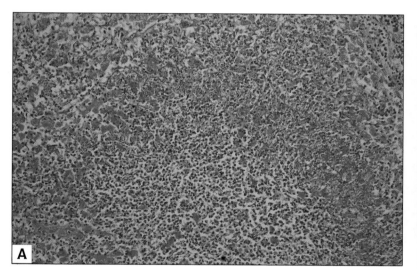

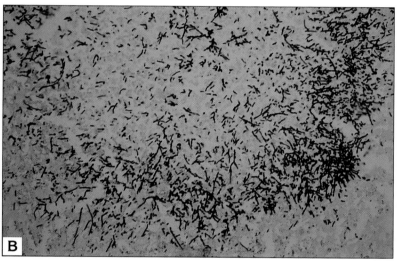

FIGURE 2-161 Disseminated candidiasis. *Candida albicans* is the most common mycotic species identified in human infections. Disseminated candidiasis is most often encountered in immuno-suppressed or debilitated patients. **A,** Liver abscess containing structures consistent with yeast forms, pseudohyphae, or hyphae.

(Hematoxylin-eosin stain.) **B,** With Gomori methenamine silver stain, many pseudohyphae and hyphae are demonstrated. The periodic acid–Schiff and Gridley stains are also excellent to demonstrate this fungus. (*Both panels,* original magnification, × 45.)

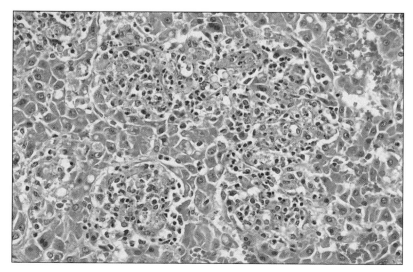

FIGURE 2-162 Disseminated candidiasis with multiple granuloma-like foci of necrosis. Many pale, round yeastlike organisms are present in the macrophage cells. (Hematoxylin-eosin stain; original magnification, × 80.)

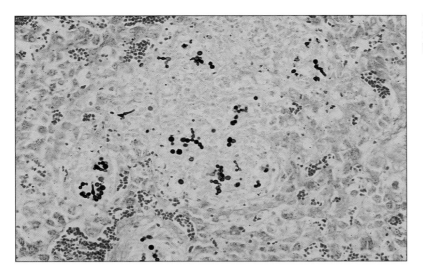

FIGURE 2-163 Gomori methenamine silver staining demonstrating mainly candidal blastospores, occasional pseudohyphae, and budding. (Original magnification, × 66.)

REFERENCES

1. Battegay M, Gust ID, Feinstone SM: Hepatitis A virus. *In* Mandell GL, Bennett JE, Dolin R (eds.): *Principles and Practice of Infectious Diseases*, 4th ed. New York: Churchill Livingstone; 1995:1637–1656.

2. Centers for Disease Control and Prevention: Recommendation of the Immunization Practices Advisory Committee (ACIP): Protection against viral hepatitis. *MMWR* 1990, 39:1–26.

3. Robinson WS: Hepatitis B virus and hepatitis D virus. *In* Mandell GL, Bennett JE, Dolin R (eds.): *Principles and Practice of Infectious Diseases*, 4th ed. New York: Churchill Livingstone; 1995:1406–1439.

4. Hsu HH, Feinstone SM, Hoofnagle JH: Acute viral hepatitis. *In* Mandell GL, Bennett JE, Dolin R (eds.): *Principles and Practice of Infectious Diseases*, 4th ed. New York: Churchill Livingstone; 1995:1136–1153.

5. Advisory Committee for Immunization Practices: Recommendations for protection against viral hepatitis. *MMWR* 1990, 38(suppl):1–26.

6. Kuhns MC: Viral hepatitis: Pt. 1. The discovery, diagnostic tests, and new viruses. *Lab Med* 1995, 26:650–659.

7. Shimizu YK, Feinstone SM, Kohara M, *et al.*: Hepatitis C virus: Detection of intracellular virus particles by electron microscopy. *Hepatology* 1996, 23:205–209.

8. Lemon SM, Brown EA: H epatitis C virus. *In* Mandell GL, Bennett JE, Dolin R (eds.): *Principles and Practice of Infectious Diseases*, 4th ed. New York: Churchill Livingstone; 1995:1474–1486.

9. Alter MJ, Hadler SC, Judson FN, *et al.*: Risk factors for acute non-A, non-B hepatitis in the United States and association with hepatitis C infection. *JAMA* 1990, 264:2231–2235.

10. Ticehurst J, Rhodes LL Jr, Krawczynski K, *et al.*: Infection of owl monkeys (*Aotus trivirgatus*) and cynomolgus monkeys (*Macaca fascicularis*) with hepatitis E virus from Mexico. *J Infect Dis* 1992, 165:835–845.

11. Lemon SM: Hepatitis E virus. *In* Mandell GL, Bennett JE, Dolin R (eds.): *Principles and Practice of Infectious Diseases*, 4th ed. New York: Churchill Livingstone; 1995:1663–1666.

12. Alter HJ: Post-transfusion hepatitis G virus infection. Presented at Hepatitis G Virus: A Newly Discovered Hepatitis Virus [symposium]. Chicago, 6 November 1995.

13. Alter MJ: Community-acquired hepatitis G virus infection. Presented at Hepatitis G Virus: A Newly Discovered Hepatitis Virus [symposium]. Chicago, 6 November 1995.

14. Yoshiba M, Okamoto H, Mishiro S: Detection of the GBV-C hepatitis virus genome in serum from patients with fulminant hepatitis of unknown etiology. *Lancet* 1995, 346:1131–1132.

15. Lemon SM, Day SP: Type A viral hepatitis. *In* Gorbach SL, Bartlett JG, Blacklow NR (eds.): *Infectious Diseases*. Philadelphia: W.B. Saunders; 1992:705–709.

16. Maddrey WC: Approach to the patient with infection of the liver. *In* Gorbach SL, Bartlett JG, Blacklow NR (eds.): *Infectious Diseases*. W.B. Saunders; 1992:699–705.

17. Ueda N, Shah SV: Apoptosis. *J Lab Clin Med* 1994, 124:169–177.

18. Krawitt EL: Chronic hepatitis. *In* Mandell GL, Bennett JE, Dolin R (eds.): *Principles and Practice of Infectious Diseases*, 4th ed. New York: Churchill Livingstone; 1995.

19. Poulsen H, Christofferson P: Abnormal bile duct epithelium in chronic aggressive hepatitis and cirrhosis. *Hum Pathol* 1972, 3:217–225.

SELECTED BIBLIOGRAPHY

Batts KP, Ludwig J: Chronic hepatitis: An update on terminology and reporting. *Am J Surg Pathol* 1995, 19:1409–1417.

Binford CH, Connor DH (eds.): *Pathology of Tropical and Extraordinary Diseases*, vol 1 and 2. Washington, DC: Armed Forces Institute of Pathology; 1976.

Ishak KG: Chronic hepatitis: Morphology and nomenclature. *Mod Pathol* 1994, 7:690–713.

Ishak KG: Granulomas of the liver. *Adv Pathol Lab Med* 1995, 8:247–361.

MacSween RNM, Anthony PP, Scheuer PJ, *et al.* (eds.): *Pathology of the Liver*, 3rd ed. New York: Churchill Livingstone; 1994.

Schiff L, Schiff ER (eds.): *Diseases of the Liver*, 7th ed. Philadelphia: J.B. Lippincott; 1993.

Schulte-Hermann R, Bursch W, Grasl-Kraupp B: Active cell death (apoptosis) in liver biology and disease. *In* Boyer JL, Ockner R (eds.): *Progress in Liver Disease*. Philadelphia: W.B. Saunders; 1995.

CHAPTER 3

Bacterial Enteritis

Richard L. Guerrant

SETTINGS AND IMPACT OF MICROBIAL DIARRHEA

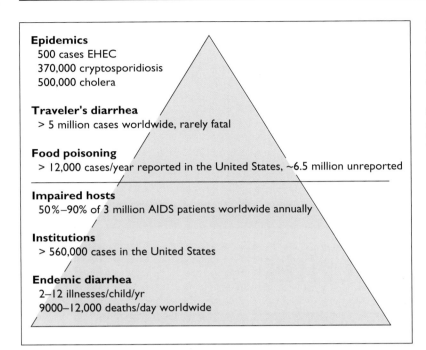

Epidemics
  500 cases EHEC
  370,000 cryptosporidiosis
  500,000 cholera

Traveler's diarrhea
  > 5 million cases worldwide, rarely fatal

Food poisoning
  > 12,000 cases/year reported in the United States, ~6.5 million unreported

Impaired hosts
  50%–90% of 3 million AIDS patients worldwide annually

Institutions
  > 560,000 cases in the United States

Endemic diarrhea
  2–12 illnesses/child/yr
  9000–12,000 deaths/day worldwide

FIGURE 3-1 Six types of microbial diarrhea. Worldwide, diarrheal diseases are second only to cardiovascular disease as a cause of death and are the leading cause of childhood death. Microbial diarrhea occurs in six settings. Reaching the greatest attention are occasional epidemics, such as those caused by enterohemorrhagic *Escherichia coli* (EHEC), water-borne cryptosporidiosis, and global spread of new cholera pandemics; traveler's diarrhea, which affects up to one third of 16 million international travelers each year; and food poisoning. Receiving considerably less attention but responsible for considerably more cases worldwide are diarrheal illnesses in impaired hosts (such as occurs in 50% to 90% of AIDS patients globally each year) and diarrhea in institutions (such as daycare centers, hospitals, and extended care facilities). Finally, there is endemic diarrhea, accounting for two to 12 illnesses per child per year and more than 9000 deaths each day globally [1].

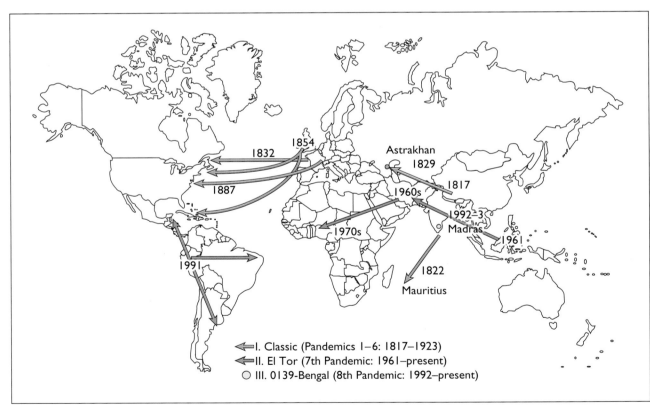

1832 1854 1887 1817 Astrakhan 1829 1960s 1970s 1992–3 Madras 1961 1991 1822 Mauritius

⇐ I. Classic (Pandemics 1–6: 1817–1923)
⇐ II. El Tor (7th Pandemic: 1961–present)
○ III. 0139-Bengal (8th Pandemic: 1992–present)

FIGURE 3-2 Collision of the 7th and 8th cholera pandemics. The first six cholera pandemics, which may have been due to classic *Vibrio cholerae* infections, occurred as six waves between 1817 and 1923. The 7th pandemic, with a distinct strain, El Tor, began in the Celebes in 1961 and continues through the present, with extensive spread in Latin America since 1991. Originating in Madras in late 1992, 0139 Bengal is yet a third strain of *V. cholerae* that has rapidly become epidemic throughout many areas of South Asia since 1993 and threatens to become the 8th pandemic. (*Adapted from* Guerrant [1].)

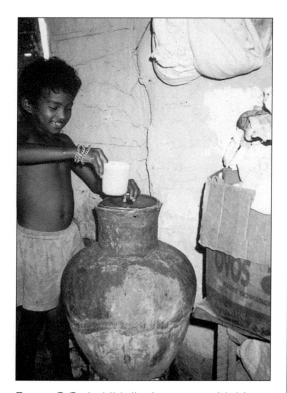

FIGURE 3-3 A child dipping a cup with his hand into the household water supply during a cholera epidemic in Fortaleza, Brazil. This common practice may contribute to the spread of cholera and is the focus of control programs designed to provide improved water sources and storage containers with narrow necks or spigots.

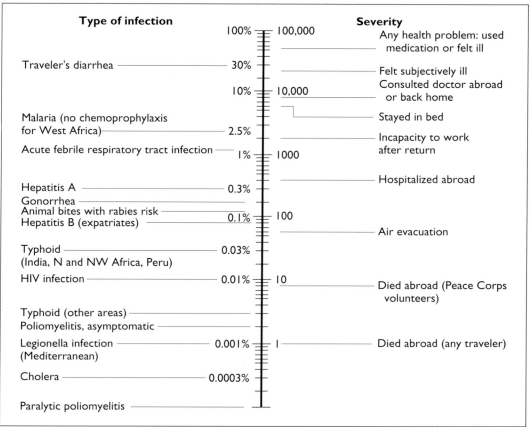

FIGURE 3-4 Incidents of selected infections per 100,000 short-term travelers to developing countries. Some 30% of travelers from developed to developing areas may expect to acquire traveler's diarrhea. This rate is approximately 10-fold the nearly 3% who develop malaria in West Africa without chemoprophylaxis, 100-fold the 0.3% who develop hepatitis A, 1000-fold the 0.03% who develop typhoid fever, and 30,000-fold the 0.001% chance of death abroad (which exceeds the 0.0003% chance of acquiring cholera, for example). (*Adapted from* Behrens *et al.* [2].)

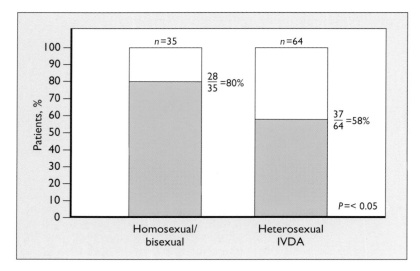

FIGURE 3-5 Diarrheal illnesses in AIDS patients. Antony and colleagues [3] noted that two thirds of patients with AIDS seen at one New York hospital had important diarrheal illness. In their study, diarrhea was more common among homosexual men than in heterosexuals with a risk factor of intravenous drug abuse (IVDA). An estimated 50% to 90% of the 100,000 AIDS patients in the United States and the 3 million worldwide suffer diarrheal illnesses, often chronically.

Nosocomial infections by site in University of Virginia Hospital

Unit	Admissions, *n*	Nosocomial diarrhea	UTI	Pulmonary	POW	BSI	Other
Medical ICU	260	7.7	2.7	3.9	0	2.7	3.9
S2 (< 5 yrs of age)	609	2.3	0.8	0.9	0.5	0.9	3.6
W2 (≥ 5 yrs of age)	545	0.7	1.1	0.5	0.9	0.5	0.9

BSI—bloodstream infection; ICU—intensive care unit; POW—postoperative wound; UTI—urinary tract infection.

FIGURE 3-6 Rates of nosocomial infections on three wards in the University of Virginia Hospital from October 1985 to March 1986. Rates per 100 admissions are presented, showing that nosocomial diarrhea often exceeds any other nosocomial infection. In addition, nosocomial diarrhea is a major predisposing factor to other nosocomial infections, such as urinary tract infections [4,5].

Attack rates in diarrhea outbreaks in daycare centers

Organism	Attack rate, %
Shigella	33–73
Campylobacter jejuni	20–50
Clostridium difficile	32
Giardia lamblia	17–90
Cryptosporidium	50–65
Rotaviruses	70–100

FIGURE 3-7 Attack rates in diarrhea outbreaks in daycare centers, according to etiologic organism. The occurrence of diarrheal illness in institutions, such as daycare centers, hospitals, and long-term care facilities, is largely dependent on personal hygiene, which often is difficult to maintain. Attack rates—the percentage of persons exposed who acquire disease—range from 17% to 100% in daycare settings, with secondary attack rates of 12% to 79% in family members. Organisms having low infectious doses, such as *Shigella, Campylobacter jejuni, Clostridium difficile, Giardia lamblia,* and *Cryptosporidium,* are particularly problematic in these settings. *C. difficile* is also emerging as an important nosocomial pathogen. (*From* Guerrant and Bobak [6].)

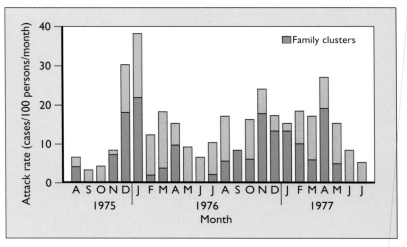

FIGURE 3-8 Monthly attack rates for acute gastrointestinal illnesses in a prospective family study conducted in Charlottesville, Virginia. The winter seasonality and family clustering of community diarrheal illnesses in Charlottesville are comparable to those seen in the Cleveland family study conducted many years before in 1964 [7]. (*Adapted from* Guerrant *et al.* [5].)

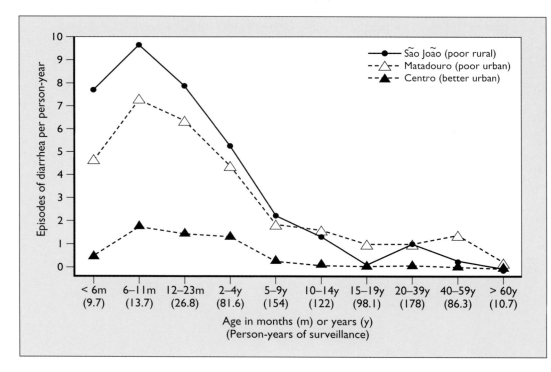

FIGURE 3-9 Age-specific attack rates of diarrheal illnesses in Pacatuba, Brazil. Striking high attack rates of diarrheal illnesses are seen in young children in the poorer areas, and lower rates, comparable to those seen in the Cleveland and Charlottesville family studies, occur in the better homes in this small community in Northwestern Brazil. The important point is that high diarrhea morbidity (as well as mortality in these poorer families) fails to control population growth. Over the 30-month prospective surveillance period, 17 of 32 poorer mothers gave birth, whereas only one of 23 mothers in the better homes gave birth to a new child [8,9]. (*Adapted from* Guerrant *et al.* [8].)

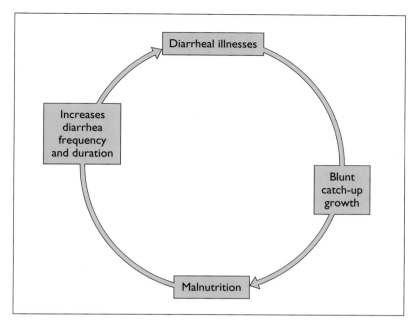

FIGURE 3-10 Vicious cycle of diarrheal illnesses and malnutrition. Not only do diarrheal illnesses blunt catch-up growth that would otherwise be seen in malnourished children or following previous diarrheal illnesses, but malnutrition also predisposes to increased frequency and duration of diarrheal illnesses. Hence, any intervention possible in this vicious cycle is important in breaking this major cause of global morbidity and impaired childhood development. (*Adapted from* Guerrant *et al.* [10].)

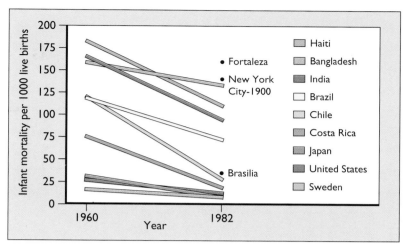

FIGURE 3-11 Comparison of infant mortalities worldwide in 1960 and 1982. Striking declines in infant mortality were seen in many areas, but a disparity remains between the different cities of Fortaleza and Brasilia in Brazil. Interestingly, the infant mortality in New York City in 1900 exceeded that seen in Bangladesh today.

PATHOGENESIS OF MICROBIAL DIARRHEA

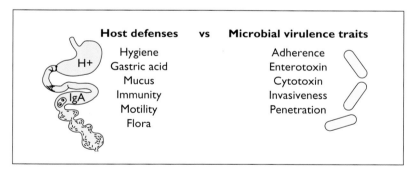

FIGURE 3-12 Host defenses and microbial virulence traits. Several specific enteric host defenses prevent many enteric infections and are often violated or bypassed in individuals who become infected. Normal hygiene usually prevents the acquisition of infectious doses of microbs in hygienic industrialized areas. The neutralization of gastric acid increases one's chances of enteric infections with many agents. Mucosal immunity, normal motility, and normal microbial flora are important barriers to colonization by enteric pathogens as well. Conversely, specific microbial virulence traits—such as adherence in an important region of the bowel, production of secretory enterotoxins or cell-damaging cytotoxins, direct invasiveness such as that seen with *Shigella*, or penetration through intact epithelial cells such as occurs with *Salmonella* infections—are key traits that enable an organism to be a pathogen.

Normal enteric microflora	
	Organisms/g feces
Anaerobes	~10^{11}
Bacteroides	
Clostridium	
Peptostreptococcus	
Peptococcus	
Others	
Aerobes	
Escherichia coli	~10^{8}
Klebsiella	10^{5-7}
Proteus	10^{5-7}
Enterococcus	10^{5-7}
Others	10^{5-7}

FIGURE 3-13 Normal enteric microflora. The normal enteric flora plays an important role in host defense by resisting colonization by pathogenic invaders. The loss of normal anaerobic flora or a shift in its balance (*eg,* due to antibiotic use) may allow replacement by organisms such as *Pseudomonas, Klebsiella, Clostridium,* and *Candida,* with an attendant risk of serious systemic infection. The normal enteric bacterial flora consists almost entirely of anaerobes (99.9%), with gram-negative aerobic coliform rods comprising most of the remainder [11].

Infectious doses of enteric pathogens

Shigella	10^{1-2}
Campylobacter jejuni	10^{2-6}
Salmonella	10^5
Escherichia coli	10^8
Vibrio cholerae	10^8
Giardia lamblia	10^{1-2} cysts
Entamoeba histolytica	10^{1-2} cysts

FIGURE 3-14 Infectious doses of enteric pathogens. Most identified enteric pathogens are acquired via the fecal-oral route, emphasizing the role of personal hygiene in host defense. For bacteria such as *Salmonella*, *Escherichia coli*, and *Vibrio cholerae*, a large number of organisms (100,000–100 million) usually must be ingested to overcome host defenses and cause disease (assuming other host defenses are intact). Some other organisms such as *Shigella*, cysts of *Giardia*, *Entamoeba histolytica*, and *Cryptosporidium*, as well as certain strains of *Campylobacter jejuni* appear to be infectious with less than a few hundred organisms or cysts and may be readily transmitted via person-to-person contact, as in daycare centers. (*From* Guerrant [11].)

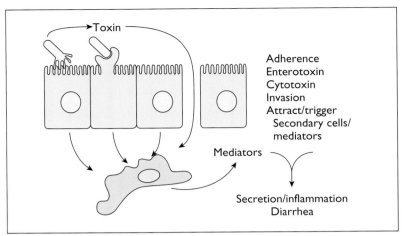

FIGURE 3-15 Mechanisms of microbial diarrhea. Microorganisms must first penetrate the gastrointestinal mucus and adhere to a relevant portion of the intestinal mucosa (often via fimbriated adhesins). Microorganisms then produce an enterotoxin (eg, choleratoxin) or cytotoxin (eg, shigalike toxin) that induces secretion and disrupts mucosal integrity. Alternatively, some microorganisms, such as invasive *Shigella* or *Salmonella*, may penetrate the epithelium. Adherence by microorganisms may attract or trigger secondary cells or mediators (eg, polymorphonuclear leukocytes, mast cells, etc.), which enhance the secretion and inflammation seen in diarrhea. Increasing evidence suggests that one or more of these virulence traits may operate in any particular type of infectious diarrhea. These traits are often encoded by transmissible genetic elements such as plasmids or bacteria phage. (*Adapted from* Guerrant [1].)

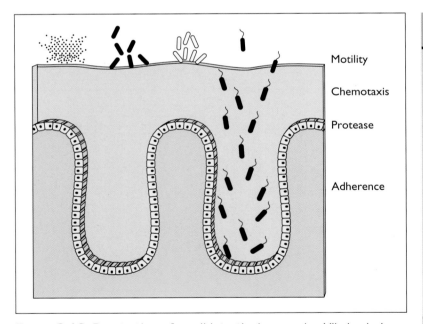

FIGURE 3-16 Penetration of small intestinal mucus by *Vibrio cholerae*. Successful colonization depends on intact *Vibrio* motility, chemotaxis, protease, and adherence in the upper small bowel, where production and delivery of the enterotoxin causes secretory diarrhea.

Enteric bacterial toxins

Neurotoxin group
Clostridium botulinum
Staphylococcus aureus
 (enterotoxin b)
Bacillus cereus (emetic toxin)
Secretory enterotoxin group
Vibrio cholerae (cAMP)
Noncholera vibrios
Escherichia coli—heat-liable
 toxin (cAMP)
E. coli—STa (cGMP)
E. coli—STb
Salmonella
Klebsiella
Clostridium perfringens (A)
Shigella dysenteriae
B. cereus

Possible enterotoxins
E. coli EIET, EAST, EALT
V. cholerae: Ace, Zot
Cytotoxin group
Shigella
C. perfringens (A)
Vibrio parahemolyticus
S. aureus
Clostridium difficile
 (A and B)
E. coli (EHEC) (certain O
 groups: 26, 39, 128, 157)
Clostridium jejuni
Helicobacter pylori

cAMP—cyclic AMP; cGMP—cyclic GMP; EALT—enteroaggregative *E. coli* heat-labile toxin; EAST—enteroaggregative *E. coli* heat-stable toxin; EHEC—enterohemorrhagic *E. coli*; EIET—enteroinvasive *E. coli* toxin.

FIGURE 3-17 Enteric bacterial toxins. Enteric bacterial toxins can be divided into those that have a predominantly neurotoxic effect, such as *Clostridium botulinum*, *Staphylococcus aureus*, and *Bacillus cereus* emetic toxins; secretory enterotoxins, including choleratoxin, *Escherichia coli* heat-labile toxin, *E. coli* heat-stable toxin, and others; possible recently described enterotoxins; and cytotoxins, such as those produced by *Clostridium difficile* and enterohemorrhagic *E. coli*. (*From* Guerrant [11].)

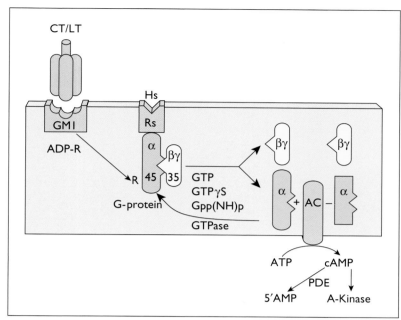

FIGURE 3-18 Mechanisms of action of choleratoxin and *Escherichia coli* heat-labile toxin on regulation of adenylate cyclase. True enterotoxins are defined as having a direct effect on intestinal mucosa to elicit net fluid secretion. The classic enterotoxin, choleratoxin (CT), causes fluid secretion by inducing adenylate cyclase (AC) to overproduce cyclic AMP (cAMP). Choleratoxin binds to GMI ganglioside on intestinal enterocytes, catalyzing ADP-ribosylation (ADP-R) of Gsα, a GTP-binding protein on the basolateral membrane of enterocytes. The resulting activation of AC results in conversion of ATP into cAMP, which in turn activates cAMP-dependent kinase (A-kinase), thereby opening chloride channels to elicit net chloride secretion and leading to loss of fluid and production of diarrhea. In a separate process, cAMP is degraded by phosphodiesterase (PDE) to 5'-AMP, a neutrophil-derived secretagogue, that may further enhance intestinal secretion. Enterotoxigenic strains of *E. coli* produce a heat-labile enterotoxin (LT) that is similar to choleratoxin and operates by the same mechanism. (Hs—hormone [stimulatory]; R—arginine residue; RS—receptor [stimulatory].) (*Adapted from* Guerrant [1].)

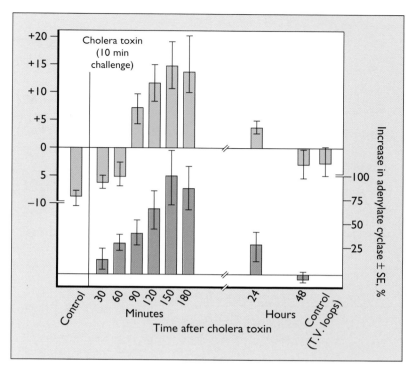

FIGURE 3-19 Time course of cholera enterotoxin effects on fluid secretion and adenylate cyclase activation. Even after a brief 10-minute exposure of canine ligated loops to choleratoxin, a lag, followed by prolonged activation of adenylate cyclase and fluid secretion ensue, lasting > 24 hours and perhaps for the life of the epithelial cell. This prolonged action of choleratoxin > 24 hours after removal of the toxin explains why continued replacement hydration therapy following initial rehydration remains imperative in controlling cholera morbidity and mortality [12]. (SE—standard error.)

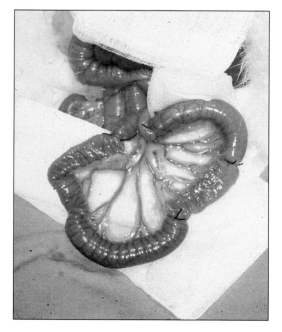

FIGURE 3-20 Gross view of small intestinal distension (rabbit) due to choleratoxin. Ligated rabbit ileal loops demonstrate the distension seen with choleratoxin after 18 hours, in contrast to the intervening loops (negative controls) in which no fluid is seen.

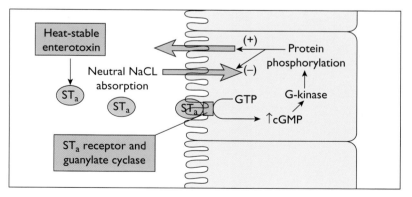

FIGURE 3-21 Mechanism of action of enterotoxigenic *Escherichia coli*–associated heat-stable enterotoxin (ST$_a$) on guanylate cyclase. As an alternative to choleratoxin and the adenylate cyclase pathway, some *E. coli* produce ST$_a$ that operates via guanylate cyclase. Binding of ST$_a$ to an intestinal receptor directly activates guanylate cyclase, which converts GTP to cyclic GMP (cGMP), causing an increase in intracellular cGMP and resulting in increased net secretion. The ST$_a$ receptor appears in normal gut and binds endogenous ST-like compounds (*eg*, guanylin) that may play key roles in normal intestinal physiology. (*Adapted from* Cho and Chang [13].)

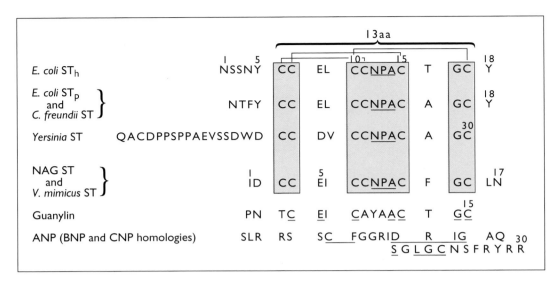

Figure 3-22 Heat-stable (ST_a) toxin family. ST_a toxin resembles the ST toxins produced by multiple bacteria, including other *Escherichia coli* (ST_h and ST_p toxins), *Citrobacter freundii*, *Yersinia*, and *Vibrio mimicus*. These compounds share much of a minimum 13 key amino acid (aa) regions that are essential to their full biologic activity and, in particular, three disulfide bonds (N-P-A, Asn–Pro–Ala), which are critical to their enterotoxic activity. (*Boxed areas* indicate the common amino acids among all ST sequences.) These toxins are biologically similar to the endogenous intestinal peptide, guanylin, and less so to atrial natriuretic factor (ANP), brain natriuretic factor (BNP), and C-type natriuretic factor (CNP) [6]. (NAG—nonagglutinable.) (*Adapted from* Guerrant [1].)

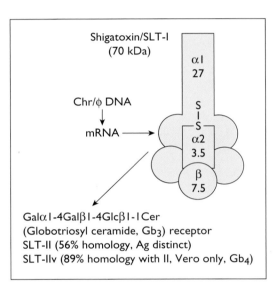

Figure 3-23 Shigatoxin and shigalike toxin. Shigatoxin, produced by *Shigella* (encoded by chromosomal DNA), and the closely related shigalike toxin I (SLT-I), produced by enterohemorrhagic *Escherichia coli* (EHEC, where it is encoded by bacteriophage DNA), are potent cytotoxins that result in colonic mucosal destruction. Shigatoxin and SLT-I toxin bind to globotriaosyl ceramide (Gb_3) receptor, cleaving an adenosine from the host-cell ribosomal RNA to inhibit protein synthesis. Subtle differences in SLT-II and SLT-IIv result in their binding to different receptors (Gb_4, globotetraosyl ceramide) with different disease manifestations. EHEC, including *E. coli* O157:H7 subtype, is implicated in numerous outbreaks of hemorrhagic colitis and in childhood hemolytic-uremic syndrome. (mRNA—messenger RNA.)

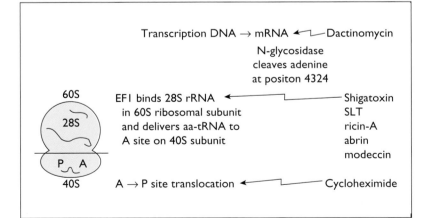

Figure 3-24 Inhibition of eukaryotic protein synthesis by shigatoxin/shigalike toxin I (SLT-I). Shigatoxin and SLT (as well as ricin-A, a plant toxin) enzymatically cleave the *N*-glycosidase bond of adenine at position 4324 in the 28S ribosomal RNA (rRNA) of the 60S ribosomal subunit. This prevents elongation factor 1 (EF1)-dependent binding of aminoacyl transfer RNA (aa-tRNA) to the ribosome, thereby halting protein synthesis. The antibiotics dactinomycin and cycloheximide also effect disruption of protein synthesis via different mechanisms. (mRNA—messenger RNA.)

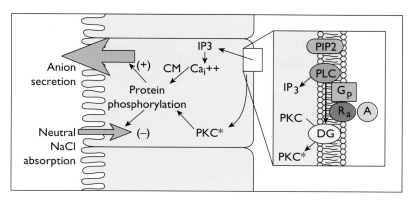

FIGURE 3-25 Mediation of intestinal secretion of cytosolic calcium and activation of protein kinase C (PKC). Some enteric pathogens, including choleratoxin, may stimulate increases in cytosolic calcium concentrations, by variable pathways, which in turn activate phosphokinase C, leading to protein phosphorylation and increased secretion. (A—agonist; CM—calmodulin; DG—diacylglycerol; G_P—PLC-associated G-protein; IP3—inositol4,5-bisphosphate; PIP2—phosphatidylinositol-4,5-bisphosphate; PKC—protein kinase C [*activated]; PLC—phospholipase C.) (*Adapted from* Cho and Chang [13].)

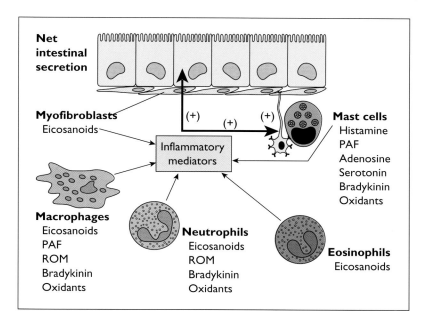

FIGURE 3-26 Immune and inflammatory mediators of net intestinal secretion. Many prostaglandins and 5-lipooxygenase inhibitors are capable of stimulating net intestinal secretion. This inflammatory response, seen with enteroinvasive infections as well as with some forms of secretory diarrhea (*eg*, choleratoxin and enterotoxigenic *Escherichia coli*, may serve to purge the gut of noxious agents and pathogens but also exacerbates the acute symptoms of diarrhea. (PAF—platelet-activating factor; ROM—reactive oxygen metabolites.) (*Adapted from* Cho and Chang [13].)

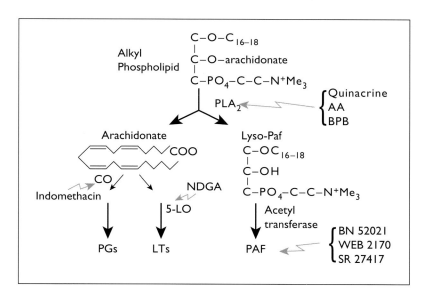

FIGURE 3-27 Alkyl phospholipid metabolism by phospholipase A_2 (PLA_2), leading to production of prostaglandins (PGs), leukotrienes (LTs), and platelet-activating factor (PAF). These pathways appear increasingly to be involved in microbial toxin-induced secretory as well as inflammatory diarrhea. Antagonists of these pathways (*shown in red*) can block these inflammatory and secretory responses at various points: quinacrine, aristolochic acid (AA), and bromophenacyl bromine (BPB) inhibit PLA_2; indomethacin blocks cyclooxygenase (CO); NDGA (nordihydroguaiaretic acid) blocks 5-lipooxygenase (5-LO); and BN 52021, WEB 2170, and SR 27417 block platelet-activating factor (PAF) [1].

DIAGNOSIS AND MANAGEMENT OF MICROBIAL DIARRHEA

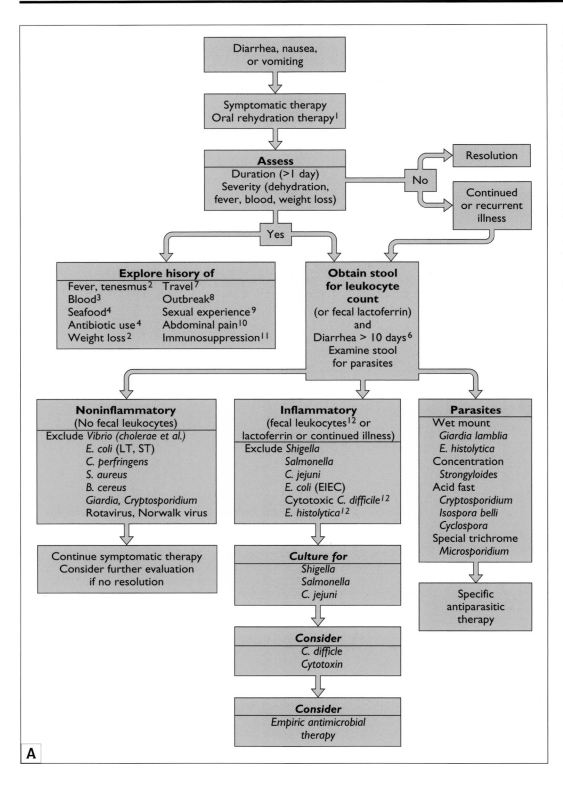

FIGURE 3-28   **A** and **B,** Selective diagnostic and therapeutic approach to diarrhea, nausea, and vomiting. Although all patients with significant gastrointestinal illnesses should receive adequate rehydration, orally if possible, further diagnostic or more specific antimicrobial therapy should be directed by specific findings in the history or stool examination. Diarrhea lasting for > 1 day or associated with severe dehydration, bloody stool, fever, or weight loss warrants additional evaluation of history and stool examination for leukocytes or a leukocyte marker (such as lactoferrin). Diarrhea lasting for 10 days should prompt examination for parasites. (*See panel 28B* for footnotes.) (EIEC—enteroinvasive *E. coli*; LT—heat-labile toxin; ST—heat-stable toxin.) (*Adapted from* Guerrant and Bobak [6].) (*Continued*)

B. Diagnosis and management of diarrhea, nausea, or vomiting

1. Oral rehydration solution can be prepared by adding 3.5 g NaCl, 2.5 g NaHCO$_3$ (or 2.9 g Na citrate), 1.5 g KCl, and 20 g glucose *or* glucose polymer (*eg*, 40 g sucrose *or* 4 tbsp sugar *or* 50–60 g cereal flour such as rice, maize, sorghum, millet, wheat, or potato) per liter (1.05 qts) of clear water. This makes approximately Na 90, K 20, Cl 80, HCO$_3$ 30, glucose 111 mmol/L.

   One level tsp of table salt and 8 level tsp of table sugar per liter makes about 86 mmol Na and 30 g sucrose/L, to which one could add 1 cup orange juice or 2 bananas for potassium (*see* Fig. 3-37).

2. Fever or tenesmus suggest an inflammatory proctocolitis.

3. Diarrhea with blood, especially without fecal leukocytes, suggests enterohemorrhagic (Shiga-like toxin–producing) *Escherichia coli* O157 or amebiasis (in which leukocytes are destroyed by the parasite).

4. Ingestion of inadequately cooked seafood should prompt consideration of infections with *Vibrio* or Norwalk-like viruses.

5. Antibiotics should be stopped if possible and cytotoxigenic *Clostridium difficile* considered. Antibiotics may also predispose to other infections, such as salmonellosis.

6. Persistence (> 10 days) with weight loss should prompt consideration of giardiasis or cryptosporidiosis.

   Whereas many stool examinations for ova and parasites are often of low yield, specific requests for *Giardia* and *Cryptosporidium* ELISA (in patients with > 10 days of diarrhea) or, in immunocompromised patients, acid fast stain for *Cryptosporidium, Isospora,* or *Cyclospora* are worth considering.

7. Travel to tropical areas increases the chance of developing enterotoxigenic *E. coli,* as well as viral (Norwalk-like or rotaviral), parasitic (*Giardia, Entamoeba, Strongyloides, Cryptosporidium*), and if fecal leukocytes are present, invasive bacterial infections.

8. Outbreaks should prompt consideration of *Staphylococcus aureus, Bacillus cereus,* anisakiasis (incubation period < 6 h), *Clostridium perfringens,* enterotoxigenic *E. coli, Vibrio, Salmonella, Campylobacter, Shigella,* or enteroinvasive *E. coli* infection. Consider saving *E. coli* for heat-labile toxin, heat-stable toxin, invasiveness, adherence testing, serotyping, and stool for rotavirus, and stool plus paired sera for Norwalk-like virus or toxin testing.

9. Sigmoidoscopy in symptomatic homosexual men should distinguish proctitis in the distal 15 cm only (caused by herpesvirus, gonococcal, chlamydial, or syphilitic infection) from colitis (*Campylobacter, Shigella, C. difficile,* or *Chlamydia* [lymphogranuloma venereum serotypes] infections) or noninflammatory diarrhea (due to giardiasis).

10. If unexplained abdominal pain and fever persist or suggest an appendicitis-like syndrome, culture for *Yersinia enterocolitica* with cold enrichment.

11. In immunocompromised hosts, a wide range of viral (cytomegalovirus, herpes simplex virus, coxsackievirus, rotavirus), bacterial (*Salmonella, Mycobacterium avium-intracellulare*), and parasitic (*Cryptosporidium, Isospora, Strongyloides, Entamoeba,* and *Giardia*) agents should be considered.

12. Some inflammatory, colonic pathogens, such as cytotoxigenic *C. difficile* or *Entamoeba histolytica,* may destroy fecal leukocyte morphology, so a reliable leukocyte marker such as fecal lactoferrin may provide a better screening test.

ELISA—enzyme-linked immunosorbent assay.

Figure 3-28 *(Continued).*

A. Noninflammatory enteric infection

Mechanism	Enterotoxin
Location	Proximal small bowel
Illness	Watery diarrhea
Stool examination	No fecal leukocytes
Examples	*Vibrio cholerae*
	Escherichia coli (LT)
	E. coli (ST)
	Clostridium perfringens
	Bacillus cereus
	Staphylococcus aureus
	Salmonella (?)
	Vibrio parahemolyticus (?)
	Giardia lamblia
	Rotavirus
	Norwalk-like viruses
	Cryptosporidium

LT—heat-labile toxin; ST—heat-stable toxin.

Figure 3-29 Types of enteric infections and pathogens. Infectious diarrheas can be divided into noninflammatory, inflammatory, and enteric fever (due to penetrating pathogens such as *Shigella typhi*). **A,** Noninflammatory diarrheas. Most diarrheal illnesses are noninflammatory, often arising from the mechanism of enterotoxin or structural impairment of absorption, usually in the upper small bowel. They cause a watery diarrheal illness characteristically without fecal leukocytes or with low amounts of a leukocyte marker such as lactoferrin [14] and typically are caused by organisms such as *Vibrio cholerae,* enterotoxigenic *Escherichia coli,* viral, or upper small bowel parasitic pathogens such as *Giardia lamblia* or *Cryptosporidium.* In addition, preformed enterotoxins, such as those seen with staphylococcal or certain *Bacillus cereus* food poisoning, are typically noninflammatory as well. *(Continued)*

B. Inflammatory enteric infection

Mechanism	Invasion, cytotoxin (?)
Location	Colon
Illness	Dysentery
Stool examination	Fecal polymorphonuclear neutrophil leukocytes
Examples	*Shigella*
	Invasive *E. coli*
	Salmonella enteritidis
	Vibrio parahemolyticus
	Clostridium difficile (?)
	Campylobacter jejuni (?)
	Entamoeba histolytica

C. Enteric fever

Mechanism	Penetrating infection
Location	Distal small bowel
Illness	Enteric fever
Stool examination	Fecal mononuclear leukocytes
Examples	*Salmonella typhi*
	Yersinia enterocolitica
	Campylobacter fetus (?)

FIGURE 3-29 *(Continued)*   **B,** Inflammatory diarrheas. In contrast, inflammatory diarrhea usually arises by invasion or cytotoxic effects in the distal small bowel or colon to cause numerous fecal polymorphonuclear leukocytes, often with fever, blood, mucus, or pus and with high levels of a neutrophil marker such as lactoferrin. These illnesses are characteristically caused by the pathogens sought in routine culture—*eg, Salmonella, Shigella,* and *Campylobacter jejuni* or cytotoxin-producing *Clostridium difficile.* Although *Entamoeba histolytica* may elicit a striking inflammatory response, neutrophils may be destroyed morphologically, leaving only the neutrophil markers [15]. **C,** Enteric fever, the third type of enteric infection, is caused by organisms, such as *Salmonella typhi, Yersinia,* and possibly *Campylobacter fetus,* that penetrate intestinal mucosa to multiply in the lymphatic and reticuloendothelial cells. It often begins with constipation early in its course, followed by a febrile systemic illness with or without diarrhea. (*From* Guerrant [11].)

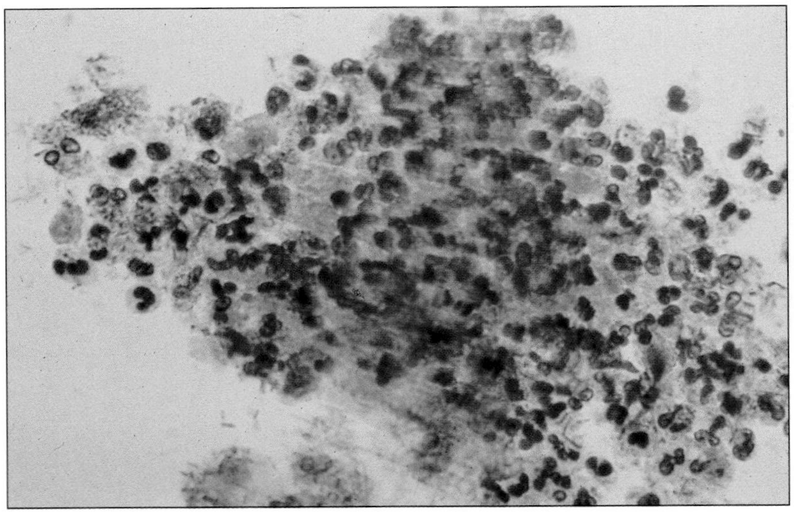

FIGURE 3-30 Fecal leukocytes on wet mount of stool specimen stained with methylene blue. Clumps of numerous polymorphonuclear leukocytes can be seen in a patient with *Shigella* infection. Examination of fresh stool is a potentially helpful screen for colonic mucosal inflammation due to invasive bacteria, such as *Shigella* or *Campylobacter jejuni,* or idiopathic inflammatory disease. However, it requires that a skilled microscopist examine a freshly stained fecal specimen to avoid false-positive and false-negative readings.

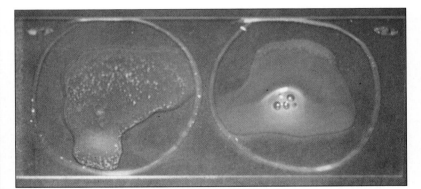

FIGURE 3-31 Latex agglutination test for leukocyte markers on fecal smear. A positive test on the left, from a patient with inflammatory diarrhea, shows agglutinated lactoferrin-antibody–coated beads, in contrast to the negative control beads on the right. This simple test for neutrophil markers is a rapid, sensitive indicator of fecal leukocytes. It can be used on swabbed or refrigerated specimens and is a suitable screening test for cytotoxic *Clostridium difficile* or *Entamoeba histolytica,* which may destroy fecal leukocytes and leave only neutrophil markers [16]. (*From* Guerrant *et al.* [14]; with permission.)

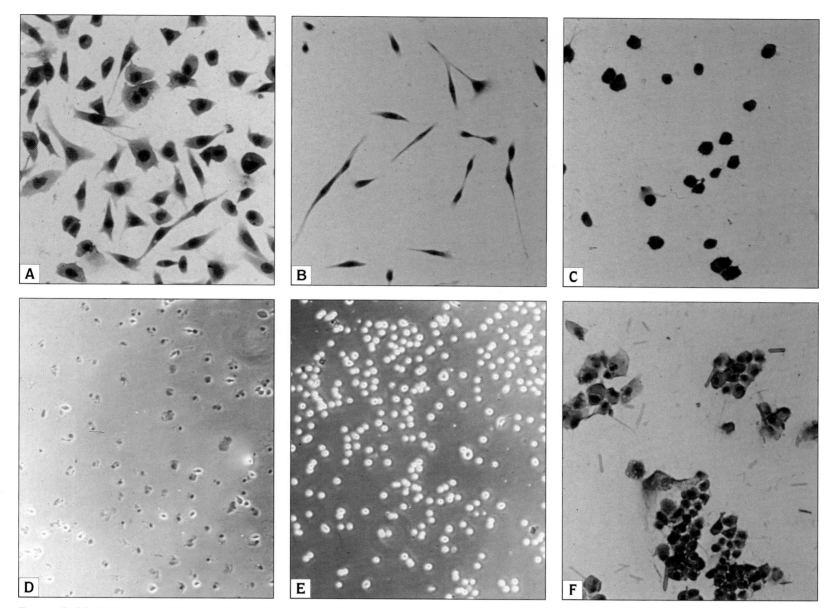

FIGURE 3-32 Effects of different microbial toxins on Chinese hamster ovary (CHO) cells in tissue culture. **A,** Normal CHO cells. **B,** Choleratoxin. **C,** *Clostridium difficile* cytotoxin. **D,** Trypan blue stain of *C. difficile* cytotoxin effects. **E,** Effects of culture super- natants of virulent *Entamoeba histolytica*, showing release of otherwise viable cells. **F,** Effects of pertussis active holotoxin. (*From* Guerrant [17]; with permission.)

Comparative costs per positive result for cultures

Culture	Cost per positive result, $
Fecal	952
Blood	279
Urine	70
Throat	50

FIGURE 3-33 Cost per positive result for fecal, blood, urine, and throat cultures. The high costs associated with stool culture are due to their insensitivity for major pathogens and poor case selection for testable pathogens. Of 2468 fecal cultures done in this study, only 2.4% were positive [18]. (*From* Guerrant *et al.* [19].)

Problems with cost-effectiveness of laboratory tests

Insensitive for major pathogens
Poor case selection for test

FIGURE 3-34 Problems with the cost-effectiveness of laboratory tests. Problems include insensitivity of tests for major pathogens and poor case selection for testable pathogens (such as *Campylobacter jejuni*, *Salmonella*, or *Shigella*) [19].

Percent yields and costs of stool cultures

Study	No.	*Salmonella* or *Shigella*, %	*Clostridium jejuni*, %	*Yersinia*, %	Total, %	Cost per positive result, $
MGH 1979	2468	2.4	—	—	2.4	952
UVH 1979–1981	2020	1.5	—	—	1.5	1200
UVH 1981–1982	1558	4.0	4.6	0.1	8.7	264
UVH POPD 1982, 1984–1986	305	11.5	6.6	0.7	18.7	118
Cup specimens with fecal PMN	30	30.0	46.7	—	76.7	30

MGH—Massachusetts General Hospital; POPD—Pediatric Outpatient Department; PMN—polymorphonuclear neutrophil leukocytes; UVH—University of Virginia Hospital.

FIGURE 3-35 Percent yields and costs of stool cultures. The high cost of stool cultures, ranging from $950 to $1200 per positive result, warrants their selective use in patients with inflammatory diarrheal disease. In patients with a suspected inflammatory process or with continued or recurrent illness, routine culture for *Salmonella*, *Shigella*, and *Campylobacter jejuni* is worthwhile, because these patients are most likely to have one of these pathogens and will benefit from empire antibiotic therapy [18,20,21].

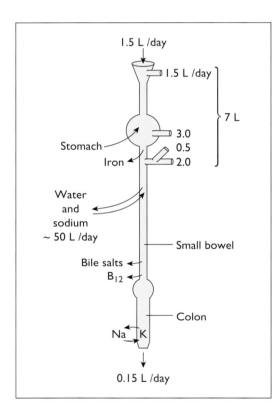

FIGURE 3-36 Fluid balance in the healthy adult gastrointestinal (GI) tract. Together with a daily oral intake of 1.5 L, salivary, gastric, biliary, and pancreatic secretions contribute a total of approximately 8.5 L of fluid that enters the upper GI tract each day. However, daily fecal fluid excretion is normally < 150 mL, indicating a net absorption of > 8 L/day by the GI tract. More than 90% of this net absorption occurs in the small bowel, where there is a massive bidirectional flux that probably exceeds 50 L/day. A relatively slight shift in the bidirectional flux can result in substantial overload of the colonic absorptive capacity, which rarely exceeds 2 to 3 L/day. Enteric disease produced by the microbe–host interaction can alter this fluid balance in three ways: disruption of the bidirectional flow by intraluminal processes in the upper small intestine, such as by enterotoxin action; inflammatory destruction of the ileal or colonic mucosa; or penetration through the mucosa to the reticuloendothelial system. (*Adapted from* Guerrant [11].)

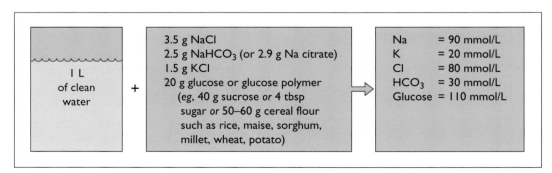

FIGURE 3-37 Formula for oral rehydration solution. The cornerstone of treatment of all diarrheal disease is replacement of lost fluid and electrolytes in quantities similar to those depleted. A simply prepared oral rehydration solution stimulates glucose-coupled sodium absorption, which remains largely intact in even the most severe diarrhea. Oral therapy is the preferred route. One simple alternative solution is made by adding 1 level tsp of table salt and 8 level tsp of table sugar to 1 L of water, which yields about 86 mmol sodium and 30 g sucrose/L; 1 cup of orange juice or two bananas may be added for potassium [22].

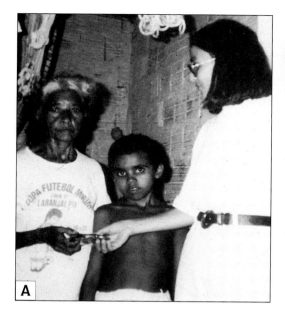 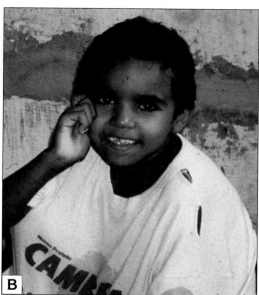

FIGURE 3-38 Effects of oral rehydration therapy in cholera. **A** and **B,** A mother in Fortaleza, Brazil, is instructed in the preparation of oral rehydration fluid from packets of salts and sugar (*panel 38A*), leading to the improvement of the child within 24 hours (*panel 38B*). Use of oral rehydration solution, called "the most important medical advance this century," has cut the mortality of cholera from > 50% to < 1%. (*Courtesy of* A.A.M. Lima, MD, and R.L. Guerrant, MD.)

Antimicrobial agents and recommended therapy in infectious diarrhea

Diagnosis	Drug	Dosage	
		Adults	Children
Shigellosis	TMP-SMX	160 mg TMP/800 mg SMX bid × 3 days	10 mg TMP/50 mg SMX/kg/d in two doses for 3 days
	Norfloxacin	400 mg bid × 3 days	Not appropriate
	Ciprofloxacin	500 mg bid × 3 days	Not appropriate
Campylobacter jejuni Enterocolitis	Norfloxacin	400 mg bid × 5 days	Not appropriate
	Ciprofloxacin	500 mg bid × 5 days	Not appropriate
	Erythromycin	500 mg qid × 5 days	50 mg/kg/d in four doses × 5 days
Traveler's diarrhea	As for *Shigella*	—	—
Giardiasis	Quinacrine*	100 mg tid × 7 days	7 mg/kg/d in three doses × 7–10 days
	Metronidazole	250 mg tid × 10 days	20 mg/kg/d in four doses/d × 10 days
	Furazolidone	100 mg tid × 7 days	5 mg/kg/d in four doses/d × 7 days
Amebiasis	Metronidazole *plus*	750 mg tid × 5 days	50 mg/kg/d in three doses/d × 10 days
	Diiodohydroxyquin	650 mg tid × 21 days	40 mg/kg/d in three doses/d × 21 days

*Availability limited.

bid—twice a day; qid—four times a day; SMX—sulfamethoxazole; tid—three times a day; TMP–trimethoprim.

FIGURE 3-39 Recommended antimicrobial therapy in infectious diarrhea. In addition to oral rehydration therapy, one should consider specific antimicrobial therapy for symptomatic patients with inflammatory or parasitic diarrheas. Antimicrobial therapy reduces the duration of diarrhea and thereby the severity of fluid loss. (*From* Bandres and DuPont [23].)

CLINICAL SYNDROMES AND ETIOLOGIES

Traveler's Diarrhea

Etiologies of traveler's diarrhea*

Characteristics	Latin America	Africa	Asia
Duration of stay, d	21 (2–42)	28 (28–35)	(28–42)
Attack rate, %	52 (21–100)	54 (36–62)	(39–57)
Percentage with			
Enterotoxigenic *Escherichia coli*	46 (28–72)	36 (31–75)	(20–34)
Shigella	0 (0–30)	0 (0–15)	(4–7)
Salmonella	—	0 (0–0)	(11–15)
Campylobacter jejuni	—	—	(2–15)
Vibrio para-haemolyticus	—	—	(1–13)
Rotavirus	23 (0–36)	0 (0–0)	—

*Data given as the median (range) from 26 studies.

FIGURE 3-40 Etiologies of traveler's diarrhea. Numerous studies of travelers to Latin America, Africa, or Asia all show a 21% to 100% attack rate over a usual 2- to 4-week travel. By far, the predominant associated pathogens in one third or more of cases are enterotoxigenic *Escherichia coli* that produce either the heat-labile or heat-stable toxins or both. Other pathogens vary with the location visited. (*From* Guerrant and Bobak [24].)

Safe and unsafe foods in developing tropical regions

Low-risk foods and beverages	High-risk foods and beverages
Any item served steaming hot (> 59° C)	Foods that are moist and served at room temperature, especially those at a buffet
Foods that are dry (*ie*, bread and crackers)	Fruits and vegetables with skin intact—strawberries, tomatoes, grapes
Items with very high sugar content (syrups and jellies)	Salads and other uncooked vegetables
Fruits and vegetables that have been peeled	Sauces and dressings in open containers on the table
Peanut butter	Milk (other than powdered milk that is constituted with previously boiled water or irradiated milk kept refrigerated after preparing or opening)
Any fresh food item properly washed and prepared by the traveler	Tap water or ice
Bottled carbonated drinks including mineral water, soft drinks, and beer	

FIGURE 3-41 Safe and unsafe foods in developing tropical regions. The usual adage of "boil it, peel it, cook it, or forget it" is the safest policy for travelers. Especially important to avoid are tap water and foods that are served at room temperature, having been left out for an unknown period. Although some authors may suggest prophylactic antimicrobial for travelers at special risk, attempts at use of prophylactic agents might provide only a false sense of security for travelers at high risk, such as those with immunocompromise, for infections that would not be prevented by prophylactic antibiotics (such as *Cryptosporidium*, which requires fastidious attention to food and water advisories). The potential risks of prophylactic antibiotics therefore might well outweigh their potential benefit in preventing only readily treatable infections. The author (RLG) recommends careful precautions with prompt treatment with either bismuth subsalicylate, other bismuth preparations, or prompt antimicrobial therapy with an agent such as a quinolone (for adults) or sulfamethoxazole-trimethoprim (for children). (*From* DuPont [25].)

Vibrio Species

Vibrio species implicated as a cause of human disease

Species	Gastrointestinal	Wound/ear	Septicemia
	Clinical presentations		
V. cholerae			
O1	++	(+)	
Non-O1	++	+	+
V. mimicus	++	+	
V. parahaemolyticus	++	+	(+)
V. fluvialis	++		
V. furnissii	++		
V. hollisae	++		(+)
V. vulnificus	+	++	++
V. alginolyticus		++	
V. damsela		++	
V. cincinnatiensis			+
V. carchariae		+	
V. metschnikovii	?		?

++—most common presentation; +—other clinical presentations; (+)—very rare presentation.

FIGURE 3-42 *Vibrio* species causing human disease. In addition to *Vibrio cholerae*, numerous other vibrios cause either noninflammatory or inflammatory diarrhea as well as wound, skin, ear, or septicemic infections. Of special concern are the associations of potentially serious septicemic infections with *V. vulnificus*, especially in impaired hosts such as those with underlying liver disease. Special risks for *Vibrio* infections are posed by consumption of raw or inadequately cooked oysters or other seafood. (*From* Morris [26].)

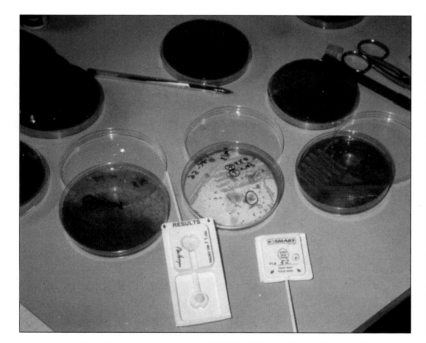

FIGURE 3-43 *Vibrio cholerae* on TCBS (thiosulfate citrate bile salt sucrose) agar plates showing yellow, sucrose-fermenting colonies. This culture was seen in the cholera outbreak in Forteleza, Brazil, in 1993.

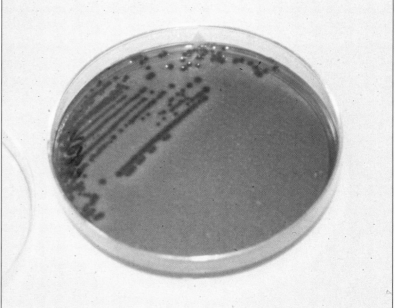

FIGURE 3-44 *Vibrio parahaemolyticus* on TCBS (thiosulfate citrate bile salt sucrose) agar showing characteristic green, nonsucrose-fermenting, halophilic vibrios. The organism was isolated from a patient who developed diarrhea after eating inadequately cooked seafood. *V. parahaemolyticus* is a common bacterial cause of diarrhea associated with ingestion of uncooked seafood. (*Courtesy of* R.L. Guerrant, MD.)

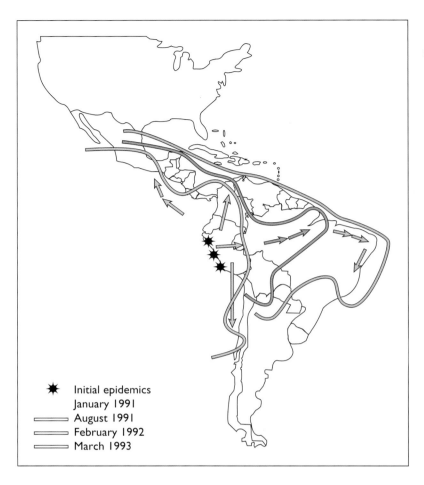

FIGURE 3-45 Spread of cholera through the Americas between 1991 and 1993. In late January 1991, *Vibrio cholerae* O1, serotype Inaba, biotype El Tor, appeared with explosive intensity in several coastal Peruvian cities, making its first appearance since 1895. The epidemic spread rapidly to other urban areas and then neighboring countries. (*Courtesy of* R.V. Tauxe, MD; *adapted from* Butterton and Calderwood [27].)

FIGURE 3-46 Cumulative cholera case totals due the El Tor epidemic in June 1993. Figures for the United States and Canada include cases unrelated to the Latin America epidemic (indicated in parentheses). (*From* Butterton and Calderwood [27].)

Cumulative cholera case totals reported to the Pan American Health Organization as of June 1993

Country	1991* Cases, *n*	1992 Cases/deaths, *n*	1993 (6 mos) Cases/deaths, *n*
Peru	322,562	206,565/709	58,565/295
Ecuador	46,320	31,870/208	3291/29
Brazil	2101	24,039/312	5103/81
Bolivia	206	21,324/383	7652/192
Guatemala	3674	15,178/207	1237/19
Colombia	11,979	15,129/23*	182/4
El Salvador	947	8109/45	3191/8
Mexico	2690	7814/99	1415/25
Nicaragua	1	3067/46	701/34
Venezuela	13	2456/62	63/3
Panama	1178	2416/49	42/4
Argentina	0	553/15	1515/24
Honduras	11	384/17	22/2
Guyana	0	290/4	58/2
Belize	0	154/4	14/0
United States	26 (8[†])	102 (11[†])/1	14 (1[†])/0
Chile	41	71/1	28/0
French Guyana	1	16/0	2/0
Surinam	0	12/1	0/0
Costa Rica	0	12/0	4/0
Paraguay	0	0/0	3/0
Canada	1[†]	0/0	0/0
Totals	391,751/4002 (1.02%)	339,561/2163 (0.64%)	83,102/722 (0.87%)

*Incomplete reporting.

[†]Not associated with the Latin American epidemic (these are included in country total).

Legend (Figure 3-45):
★ Initial epidemics January 1991
— August 1991
— February 1992
— March 1993

A. Antigenic determinants of *Vibrio cholerae* O1

Serotype	O Antigens
Ogawa	A, B
Inaba	A, C
Hikojima	A, B, C

FIGURE 3-47 Classification of *Vibrio cholerae* serotypes and biotypes. **A,** Antigenic determinants of *V. cholerae* O1. **B,** Differentiation of the classic and El Tor biotypes of *V. cholerae* O1. The serotypes of *V. cholerae* that cause epidemic human disease have three determinants, which are the O or somatic antigens. Whereas serotypes are determined by O antigens, biotypes (classic and El Tor) are determined by characteristic hemolysis, chicken red cell agglutination, polymyxin sensitivity, Voges-Proskauer reaction, and phage sensitivity. (Panel 47A *from* Greenough [28]; panel 47B *from* Butterton and Calderwood [27].)

B. Differentiation of the classic and El Tor biotypes of *Vibrio cholerae* O1

Characteristics	Classic	El Tor
Hemolysis	–	+
Agglutination of chicken red cells	–	+
Susceptibility to polymyxin B (50 intrauterine)	+	–
Voges-Proskauer reaction	–	+
Susceptibility to bacteriophages		
IV	+	–
V	–	+

Electrolyte composition of cholera stool*

	Concentration, *mmol/L*			
	Na⁺	K⁺	Cl⁻	HCO₃⁻
Adults	135	15	100	45
Children	105	25	90	30

*When purging rate is 50 mL/kg/24 hrs or more.

FIGURE 3-48 Electrolyte composition of cholera stool. In the isotonic diarrhea seen with cholera, the more severe the diarrhea, the closer to typical serum electrolyte compositions becomes the cholera stool (with somewhat more potassium and bicarbonate losses). This composition provides an important guide to electrolytes in need of replacement. (*From* Greenough [28].)

Oral replacement solutions

	Salts to add to 1 L of drinking water, g	Concentration, *mmol/L*				
		Na⁺	K⁺	Cl⁻	HCO₃⁻	Glucose
WHO solution		90	20	80	30	111
NaCL	3.5					
NaHCO₃	2.5					
KCl	1.5					
Glucose	20					
Household solution		85				
NaCl	5					
Precooked rice*	50–80					

*May substitute sucrose 40 g/L.

WHO—World Health Organization.

FIGURE 3-49 Oral replacement solutions for cholera. Treatment of cholera is based, simply enough, on rehydration. The water and salts lost in cholera stool must be replaced in comparable amounts and concentrations, and this can usually be accomplished orally. The availability of oral rehydration solution has reduced mortality from > 50% to < 1%. (*From* Greenough [28].)

Clinical findings to estimate fluid volume depletion in cholera

	Depletion (% body weight)		
Finding	0%–3%	4%–8%	8%–12%
Central pulses (femoral, carotid)	Full	Full	Weak
Peripheral pulses (radial, pedal)	Full	Weak	Absent
Skin turgor	Normal	Decreased	Poor
Eyes	Normal	Slightly sunken	Sunken
Muscles	Normal	Some cramps	Severe cramps
Appearance	Alert, slight thirst	Alert, thirsty	Restless, very thirsty
Urine flow	Normal	Reduced	Absent

FIGURE 3-50 Signs and symptoms of cholera correlated with degree of dehydration. Treatment of clinical cholera is rapid, appropriate rehydration. The signs and symptoms can provide a quick assessment of the degree of dehydration and serve as a guide to the course of treatment. (*From* Greenough [28].)

Intravenous replacement solutions

	Concentration, *mmol/L*				
	Na$^+$	K$^+$	Cl$^-$	HCO$_3^-$	Glucose
Diarrhea treatment solution	118	13	83	48	50
Dhaka solution (5/4/1) 5 g NaCl 4 g NaHCO$_3$* 1 g KCl	134	13	99	48*	0
Ringer's lactate solution	131	4	109	29	0

*Acetate may be substituted for bicarbonate for a more stable solution; sodium acetate anhydrous 3.9 g/L, or if the triple hydrate is used, 6.5 g/L.

FIGURE 3-51 Intravenous replacement solution. Patients who are severely dehydrated (< 10% of body weight) or in whom mental status changes or vomiting preclude the use of oral therapy should be treated with intravenous solutions such as Ringer's lactate, which is the only generally available solution with the appropriate electrolyte composition. In the Dhaka 5/4/1 solution, sodium acetate anhydrous, 3.9 g/L (or triple hydrate, 6.5 g/L), may be substituted for bicarbonate to make a more stable solution. (*From* Greenough [28].)

Antibiotics for treatment of cholera

	Dosage		
	Children	Adults	Schedule
First choices			
Tetracycline*	12.5 mg/kg	500 mg	Four times a day × 3 days
Doxycycline*	6 mg/kg	300 mg	Single dose
Alternatives (tetracycline-resistant strains)			
Erythromycin	10 mg/kg	250 mg	Adults: four times a day × 3 days Children: three times a day × 3 days
TMP-SMX	5 mg/kg TMP/25 mg/kg SMX	160 mg TMP/800 mg SMX	Twice a day × 3 days
Furazolidone	1.25 mg/kg	100 mg	Four times a day × 3 days

*Some physicians prefer to avoid tetracycline use in children because of tooth staining.

SMX—sulfamethoxazole; TMP—trimethoprim.

FIGURE 3-52 Antibiotic therapy for cholera. Although rehydration is the only therapy necessary to treat cholera, antibiotics will diminish the duration of diarrhea and thereby the fluid loss. The tetracyclines are the drugs of choice, but some antibiotic resistance has been seen among *Vibrio cholerae* isolates. (*Adapted from* Swerdlow and Ries [29].)

Escherichia coli

Types and mechanisms of *Escherichia coli* enteropathogens

	Genetic code	Mechanism	Model	Type of diarrhea
Enterotoxigenic				
Heat-labile toxin	Plasmid	CFA/I–V → colonize	MRHA	Acute watery
	Plasmid/chromosomal	Adenylate cyclase secretion	18-hr rabbit ileal loop	
			Chinese hamster ovary cell, Y1 cells	
heat-stable toxin (ST$_a$)	Plasmid	Guanylate cyclase secretion	4–8-hr rabbit ileal loop	Acute watery
			Suckling mice	
ST$_b$	Plasmid	Cyclic nucleotide-independent HCO$_3$ secretion	Piglet loop	?
Enterohemorrhagic				
Shigella-like toxin	Phage/plasmid(?)	Glycosidase cleaves ribosomal RNA to halt protein synthesis	HeLa cell cytotoxicity	Bloody (hemolytic-uremic syndrome)
Enteroinvasive	Plasmid (140 MDa) + chromosomal	Cell invasion and spread 58–80-KDa EIET (chromosomal)	Sereny test	Acute dysenteric
Enteropathogenic	Plasmid (60 MDa; EAF, *bfpA*)	BFP → localized adherence	Localized adherence to HEp-2 cells	Acute + persistent
	Chromosomal (*cfm*)	Tyrosine kinase- and intracellular Ca^{2+}-dependent actin condensation	Fluorescence actin staining	
	Chromosomal (*eaeA*)	94-kDa intimin → effacing adherence		
Enteroaggregative	Plasmid (60 MDa)	BFP → aggregative adherence	Aggregative adherence to HEp-2 cells	Persistent (acute[?])
		2–5-kDa, EAST-1, guanylate cyclase, EALT pore forming Ca^{2+} inonophore	Ussing chambers	
Diffusely adherent	Chromosomal	Fimbial adhesion (F1845)	Diffuse adherence to HEp-2 cells	Acute(?), persistent(?)
	Plasmid	Afimbrial adhesin (homologous to *Shigella* IcsA)		
Normal enteric colonizing	Plasmid	CFA/I–V → colonize Hydrophobic(?)	MRHA (NH$_1$)$_2$SO$_4$ hydrophobicity	Persistent(?)
Genitourinary/central nervous system/normal flora	Chromosomal/plasmid	Type I pili (P-fimbriae, S-fimbriae, AFA-I)	MRHA, binds P blood group antigen	None

AFA—afimbrial adhesion; BFP—bundle-forming pili; CFA—colonization factor antigen; EAF—enteropathogenic *E. coli* adherence factor; EALT—enteroaggregative *E. coli* heat-labile toxin; EAST—enteroaggregative *E. coli* heat-stable toxin; EIET—enteroinvasive *E. coli* enterotoxin; MRHA—mannose-resistant hemagglutination.

FIGURE 3-53 Types and mechanisms of *Escherichia coli* enteropathogens. *E. coli* can cause diarrhea in a variety of ways. This versatile organism can produce either a heat-labile or heat-stable enterotoxin, to cause watery endemic or traveler's diarrhea; produce shigalike toxin to cause enterohemorrhagic illness; be invasive to cause *Shigella*-like illness; or adhere via carefully orchestrated attaching and effacing mechanisms, such as those seen with classic enteropathogenic *E. coli*, or via poorly understood enteroaggregative or diffuse adherence patterns. (*Adapted from* Guerrant and Thielman [30].)

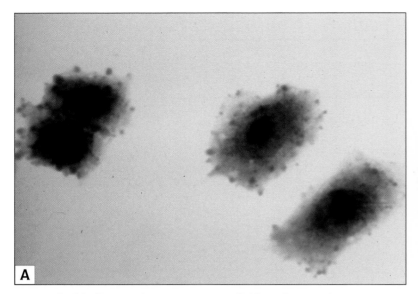

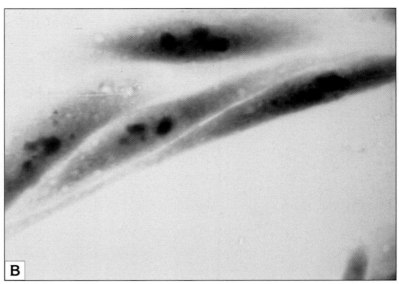

FIGURE 3-54 Chinese hamster ovary (CHO) cell assay for *Escherichia coli* heat-labile (LT) enterotoxin or choleratoxin.

A, Normal control CHO cells. **B,** *E. coli* LT enterotoxin produces CHO cell elongation. (*From* Guerrant *et al.* [31]; with permission.)

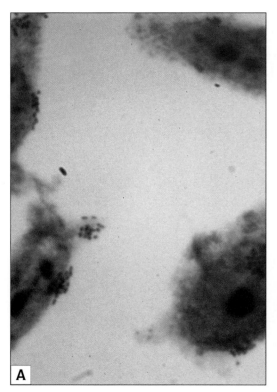

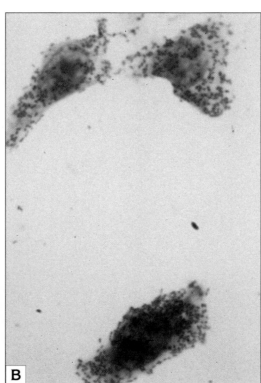

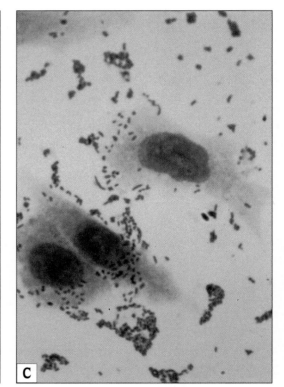

FIGURE 3-55 Patterns of *Escherichia coli* HEp-2 cell adherence. **A,** Localized (or focal) adherence for classic localized adherence *E. coli*

(enteropathogenic *E. coli*). **B,** Diffusely adherent *E. coli*. **C,** Enteroaggregative *E. coli*. (*Courtesy of* R.L. Guerrant, MD.)

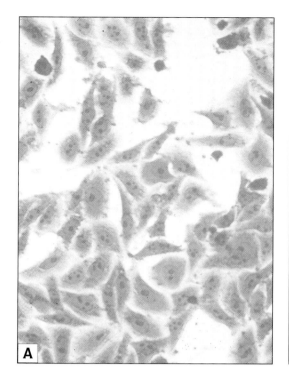
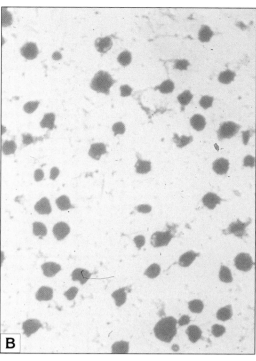

FIGURE 3-56 **A** and **B**, Normal HeLa cells (*panel 56A*) compared with the effect of shigalike toxin of enterohemorrhagic *Escherichia coli* O157 on HeLa cells (*panel 56B*).

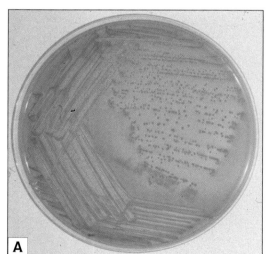
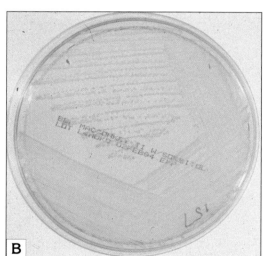

FIGURE 3-57 **A** and **B**, *Escherichia coli* O157:H7 on regular (*panel 57A*) and sorbitol (*panel 57B*) MacConkey agar plates. This organism, which is a major cause of bloody diarrhea/hemorrhagic colitis and occasional hemolytic-uremic syndrome, is sorbitol negative (*Courtesy of* B. Strain, MD, D. Gröschel, MD, and R.L. Guerrant, MD.)

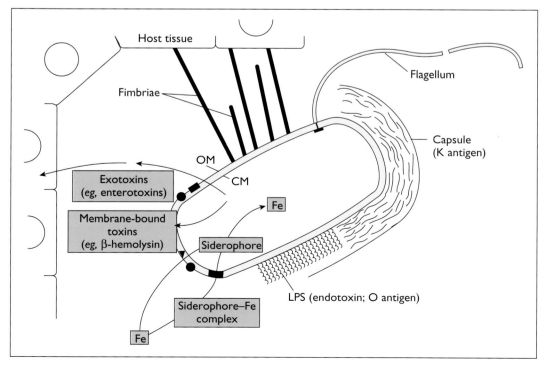

FIGURE 3-58 Virulence factors of *Escherichia coli*. Surface fimbriae, with colonization factor antigens (CFA) I to V, are critical to the organism's ability to colonize the small bowel. Lipopolysaccharide (LPS) of the outer membrane (OM) possesses endotoxin function, and some possess O antigenicity. *E. coli* secretes siderophore, a high-affinity iron-chelating compound, which the bacteria uses to capture extracellular iron. Exotoxin (*eg*, enterotoxin) and membrane-bound hemolysins present in some *E. coli* are enterotoxic or cytotoxic. (CM—cytoplasmic membrane.) (*Adapted from* Eisenstein and Jones [32].)

Frequency of enterotoxigenic *Escherichia coli* in association with traveler's diarrhea

Feature	Study				Total
	Gastroenterologists in Mexico [36]	Peace Corps volunteers in Kenya [37]	Yale Glee Club in Latin America [38]	Japanese travelers returning to Tokyo from India, Southeast Asia, Orient [39]	
Illness attack rate	49% in 16 days	69% in 5 wks	74% in 1 mo	—	—
Type of enterotoxin					
LT only	16%	33%	25%	4.8%	21%
LT and ST	16%	15%	12.5%	11.8%	38%
ST only	9.8%	2%	19%	13.6%	41%
Total	21/51 cases	14/27 cases	9/16 cases	226/749 cases	270/843 cases
Percentage of illness with ETEC	41%	52%	56%	30.2%	32%

ETEC—enterotoxigenic *E. coli*; LT—heat-labile toxin; ST—heat-stable toxin.

FIGURE 3-59 Frequency of enterotoxigenic *Escherichia coli* (ETEC) in association with traveler's diarrhea. ETEC is found in approximately 50% of cases of traveler's diarrhea in Latin America, Africa, and Asia [33–39]. (*From* Guerrant and Bobak [24].)

Reported outbreaks of *Escherichia coli* O157:H7 infections in the United States, 1982–1993

Month and year	State	Setting	Affected/ hospitalized, *n*	HUS or TTP, *n*	Deaths, *n*	Likely vehicle of spread
Feb 1982	OR	Community	26/19	0	0	Ground beef
May 1982	MI	Community	21/14	0	0	Ground beef
Sep 1984	NE	Nursing home	34/14	1	4	Ground beef
Sep 1984	NC	Daycare center	36/3	3	0	Person-to-person
Oct 1986	WA	Community	37/17	4	2	Ground beef/ranch dressing
Jun 1987	UT	Custodial institutions	51/8	8	4	Ground beef/person-to-person
May 1988	WI	School	61/2	0	0	Roast beef
Aug 1988	MN	Daycare center	19/NR	3	0	Person-to-person
Oct 1988	MN	School	54/4	0	0	Precooked ground beef
Dec 1989	MO	Community	243/32	2	4	Municipal water
Jul 1990	ND	Community	65/16	2	0	Roast beef
Nov 1990	MT	School	10/2	1	0	School lunch
Jul 1991	OR	Community	28/7	3	0	Swimming water
Nov 1991	MA	Community	23/7	3	0	Apple cider
Jul 1992	NV	Daycare center	57/1	0	0	Person-to-person
Sep 1992	ME	Family	4/3	1	1	Vegetable/person-to-person
Dec 1992	OR	Community	8/2	0	0	Raw milk
Jan 1993	WA, ID, NV, CA	Community	732/195	55	4	Ground beef
Mar 1993	OR	Community	48/12	0	0	Mayonnaise-containing dressing/sauces
Total	—	—	1557/358	86	19	—

HUS—hemolytic-uremic syndrome; NR—not reported; TTP—thrombotic thrombocytopenic purpura.

FIGURE 3-60 Reported outbreaks of *Escherichia coli* O157:H7 infections in the United States between 1982 and 1993. The enterohemorrhagic *E. coli* O157:H7, which produces a cytotoxic shigalike toxin, was first associated with a multistate outbreak of hemorrhagic colitis in 1982 and more recently has been associated with additional outbreaks of hamburger-related food poisoning. Unlike classic *Shigella* dysentery, there is less mucosal invasion and patients are often afebrile. Hemolytic-uremic syndrome, especially in children, and thrombocytopenic purpura have been associated with these strains. (*From* Griffin [40].)

Shigella Species

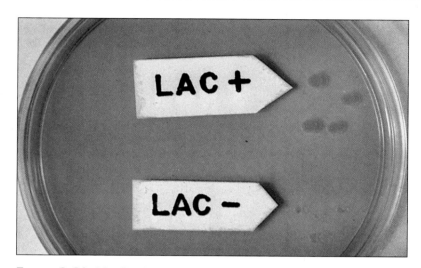

FIGURE 3-61 MacConkey agar plate showing appearance of non-lactose–fermenting colonies, typical of *Shigella*. Shigella produces an acute inflammatory colitis, often as bacillary dysentery. The pathogenic species (*S. dysenteriae, flexneri, boydii,* and *sonnei*) are mostly lactose-negative and are characterized by their ability to invade intestinal epithelium and produce highly potent shigatoxins that halt eukaryotic protein synthesis. Shigellosis is highly communicable because of its low infectious dose (10^1–10^2 organisms). (*From* Finegold and Baron [41]; with permission.)

Antimicrobial therapy for bacillary dysentery	
First choice	
Children	TMP, 10 mg/kg/d, *plus* SMX, 50 mg/kg/d, in two equal doses every 12 hrs orally × 3–5 days
Adults	TMP, 160 mg, *plus* SMX, 800 mg, every 12 hrs orally × 3–5 days
Alternate	
Children	Nalidixic acid, 55 mg/kg/d, in four equal doses orally × 5 days
Adults	Ciprofloxacin, 500 mg bid orally × 3–5 days* Norfloxacin, 400 mg bid orally × 3–5 days* Ofloxacin, 300 mg bid orally × 3–5 days*

*For mild to moderately ill persons, single-dose therapy is adequate.

bid—twice a day; SMX—sulfamethoxazole; TMP—trimethoprim.

FIGURE 3-62 Antibiotic therapy for bacillary dysentery. If dehydration is present, the patient should receive oral rehydration. Antibiotics, usually trimethoprim-sulfamethoxazole, are useful in shigellosis in shortening the duration of diarrhea and in limiting the course of illness. The quinolones represent a good alternative for adults, especially with the increasing resistance to sulfamethoxazole and trimethoprim. (*Adapted from* DuPont [42].)

Campylobacter Species

Campylobacter, Helicobacter, and *Arcobacter* species associated with different clinical manifestations of infection		
Disease syndrome	**Enteric**	**Extraintestinal**
Major pathogen	*C. jejuni*	*C. fetus*
Minor pathogens	*C. coli*	*C. jejuni*
	C. lari	*C. coli*
	C. fetus	*C. lari*
	H. fennelliae	*H. fennelliae*
	H. cinaedi	*H. cinaedi*
	C. upsaliensis	*C. sputorum*
	Nitrate-negative *Campylobacter*	*C. hyointestinalis*
	A. butzleri	
	A. skirrowi	
	X. cryaerophila	

FIGURE 3-63 *Campylobacter* species and related organisms associated with clinical illness. Campylobacters cause both diarrheal and systemic illness. The prototypical enteric pathogen is *Campylobacter jejuni*, and for extraintestinal infection, the major pathogen is *C. fetus*. (*From* Blaser [43].)

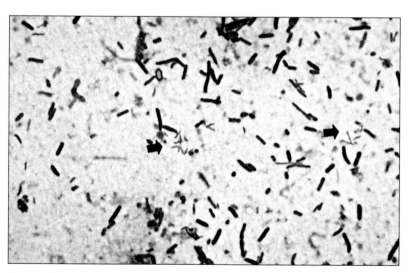

FIGURE 3-64 Gram stain of fecal specimen from a patient with *Campylobacter* enteritis. Typical gram-negative, fine, small, spiral and *Vibrio*-like organisms are seen. The finding of vibrio forms on Gram stain of stools is a reasonably specific means for making a diagnosis of *Campylobacter* enteritis, although the sensitivity of this technique is only 50% to 70%. (Original magnification, × 1024.) (*From* Blaser [43]; with permission.)

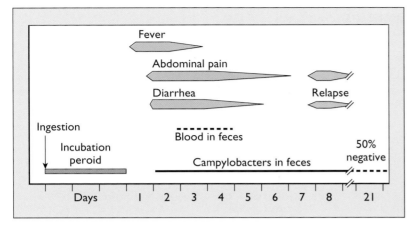

FIGURE 3-65 Symptoms and clinical course of *Campylobacter* enteritis. *Campylobacter* enteritis is essentially an acute inflammatory diarrheal disease that is clinically indistinguishable from that due to *Salmonella*, *Shigella*, or other bacterial enteropathogens. The illness usually lasts 4 to 5 days [44]. (*Adapted from* Skirrow [45].)

Frequency of clinical features in community outbreaks of *Campylobacter* enteritis

Feature	Outbreaks, *n*	Mean (range)
Diarrhea	44	86% (27–100)
Abdominal pain	43	78% (39–100)
Fever	42	53% (6–90)
Headache	35	39% (0–72)
Myalgia	8	40% (27–59)
Vomiting	34	15% (0–44)*
Blood in feces	11	14% (0.5–32)

*Excludes water-borne outbreaks.

FIGURE 3-66 Frequency of clinical features in community outbreaks of *Campylobacter* enteritis. The proportion of patients hospitalized averages about 5% in community outbreaks but ranges from 9.4% to 32% in sporadic cases. (*From* Blaser [44].)

Salmonella Species

Clinical syndromes due to *Salmonella* infection

Syndrome	Most common causative serotypes	Symptoms and findings
Gastroenteritis	S. typhimurium S. enteritidis S. newport S. anatum	Moderate fever, nausea, vomiting, diarrhea, variable abdominal discomfort
Enteric fever	S. typhi S. paratyphi A S. schottmuelleri S. hirschfeldii	Prolonged fever, headache, myalgias, nausea, constipation or diarrhea, hypertrophy of reticuloendothelial system, possible metastatic infection, possible immune complex deposition
Bacteremia, with or without metastatic disease	S. typhimurium S. choleraesuis S. heidelberg	Fever, possible nausea, vomiting, possible diarrhea, abdominal discomfort, possible cardiovascular infection, possible metastatic infection
Chronic carrier state	S. typhimurium	Asymptomatic

FIGURE 3-67 Clinical syndromes due to *Salmonella* infection. The most commonly recognized clinical syndrome caused by *Salmonella* is gastroenteritis. Typically, the symptoms of nausea and vomiting begin 8 to 48 hours after ingestion of contaminated food, followed by diarrhea and colicky abdominal pain. However, overlap is seen among the syndromes such that a patient with enteric fever may also have diarrhea and those with gastroenteritis may also have high fever. *Salmonella typhimurium* is the most common cause of the gastroenteritis as well as bacteremia syndromes. (*From* Goldberg and Rubin [46].)

Frequency of isolation of non-*typhi Salmonella* serotypes in the United States, 1991

Serotype	Isolates, *n*	%
S. typhimurium*	8878	22.2
S. enteritidis	7712	19.3
S. heidelberg	2927	7.3
S. hadar	1945	4.9
S. newport	1790	4.5
S. agona	988	2.5
S. montevideo	861	2.2
S. poona	787	2.0
S. javiana	780	1.9
S. thompson	705	1.8
Subtotal	27,373	68.4
Total non-*typhi* cases	40,012	100

*Includes variant Copenhagen.

FIGURE 3-68 Frequency of isolation of non-*typhi Salmonella* serotypes in the United States in 1991. The incidence of nontyphoidal *Salmonella* increased rapidly in the United States in the 1980s, but the illness is still likely to be underreported. Most outbreaks are related to food products, often poultry and eggs. (*From* Miller *et al.* [47].)

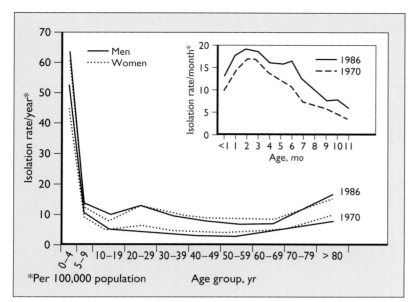

FIGURE 3-69 *Salmonella* isolation rates by age and sex of patient in the United States between 1970 and 1986. There is a marked seasonal variation in the occurrence of *Salmonella* infection, with peak incidences in the summer and fall due to many small outbreaks of picnic-related poisonings (*Salmonella* accounts for 10% of all food poisonings). The highest rates of *Salmonella* infection are seen in children younger than 5 years of age (particularly infants), persons aged 20 to 30, and the elderly over 70 years of age. If one household member becomes infected, the probability that another will become infected approaches 60%. (*Adapted from* Hargrett-Bean *et al.* [48].)

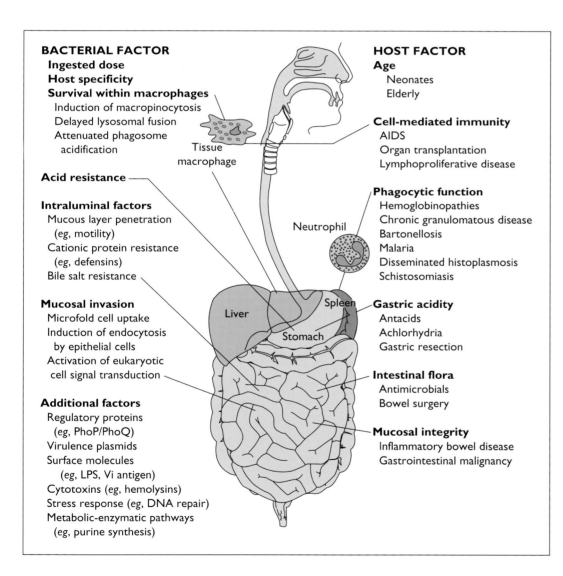

BACTERIAL FACTOR
Ingested dose
Host specificity
Survival within macrophages
  Induction of macropinocytosis
  Delayed lysosomal fusion
  Attenuated phagosome
    acidification

Acid resistance

Intraluminal factors
  Mucous layer penetration
    (eg, motility)
  Cationic protein resistance
    (eg, defensins)
  Bile salt resistance

Mucosal invasion
  Microfold cell uptake
  Induction of endocytosis
    by epithelial cells
  Activation of eukaryotic
    cell signal transduction

Additional factors
  Regulatory proteins
    (eg, PhoP/PhoQ)
  Virulence plasmids
  Surface molecules
    (eg, LPS, Vi antigen)
  Cytotoxins (eg, hemolysins)
  Stress response (eg, DNA repair)
  Metabolic-enzymatic pathways
    (eg, purine synthesis)

HOST FACTOR
Age
  Neonates
  Elderly

Cell-mediated immunity
  AIDS
  Organ transplantation
  Lymphoproliferative disease

Phagocytic function
  Hemoglobinopathies
  Chronic granulomatous disease
  Bartonellosis
  Malaria
  Disseminated histoplasmosis
  Schistosomiasis

Gastric acidity
  Antacids
  Achlorhydria
  Gastric resection

Intestinal flora
  Antimicrobials
  Bowel surgery

Mucosal integrity
  Inflammatory bowel disease
  Gastrointestinal malignancy

Tissue macrophage

Neutrophil

Liver   Spleen   Stomach

FIGURE 3-70 Pathogenic bacterial properties and host factors involved in the susceptibility to *Salmonella* infection. (LPS—lipopolysaccharide.) (*Adapted from* Pegues *et al.* [49].)

Currently available *Salmonella typhi* vaccines

Vaccine	Efficacy	Administration	Adverse reactions
Acetone inactivated	55%–85% for 2.5–5 yrs	Two 0.5-mL subcutaneous injections, 4–8 wks apart, booster every 3 yrs	Pain at injection site, headache, fever, malaise
Live attenuated Ty21a	0%–95% for 3 yrs or longer	Three doses of capsule or reconstituted liquid orally	None
Vi capsular polysaccharide	75% for ≥ 17 mos	One intramuscular injection	Local pain (25%), tenderness (25%), fever (9%), malaise (9%)

FIGURE 3-71 Currently available vaccines against *Salmonella typhi*. No vaccine is currently approved for use against non-*typhi Salmonella* in the United States. Three vaccines for *S. typhi* are currently used worldwide. In the United States, vaccination is recommended for travel to regions where there is a recognized risk of exposure, which includes many developing countries. (*From* Goldberg *et al.* [50].)

Yersinia Species

Selected outbreaks of *Yersinia enterocolitica* infection with identified sources

Location	Cases, *n*	Source or common vehicle	Predominant serotype
North Carolina	16	Dog	O:8
Canada	138	Raw milk (?)	O:5,27
New York	38	Chocolate milk	O:8
Japan	1051	Milk	O:3
New York	159	Powdered milk, chow mein	O:8
Washington	50	Tofu, spring water	O:8
Pennsylvania	16	Bean sprouts, well water	O:8
Southern United States	172	Pasteurized milk	O:13a,13b
Georgia	15	Chitterlings	O:3

FIGURE 3-72 Outbreaks of *Yersinia enterocolitica* infection and sources. *Y. enterocolitica* is a relatively infrequent cause of diarrhea and abdominal pain in the United States, but its recognition has grown over the past decade. Children are more often affected than adults. Transmission occurs by ingestion of contaminated food or water and, less commonly, by direct contact with infected animals (farm animals, dogs, cats, rabbits, rodents) and patients. (*From* Cover [51].)

Clinical manifestations of *Yersinia enterocolitica* infection

Syndrome	Typical age of patient	Predisposing host factors
Enterocolitis	Child or adult	Young age
Pseudoappendicitis syndrome	Older child or adult	None
Septicemia	Child or adult	Iron overload, deferoxamine therapy, immunocompromise
Reactive arthritis	Adult	HLA-B27, residence in Scandinavia
Erythema nodosum	Adult	Residence in Scandinavia, female gender

FIGURE 3-73 Clinical manifestations of *Yersinia enterocolitica* infection. *Y. enterocolitica* infection may result in a variety of syndromes, depending on the age and physical state of the host. Illness is most common among children. Enterocolitis, the most common presentation, is characterized by diarrhea, low-grade fever, and abdominal pain, with bloody stools evident in one fourth of patients. The illness typically lasts 14 to 22 days, but symptoms may persist for months. Most infections are self-limited. (*From* Cover [52].)

Food-Borne Disease

Food-borne disease outbreaks of known etiology, United States, 1973–1987

Etiologic agent	Outbreaks		Cases	
	No.	%	No.	%
Bacterial		66		87
Bacillus cereus	58	2	1123	1
Campylobacter	53	2	1547	1
Clostridium botulinum	231	8	494	0
Clostridium perfringens	190	7	12,234	10
Escherichia coli	10	0	1187	1
Salmonella	790	28	55,864	45
Shigella	104	4	14,399	12
Staphylococcus aureus	367	13	17,248	14
Vibrio cholerae O1	6	0	916	1
Vibrio cholerae non-O1	2	0	11	0
Vibrio parahaemolyticus	23	1	535	0
Yersinia enterocolitica	5	0	767	1
Other bacterial	30	1	2581	2
Chemical		24		3
Ciguatera	234	8	1052	1
Heavy metals	46	2	753	1
Histamine fish poisoning	202	7	1046	1
Monosodium glutamate	18	1	58	0
Mushrooms	61	2	169	0
Paralytic shellfish poisoning	21	1	160	0
Other chemical	115	4	1046	1
Parasitic		5		1
Giardia	5	0	131	0
Trichinella spiralis	128	5	843	1
Other parasitic	7	0	30	0
Viral		5		9
Hepatitis A	110	4	3133	3
Norwalk virus	15	1	6474	5
Other viral	10	0	1023	1
Total	2841	100	124,824	100

FIGURE 3-74 Food-borne disease outbreaks of known etiology in the United States between 1973 and 1987. More than 16,000 cases of food-borne disease occur in 400 to 600 outbreaks annually in the United States. However, because most cases are not reported, truer numbers probably approach 6.5 to 8.1 million illnesses annually, with 7000 deaths. Bacterial agents are the most important etiologic factor, accounting for 66% of outbreaks in which the etiology is known (and 87% of sporadic cases), but a cause cannot be determined in 62% of outbreaks. (*From* Tauxe and Hughes [52].)

Factors contributing to food-borne disease outbreaks

Factor	% Implicated*
Inadequate refrigeration	47
Food prepared too far in advance of service	21
Infected food handler with poor personal hygiene	21
Inadequate cooking	16
Improper holding temperature	16
Inadequate reheating	12
Contaminated raw ingredients	11
Cross-contamination	7
Dirty equipment	7

*More than one factor may contribute to a food-borne outbreak.

FIGURE 3-75 Factors contributing to food-borne disease outbreaks. The common theme that ties all food-borne illness together is the presence of an improper food-handling procedure, usually inadequate refrigeration or cooking. (*From* Snydman and Gorbach [53].)

Etiology of food-borne disease outbreaks by food, season, and geographic predilection

Biology	Foods	Season	Geographic predilection
Bacterial			
Salmonella	Beef, poultry, eggs, dairy products	Summer	None
Staphylococcus aureus	Ham, poultry, egg salads, pastries	Summer	None
Campylobacter jejuni	Poultry, raw milk	Spring, summer	None
Clostridium botulinum	Vegetables, fruits, fish, honey (infants)	Summer, fall	West, Northeast
Clostridium perfringens	Beef, poultry, gravy, Mexican food	Fall, winter, spring	None
Shigella	Egg salads, lettuce	Summer	None
Vibrio parahaemolyticus	Crabs	Spring, summer, fall	Coastal states
Bacillus cereus	Fried rice, meats, vegetables	Year round	None
Yersinia enterocolitica	Milk, tofu, pork	Winter	Unknown
V. cholerae O1	Shellfish	Variable	Tropical, Gulf Coast, Latin America
V. cholerae non-O1	Shellfish	Unknown	Tropical, Gulf Coast
Verotoxigenic *Escherichia coli*	Beef, raw milk	Summer, fall	Unknown
Viral			
Norwalk agent	Shellfish, salads	Year round	Northeast
Chemical			
Ciguatera	Barracuda, snapper, amberjack, grouper	Spring, summer (in Florida)	Tropical
Histamine fish poisoning (scombroid)	Tuna, mackerel, bonito, skipjack, mahi-mahi	Year round	Coastal
Mushroom poisoning	Mushrooms	Spring, fall	Temperate
Heavy metals	Acidic beverages	Year round	None
Monosodium-L-glutamate	Chinese food	Year round	None
Paralytic shellfish poisoning	Shellfish	Summer, fall	Temperate
Neurotoxic shellfish poisoning	Shellfish	Spring, fall	Subtropical

FIGURE 3-76 Etiology of food-borne disease outbreaks, by food, season, and geographic predilection. Clues to the etiology of an outbreak of food-borne disease may be provided by the type of food consumed, season, and sometimes geographic region. (*From* Tauxe and Hughes [52].)

Water-borne disease outbreaks of known etiology, United States, 1972–1990

	Outbreaks	
Etiologic agent	No.	%
Giardia lamblia	100	39.5
Shigella	29	11.5
Hepatitis A	20	7.9
Norwalk-like agents	16	6.3
Campylobacter jejuni	12	4.7
Nontyphoid salmonella	12	4.7
Salmonella typhi	5	2.0
Enterotoxigenic *Escherichia coli*	1	0.4
E. coli O157:H7	1	0.4
Vibrio cholerae O1	1	0.4
Yersinia enterocolitica	1	0.4
Rotavirus	1	0.4
Cryptosporidium	2	0.8
Entamoeba histolytica	1	0.4
Miscellaneous chemicals	51	20.2
Total	253	100

FIGURE 3-77 Water-borne disease outbreaks of known etiology in the United States between 1972 and 1990. Occasional cluster of water-borne disease are reported that mimic a food-borne epidemic. The pathogenic agents in water-borne disease differ from those involved in food-borne disease, but again, the majority of water-borne outbreaks are of unknown etiology. (*From* Tauxe and Hughes [52].)

Clinical diagnosis of food poisoning by onset and symptoms

Symptoms	Incubation period, *hrs*	Possible agents
Acute upper gastrointestinal symptoms, nausea, vomiting	6	Preformed heat-stable toxins of *Staphylococcus aureus* and *Bacillus cereus*; also *Diphyllobothrium latum*, *Anisakis*, heavy metals
Upper-small-bowel symptoms; watery noninflammatory diarrhea	6–72	*Clostridium perfringens* type A, *Bacillus cereus*, enterotoxigenic *Escherichia coli*, *Vibrio cholerae*, *Giardia lamblia*
Inflammatory ileocolitis	16–72	*Salmonella*, *Shigella*, *Campylobacter jejuni*, *Vibrio parahaemolyticus*, enteroinvasive *E. coli*, *Yersinia*, *Aeromonas*
Sensory or motor neurologic symptoms with or without gastrointestinal symptoms, suggesting botulism, fish or shellfish poisoning, or chemical poisoning	1–8	Histamine-like scombrotoxin, dinoflagellate neurotoxin, monosodium glutamate, mushroom, solanine, pesticides

FIGURE 3-78 Clinical diagnosis of food poisoning by onset and symptoms. The pathogenic mechanisms by which the bacterial agents produce disease determines the incubation period seen with each disease. Illness having a rapid onset, within 1 to 6 hours after consumption, indicates a preformed enterotoxin, usually due to *Staphylococcus*; it presents with vomiting and generally lasts < 12 hours. Intermediate-onset diarrhea, starting 6 to 16 hours after consumption, suggests a toxin that is produced by bacteria within the upper small bowel, such as *Clostridium perfringens* type A or *Escherichia coli*. Longer incubation periods and systemic symptoms suggest tissue invasion and inflammatory colitis. (*From* Guerrant and Bobak [6].)

Deaths in food-borne disease outbreaks, United States, 1973–1987

Etiologic agent	Deaths, *n*	Death-to-case ratio*
Bacterial		
Bacillus cereus	0	0
Campylobacter	2	2
Clostridium botulinum	47	192
Clostridium perfringens	12	1
Escherichia coli	4	3
Listeria monocytogenes	70	317
Salmonella	88	2
Shigella	4	1
Staphylococcus aureus	4	< 1
Vibrio cholerae O1	12	13
Vibrio cholerae non-O1	0	0
Yersinia enterocolitica	0	0
Other bacterial	4	2
Chemical		
Mushrooms	8	49
Paralytic shellfish poisoning	1	6
Other chemical	12	3
Parasitic		
Trichinella spiralis	5	8
Other parasitic	0	0
Viral	2	< 1
Unknown	26	< 1

*Per 1000 cases.

FIGURE 3-79 Mortality rates in food-borne disease outbreaks in the United States between 1973 and 1987. Most cases of food poisoning are self-limited, but fatalities may occur in previously healthy people due to botulism, mushrooms, or paralytic shellfish poisoning. Listeriosis is most often fatal in neonates and immunocompromised persons. Deaths from salmonellosis and other causes are seen mostly in infants, the elderly, and the debilitated. (*From* Tauxe and Hughes [52].)

Symptoms and signs in food-borne botulism outbreaks 1953–1973	
Symptoms	
Blurred vision, diplopia, photophobia	90.4%
Dysphagia	76.0%
Generalized weakness	57.7%
Nausea and/or vomiting	55.8%
Dysphonia	54.8%
Dizziness or vertigo	30.8%
Abdominal pain, cramps, fullness	20.2%
Diarrhea	15.4%
Urinary retention or incontinence	6.7%
Sore throat	6.7%
Constipation	5.8%
Paresthesias	1.0%
Signs	
Respiratory impairment	73.1%
Specific muscle weakness or paralysis	46.2%
Eye muscle involvement, including ptosis	44.2%
Dry mouth, throat, or tongue	21.2%
Dilated, fixed pupils	15.4%
Ataxia	8.7%
Postural hypotension	2.9%
Nystagmus	2.9%
Somnolence	1.0%

FIGURE 3-80 Symptoms and signs in food-borne botulism outbreaks between 1953 and 1973. Botulism is a neuroparalytic disease that principally affects the nerves stimulating skeletal muscle, often by blocking acetylcholine release. The classic presentation is the development of acute, bilateral cranial neuropathies associated with symmetric descending weakness. Serotypes A, B, E, and (rarely) F are associated with human disease (*Adapted from* Hatheway [54].)

Clostridium and Antibiotic-Related Colitis

Rates of isolation of *Clostridium difficile* and cytotoxin in stools		
Patient category	Culture positive rates, %	Toxin positive rates (tissue culture assay), %
Antibiotic-associated diarrhea or colitis with positive toxin assay	95–100	—
Antibiotic-associated pseudo-membranous colitis	95–100	95–100
Antibiotic-associated diarrhea	15–25	10–25
Antibiotic-exposure without diarrhea	20	2–8
Hospitalized patients	10–25	?
Gastrointestinal disease unrelated to antibiotic exposure	2–3	0.5
Healthy adults	2–3	0
Healthy neonates	5–70	5–63

FIGURE 3-81 Rates of isolation of *Clostridium difficile* and cytotoxin in stools. *C. difficile* is part of the normal fecal flora. Antibiotic use may inhibit the growth of other gastrointestinal flora, allowing the proliferation of *C. difficile* or production of its toxin. *C. difficile* is recognized as the most frequent cause of antibiotic-related colitis and pseudomembranous colitis. (*From* Bartlett [55].)

Antimicrobial agents associated with *C. difficile*–associated diarrhea and pseudomembranous colitis

Frequent	Infrequent	Rare
Ampicillin	Tetracyclines	Parenteral
Amoxicillin	Sulfonamides	aminoglycosides
Cephalosporins	Erythromycin	Bacitracin
Clindamycin	Chloramphenicol	Metronidazole
	Trimethoprim	Vancomycin
	Quinolones	

FIGURE 3-82 Antimicrobial agents associated with *Clostridium difficile*–related diarrhea and pseudomembranous colitis [56]. (*Adapted from* Kelly *et al.* [57].)

Methods and tests for detecting *Clostridium difficile* and its toxins

Method	Protein detected	Advantages	Limitations
Stool culturing	Organism	Classic microbiology	Inconsistent; does not distinguish toxigenic and nontoxigenic isolates
Latex agglutination/ELISA	Glutamate dehydrogenase	Rapid and simple	Not extremely sensitive; does not distinguish toxigenic and nontoxigenic isolates
Tissue culture assay	Toxin B	Sensitive, specific, and adaptable	Requires 24–48 hrs; noncommercial versions are not standardized; tedious; often done incorrectly
ELISA	Toxin A Toxins A and B	Rapid, sensitive, and simple	Possibly higher number of indeterminate readings and unconfirmed positive results

ELISA—enzyme-linked immunosorbent assay.

FIGURE 3-83 Methods and tests for detecting *Clostridium difficile* or its toxins. Stool culture can reliably detect *C. difficile*, but a positive culture does not prove that enteric disease is due to this organism. Several tests are available for detecting *C. difficile* toxins. (*Adapted from* Lyerly and Wilkins [58].)

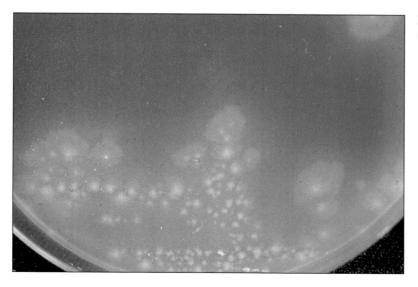

FIGURE 3-84 *Clostridium difficile* growing on selective CCFA (cycloserine, cefoxitin fructose agar).

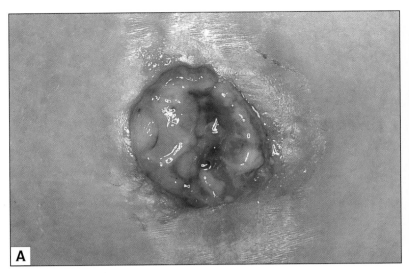

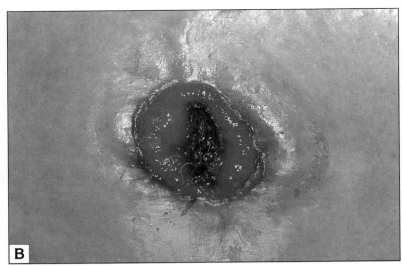

FIGURE 3-85 Antibiotic-related colitis due to *Clostridium difficile*. **A,** Endoscopic view of the colonic mucosa demonstrating pseudomembranous polypoid lesions in antibiotic-related colitis. A woman aged 36 years was evaluated for fever after extensive surgery for a pelvic malignancy. Postoperative antibiotics included ampicillin, clindamycin, and gentamicin. Examination demonstrated pseudomembranes covering her colostomy. Stool obtained through the colostomy demonstrated *C. difficile* toxin. **B,** Colostomy after 72 hours of oral vancomycin therapy showing complete resolution of pseudomembranes. (*Courtesy of* R. Fagerburg, MD.)

Treatment of *Clostridium difficile*–associated diarrhea and colitis

Nonspecific measures
  1. Discontinue or change implicated antimicrobial agent
  2. Supportive measures
  3. Avoid antiperistaltic agents
  4. Enteric precautions for hospitalized patients (until diarrhea resolves)
Antimicrobial treatment
  1. Metronizadole: 250 mg orally three times a day × 7–14 days
  2. Vancomycin: 125 mg orally four times a day × 7–14 days
  3. Metronidazole: 500 mg intravenously every 6 hrs (only until oral agents are tolerated)

FIGURE 3-86 Treatment of *Clostridium difficile*–associated diarrhea and colitis. Treatment of antibiotic-related colitis begins with discontinuation of the offending agent and any necessary supportive measures. The preferred oral agent is metronidazole because there is a *potential risk for vancomycin-resistant enterococcal colonization*, which may pose serious health risks. Intravenous metronidazole may be used if the patient cannot take oral agents, but oral therapy should be begun as soon as possible. Vancomycin may be given via catheter or enema in this setting. (*From* Bartlett [55].)

Management of relapses of *Clostridium difficile*–associated diarrhea or colitis

1. Metronidazole or vancomycin po × 10– days followed by cholestyramine (4 g tid) ± lactobacilli (as Lactinex, 1 g po qid) × 3 wks
2. Vancomycin, 125 mg po qid × 10–14 days, followed by vancomycin, 125 mg po every other day × 3 wks
3. Vancomycin, 125 mg po qid × 4–6 wks, then taper over 4–8 wks
4. Vancomycin, 125 mg po qid, plus rifampin, 600 mg po every day, × 10–14 days
5. Vancomycin, 125 mg po qid, plus *Saccharomyces boulardii* × 10–14 days, then *S. boulardii* for 4 wks
6. Intravenous gammaglobulin, 400 mg/kg every 3 wks (in children)
7. Rectal instillation of feces (50 g fresh stool from healthy donor in 500 mL of saline, delivered by enema)
8. Broth cultures of bacteria from healthy donors (stool culture using stool from healthy donor, 10 strains selected based on *in vitro* inhibition of *C. difficile* grown in broth culture 10^9/mL, 2 mL of each mixed in anaerobic glovebox with 180 mL saline and given by enema)
9. Lactobacillus G-G, 1 g po qid × 3 wks

po—orally; qid—four times a day; tid—three times a day.

FIGURE 3-87 Management of relapses of *Clostridium difficile*–associated diarrhea and colitis. Recurrences are seen in 10% to 20% of treated patients but usually respond promptly to metronidazole. As with primary treatment, metronidazole is given as the preferred oral agent, because of the *potential risk for vancomycin-resistant enterococcal colonization*. A few patients will have multiple relapses and tend to have a high rate of recurrences. Options for these patients include longer courses of antibiotic treatment, intermittent short-course antibiotics, and additional cholestyramine or rifampin instillation. *Lactobacillus* and *Saccharomyces* are under current study as possible inhibitors of *C. difficile* or its toxin in the gut. (*From* Bartlett [55].)

Bacterial Overgrowth Syndrome

Normal bacterial flora within the gastrointestinal tract				
	Stomach	**Jejunum**	**Ileum**	**Cecum**
Total bacterial counts*	10^{0-3}	10^{0-4}	10^{5-8}	10^{10-12}
Aerobes and facultative anaerobes	10^{0-3}	10^{0-4}	10^{2-5}	10^{2-9}
Anaerobes	0	0	10^{3-7}	10^{9-12}
*Per gram of contents.				

FIGURE 3-88 Normal bacterial flora within the gastrointestinal tract. Malabsorption in a patient may result from the overgrowth of bacteria within the small intestine, in which the overgrown flora successfully compete with the host for normal ingested nutrients. Normally, the upper portion of the small bowel has relatively few bacteria ($< 10^5$/mL), which are predominantly facultative gram-positive organisms (*eg*, diphtheroids, *Strepto-coccus*, and *Lactobacillus*). The organisms often implicated in overgrowth syndromes in the small bowel are aerobic enteric coliforms (Enterobacteriaceae) and anaerobic gram-negative fecal flora (*eg*, *Bacteroides* and *Clostridium*). (*From* Toskes and Donaldson [59].)

Clinical conditions associated with bacterial overgrowth

Gastric proliferation
  Hypo- or achlorhydria, especially when combined with motor or anatomic disturbances
  Sustained hypochlorhydria induced by omeprazole
Small intestinal stagnation
Anatomic
  Afferent loop of Billroth II partial gastrectomy
  Duodenal–jejunal diverticulosis
  Surgical blind loop (end-to-side anastomosis)
  Surgical recirculating loop (end-to-side anastomosis)
  Obstruction (stricture, adhesion, inflammation, neoplasm)
Motor
  Scleroderma
  Idiopathic intestinal pseudoobstruction
  Absent or disordered migrating motor complex
  Diabetic autonomic neuropathy
  Amyloidosis
  Hypothyroidism
Abnormal communication between proximal and distal gastrointestinal tract
  Gastrocolic or jejunocolic fistula
  Resection of diseased ileocecal valve
Miscellaneous
  Chronic pancreatitis
  Immunodeficiency syndromes
  Cirrhosis

FIGURE 3-89 Clinical conditions associated with small intestinal bacterial overgrowth. In the past, bacterial overgrowth was associated with gastrointestinal surgery, including Bilroth II gastrectomies and other anastomoses, which created intestinal blind loops. Now, it is appreciated that bacterial overgrowth may occur with no definable blind loop. Both normal intestinal motility and normal gastric acid secretion are important factors in preventing this condition. (*From* Toskes [60].)

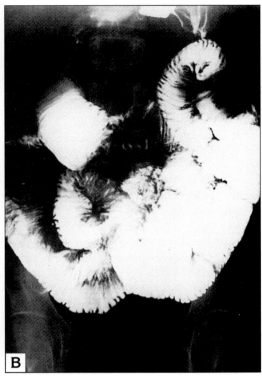

FIGURE 3-90 Barium enemas in bacterial overgrowth. **A,** Multiple duodenal and jejunal diverticuli in a patient with malabsorption due to bacterial overgrowth. Associated hypo- or achlorhydria are additional risk factors in the setting of anatomic abnormalities. **B,** Diffusely dilated small intestine in a patient with scleroderma and malabsorption due to bacterial overgrowth. Abnormalities in intestinal motility, often combined with decreased gastric acid secretion, resulting from conditions such as scleroderma, intestinal pseudoobstruction, or diabetic autonomic neuropathy predispose to bacterial growth. (Panel 90A *from* Toskes [61]; with permission. Panel 90B *from* Toskes [62]; with permission.)

Tests for small intestinal bacterial overgrowth

Test	Simplicity	Sensitivity	Specificity	Safety
Culture	–	+++	+++	++
Urinary indican	++	–	–	+++
Jejunal fatty acids	–	++	+++	++
Jejunal bile acids	–	++	+++	++
Fasting breath H_2	+++	–	++	+++
^{14}C-bile acid BT	+++	+	–	++
^{14}C-xylose BT	+++	+++	+++	++
Lactulose-H_2 BT	+++	+	+–++	+++
Glucose-H_2 BT	+++	++	+–++	+++

– —poor; + —fair; ++ —good; +++ —excellent.

BT—breath test.

FIGURE 3-91 Tests for small intestinal bacterial overgrowth. The excellent sensitivity and specificity of the 1-g ^{14}C-xylose breath test makes it the test of choice to screen for bacterial overgrowth. (*Adapted from* Toskes and Donaldson [59].)

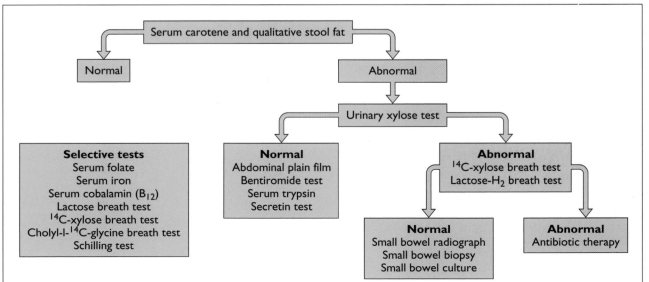

FIGURE 3-92 Algorithm for evaluation of malabsorption. Clinicians should have a low threshold for suspecting bacterial overgrowth as the cause of malabsorption in a given patient because the condition is rather common and readily treatable. Noninvasive tests, such as the breath tests, are preferable to the invasive intestinal biopsy. (*Adapted from* Toskes [63].)

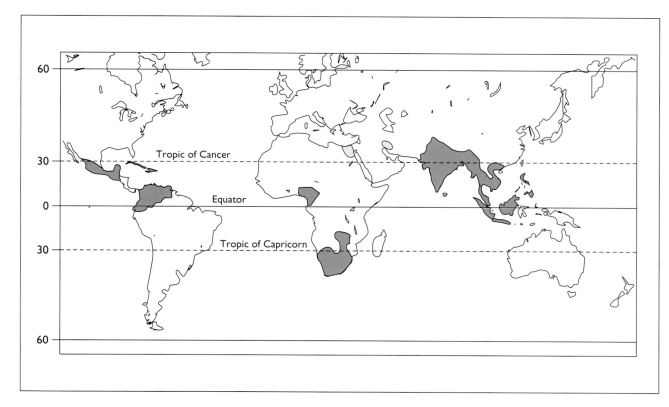

FIGURE 3-93 Geographic distribution of tropical sprue. Tropical sprue, also called *postinfectious tropical malabsorption*, is a syndrome of unclear etiology characterized by prolonged diarrheal illness and malabsorption affecting persons (mostly adults) in the tropics who have no other reason for malabsorption. An enteric infection is suspected, and the condition may involve bacterial overgrowth combined with other poorly understood factors. The *red areas* are endemic regions where sprue is known to occur. The *yellow areas* indicate where only subclinical malabsorption (tropical enteropathy) is present. (*Adapted from* Klipstein [64].)

Mycobacterial Enteritis

Location of tuberculous lesions of the gastrointestinal tract in 184 cases	
Location	**No. (%)**
Tongue	1 (0.6)
Stomach	1 (0.6)
Duodenum	7 (3.8)
Jejunum	39 (21.2)
Ileum	153 (83.2)
Cecum	160 (87.0)
Appendix	72 (39.1)
Colon	132 (71.7)
Sigmoid/rectum	30 (16.3)

FIGURE 3-94 Location of tuberculous lesions of the gastrointestinal tract in 184 cases. Many swallowed or ingested bacilli are destroyed in the acid environment of the stomach, but some pass through the mucosa where they are phagocytized and carried to Peyer's patches, lymphoid follicles in the mucosa, or mesenteric lymph nodes. The most common sites of infection are areas having the greatest concentration of lymphoid tissue and slowest transit time. Most infections occur in the ileocecal region, where 50% to 90% of lesions are observed, but multiple lesions are common. (*From* Horsburgh and Nelson [65].)

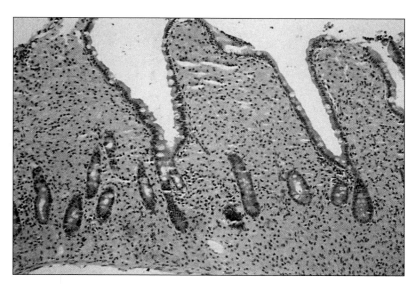

FIGURE 3-95 *Mycobacterium avium* complex enteritis. Histologic section of the intestine shows marked expansion of villi and submucosa by a diffuse infiltrate of foamy histiocytes. (Hematoxylin-eosin stain; × 100.) (*Courtesy of* C.M. Wilcox, MD; *from* Horsburgh and Nelson [65]; with permission.)

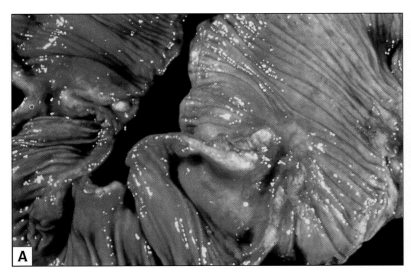
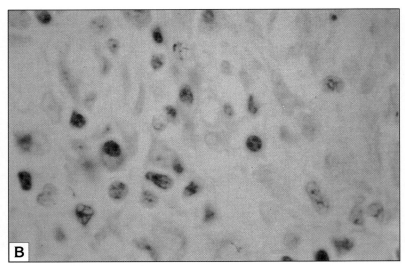

FIGURE 3-96 Tuberculous enteritis. **A,** Tuberculous enteritis in an ulcerative ileocolostomy specimen shows multiple ulcerations with focal thickening at the ileocecal junction. **B,** A Ziehl-Neelsen–stained section of intestinal wall shows loosely formed granuloma with numerous acid-fast bacilli. (× 600.) (*Courtesy of* Mount Sinai Hospital; *from* Horsburgh and Nelson [65]; with permission.)

AIDS-Associated Diarrhea

Possible causes of diarrhea in AIDS patients

Pathogen	Diarrhea, % (*n* = 181)	No diarrhea, % (*n* = 28)
Cytomegalovirus	12–45	15
Cryptosporidium	14–26	0
Microsporidium	7.5–33	0
Entamoeba histolytica	0–15	0
Giardia lamblia	2–15	5
Salmonella spp	0–15	0
Campylobacter spp	2–11	8
Shigella spp	5–10	0
Clostridium difficile toxin	6–7	0
Vibrio parahaemolyticus	4	0
Mycobacterium spp	2–25	0
Isospora belli	2–6	0
Blastocystis hominis	2–15	16
Candida albicans	6–53	24
Herpes simplex	5–18	40
Chlamydia trachomatis	11	13
Strongyloides	0–6	0
Intestinal spirochetes	11	11
One or more pathogens	55–86	39

FIGURE 3-97 Possible causes of diarrhea in patients with AIDS. One or more identifiable pathogens can usually be identified in 65% to 86% of patients with diarrhea and AIDS. This list is led by cytomegalovirus, followed by *Cryptosporidium*, *Microsporidium*, and numerous other potential pathogens, some of which may respond to specific therapy and should be sought. This diagnosis usually can be accomplished by noninvasive special methods. (*From* Guerrant and Bobak [24].)

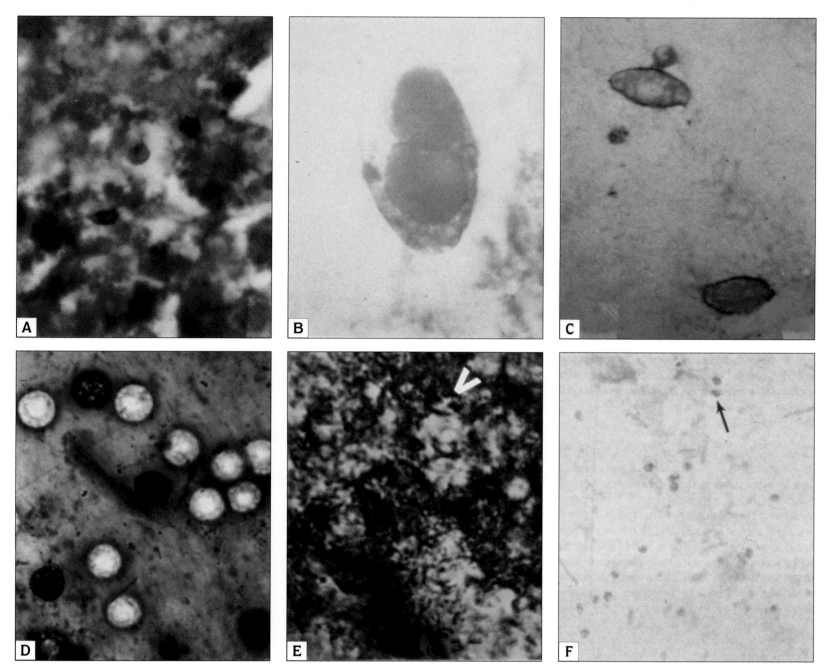

FIGURE 3-98 Causes of diarrhea in AIDS. Four different acid-fast organisms may cause diarrhea in AIDS patients. **A**, *Cryptosporidium* oocysts in a fecal specimen stained with modified Kinyoun acid-fast stain. **B**, *Isospora belli* oocyst with bilobed nuclei in a stool smear. **C**, *Cryptosporidium* and *I. belli* together in stool specimen. **D**, *Cyclospora* (also previously called cyanobacterium-like bodies) seen in a specimen of diarrhea. Some of the organisms are completely resistant to the acid-fast stain, showing only internal granularity. **E**, *Mycobacterium avium* complex (or *M. tuberculosis*). **F**, *Microsporidium*, which stains with a modified trichrome stain, also should be considered [66]. (*From* Guerrant and Bobak [6]; with permission.)

Whipple's Disease

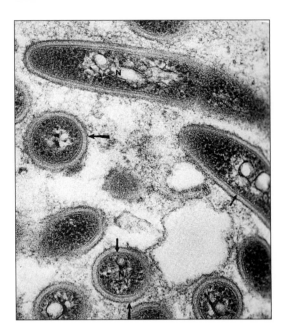

FIGURE 3-99 Electron micrograph showing the characteristic appearance of the Whipple bacillus, *Tropheryma whippelii.* Whipple's disease is a systemic bacterial illness that is characterized morphologically by an infiltrate of macrophages intensely stained by periodic acid–Schiff in virtually all organ systems. The greatest involvement occurs in the lamina propria of the small intestine and its lymphatic drainage, in the heart, and central nervous system. The patient is typically a white, middle-aged man with a history of intermittent arthralgias involving multiple joints over a period of years. The actual illness develops gradually, with diarrhea followed by steatorrhea, weight loss, and a progressive downhill course. (× 100,000.) (*From* Dobbins [67]; with permission.)

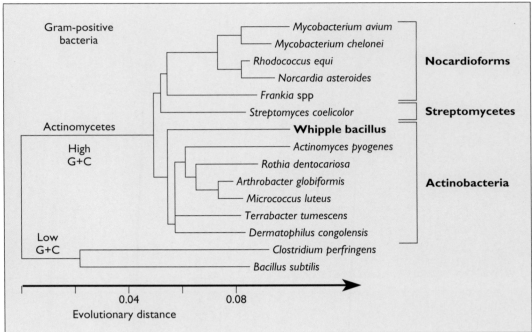

FIGURE 3-100 Phylogenic tree of the Whipple's disease bacillus. *Tropheryma whippelii* is a novel gram-positive actinomycetes that is not closely related to any other characterized organism. This phylogenic tree is based on comparative analysis of 16S ribosome RNA sequences; evolutionary distance (*abscissa*) is proportional to the sum of the horizontal line segments connecting any two organisms (point mutations per sequence position) [68]. (C—cytosine; G—guanosine.) (*Adapted from* Relman [69].)

FIGURE 3-101 Endoscopic appearance of Whipple's disease. Note the characteristic coarsening of the villous pattern and pale, yellow, shaggy mucosa. (*From* Silverstein and Tytgat [70]; with permission.)

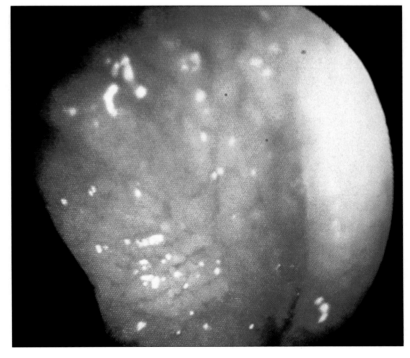

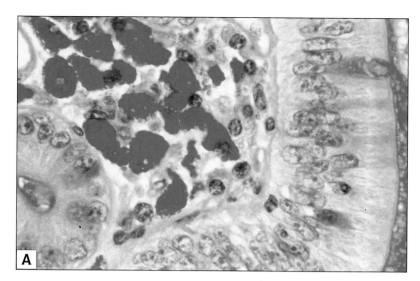

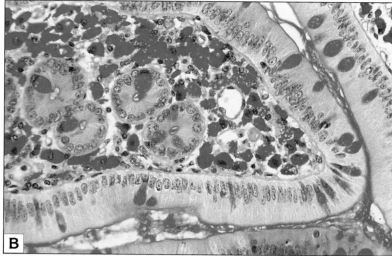

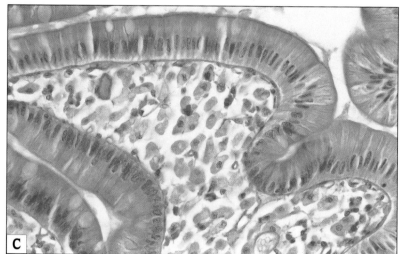

FIGURE 3-102 Typical histology of the duodenal mucosa in Whipple's disease. **A,** Numerous vacuolated macrophages crowd the lamina propria. (Hematoxylin-eosin stain; × 300.) **B,** On periodic acid–Schiff (PAS) stain, vacuoles of the macrophages within the lamina propria react intensely and appear purple, indicating the presence of glycoprotein (in this case, the bacterial cell wall). Epithelial globlet cells are also PAS-positive. (× 300.) **C,** Higher power view of PAS-stained tissue. (× 750.) (*Courtesy of* D.A. Relman, MD.)

Inflammatory Bowel Disease

Enteric pathogens causing inflammation resembling inflammatory bowel disease	
Resemble ulcerative colitis	**Resemble Crohn's disease**
Campylobacter jejuni	*Mycobacterium tuberculosis*
Salmonella spp	*Yersinia enterocolitica*
Shigella spp	Cytomegalovirus
Clostridium difficile	*Entamoeba histolytica*
Escherichia coli O157:H7	*Chlamydia trachomatis*
Aeromonas spp	*Histoplasma capsulatum*
Plesiomonas spp	*Actinomyces* spp
Vibrio noncholera spp	*Cryptococcus neoformans*
Neisseria gonorrhoeae	*Mycobacterium avium*
Legionella spp	complex
Treponema pallidum	
Herpes simplex virus type II	
Blastocystis hominis	

FIGURE 3-103 Enteric pathogens causing inflammation resembling inflammatory bowel disease (IBD). IBD refers to a group of chronic inflammatory disorders of unknown cause involving the gastrointestinal tract, which includes Crohn's disease and ulcerative colitis. Many enteric pathogens can produce an acute colitis resembling IBD, but fewer produce the chronic inflammation characteristic of IBD. (*From* Sartor [71].)

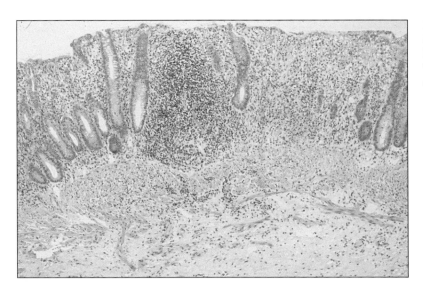

FIGURE 3-104 Colon biopsy specimen showing intraepithelial abscess suggestive of inflammatory bowel disease (IBD). IBD can be mimicked by *Campylobacter jejuni* (as seen in this patient) as well as by other treatable enteric infections, such as amebiasis, and other invasive causes of inflammatory diarrhea.

Pathogens associated with inflammatory bowel disease relapse

Viral	Bacterial	Parasitic
Cytomegalovirus	*Clostridium difficile*	*Entamoeba histolytica*
Rotavirus	*Salmonella* spp	*Giardia lamblia*
Norwalk agent	*Shigella* spp	*Blastocystis hominis*
Respiratory syncytial virus	*Campylobacter jejuni*	
Influenza A and B	*Yersinia* spp	
Parainfluenza	Enteropathogenic	
Rubella	*Escherichia coli*	
Epstein-Barr virus	*Aeromonas* spp	
Herpes simplex virus		
Adenovirus		

FIGURE 3-105 Pathogens associated with inflammatory bowel disease (IBD) relapse. Evidence indicates that enteric infections are associated with relapses of established ulcerative colitis and Crohn's disease, but whether these infections have a primary or secondary role in the inflammation associated with relapse remains unresolved. Between 4% and 32% of patients with an acute relapse of IBD are infected with enteric bacterial or protozoal pathogens, most commonly *Clostridium difficile*. (*From* Sartor [71].)

Infectious complications of inflammatory bowel disease

Abscess: Intra-abdominal, perianal, retroperitoneal abdominal wall, hepatic
Fistula: Enteroenteric, enterovesicular, enterocutaneous, perianal
Postoperative infection: Intra-abdominal abscesses, wound infections
Hematogenous infection: Sepsis, endocarditis
Opportunistic infection: Secondary to immunosuppressive therapy
Bacterial overgrowth: Small bowel, pouchitis

FIGURE 3-106 Infectious complications of inflammatory bowel disease (IBD). Extraluminal spread of ubiquitous enteric bacteria account for some of the frequent complications of IBD. These infectious complications are particularly prevalent in patients with Crohn's disease, in whom deep fissures, ulcers, increased luminal pressures due to stenoses, and chronic immunosuppressive therapy may enhance translocation of luminal bacteria. (*From* Sartor [71].)

REFERENCES

1. Guerrant RL: Lessons from diarrheal diseases: Demography to molecular pharmacology. *J Infect Dis* 1994, 169:1206–1218.

2. Behrens RH, Steffan R, Looke DFM: Travel medicine: I. Before departure. *Med J Austr* 1994, 160:144.

3. Antony MA, Brandt LJ, Klein RS, Bernstein LH: Infectious diarrhea in patients with AIDS. *Dig Dis Sci* 1988, 33:1141–1146.

4. Lima NL, Guerrant RL, Kaiser DL, *et al.*: A retrospective cohort study of nosocomial diarrhea as a risk factor for nosocomial infection. *J Infect Dis* 1990, 161:948–952.

5. Guerrant RL, Hughes JM, Lima NL, Crane JK: Diarrhea in developed and developing countries: Magnitude, special settings, and etiologies. *Rev Infect Dis* 1990, 12(suppl 1):S41–S50.

6. Guerrant RL, Bobak DA: Bacterial and protozoal gastroenteritis. *N Engl J Med* 1991, 325:327–340.

7. Dingle JH, Badger DG, Jordan SW Jr: *Illness in the Home: A Study of 25,000 Illnesses in a Group of Cleveland Families.* Cleveland: Case Western Reserve University Press; 1964.

8. Guerrant RL, Kirchoff LV, Shields DS, *et al.*: Prospective study of diarrheal illnesses in northeastern Brazil: Patterns of disease, nutritional impact, etiologies, and risk factors. *J Infect Dis* 1983, 148:986–997.

9. Guerrant RL: Twelve messages from diarrheal diseases for science and society. *Am J Trop Med Hyg* 1992, 47:28–35.

10. Guerrant RL, Schorling JB, McAuliff JF, de Souza MA: Diarrhea as a cause and effect of malnutrition: Diarrhea prevents catch-up growth and malnutrition increases diarrhea frequency and duration. *Am J Trop Med Hyg* 1992, 47:28–35.

11. Guerrant RL: Principles and syndromes of enteric infection. *In* Mandell GL, Bennett JE, Dolin R (eds.): *Principles and Practice of Infectious Diseases*, 4th ed. New York: Churchill Livingstone; 1995:945–962.

12. Guerrant RL: Intestinal adenyl-cyclase activity in canine cholera: Correlation with fluid accumulation. *J Infect Dis* 1972, 125:377–381.

13. Cho JH, Chang EB: Intracellular mediators and mechanisms of pathogen-induced alterations in intestinal electrolyte transport. *In* Blaser MJ, Ravdin JI, Smith PD, *et al.* (eds.): *Infections of the Gastrointestinal Tract.* New York: Raven Press; 1995:635–648.

14. Guerrant RL, Araujo V, Cooper WH, Lee AG: Measurement of fecal lactoferrin as a marker of fecal leukocytes and inflammatory enteritis. *J Clin Microbiol* 1992, 30:1238–1242.

15. Guerrant RL, Brush J, Ravdin JI, *et al.*: Interaction between *Entamoeba histolytica* and human polymorphonuclear leukocytes. *J Infect Dis* 1981, 143:83–93.

16. Young WH, *et al.*: Comparison of fecal lactoferrin latex agglutination assay and methylene blue microscopy for detection of fecal leukocytes in *Clostridium difficile*-associated disease. *J Clin Microbiol* 1994, 32:1360–1361.

17. Guerrant RL: Introduction and overview: Microbial toxins and diarrheal disease. *Ciba Found Symp* 1984, 112.

18. Koplan JP, Fineberg HV, Ferraro MJB, Rosenberg ML: Value of stool cultures. *Lancet* 1980, 2:413–416.

19. Guerrant RL, *et al.*: A cost effective and effective diagnosis and management of acute infectious diarrhea. *Bull NY Acad Sci* 1987, 63:484–499.

20. Guerrant RL, Shields DS, Thorson SM, *et al.*: Evaluation and diagnosis of acute infectious diarrhea. *Am J Med* 1985, 78:91–98.

21. Thorson SM, *et al.*: Value of methylene blue examination, darkfield microscopy, and carbol-fuchsin Gram stain in the detection of *Campylobacter enteritis. J Pediatr* 1985, 106:941–943.

22. Water with sugar and salt [editorial]. *Lancet* 1978, 2:300–301.

23. Bandres JC, DuPont HL: Approach to the patient with diarrhea. *In* Gorbach SL, Bartlett JG, Blacklow NR (eds.): *Infectious Diseases.* Philadelphia: W.B. Saunders; 1992: 574.

24. Guerrant RL, Bobak DA: Nausea, vomiting, and noninflammatory diarrhea. *In* Mandell GL, Bennett JE, Dolin R (eds.): *Principles and Practice of Infectious Diseases*, 4th ed. New York: Churchill Livingstone; 1995:965–978.

25. DuPont HL: Traveler's diarrhea. *In* Blaser MJ, Ravdin JI, Smith PD, *et al.* (eds.): *Infections of the Gastrointestinal Tract.* New York: Raven Press; 1995:302.

26. Morris JG Jr: Noncholera *Vibrio* species. *In* Blaser MJ, Ravdin JI, Smith PD, *et al.* (eds.): *Infections of the Gastrointestinal Tract.* New York: Raven Press; 1995:672.

27. Butterton JR, Calderwood SB: *Vibrio cholerae* O1. *In* Blaser MJ, Ravdin JI, Smith PD, *et al.* (eds.): *Infections of the Gastrointestinal Tract.* New York: Raven Press; 1995:652.

28. Greenough WB III: *Vibrio cholerae* and cholera. *In* Mandell GL, Bennett JE, Dolin R (eds.): *Principles and Practice of Infectious Diseases*, 4th ed. New York: Churchill Livingstone; 1995:1935.

29. Swerdlow DL, Ries AA: Cholera in the Americas. *JAMA* 1992, 267:1495–1499.

30. Guerrant RL, Thielman NM: Types of *Escherichia coli* enteropathogens. *In* Blaser MJ, Ravdin JI, Smith PD, *et al.* (eds.): *Infections of the Gastrointestinal Tract.* New York: Raven Press; 1995:688.

31. Guerrant RL, Brunton LL, Schnaitman TC, *et al.*: Cyclic adenosine monophosphate and alteration of Chinese hamster ovary cell morphology: A rapid, sensitive in vitro assay for the enterotoxins of *Vibrio cholerae* and *Escherichia coli. Infect Immun* 1974, 10:320–327.

32. Eisenstein BI, Jones GW: The spectrum of infectious and pathogenic mechanisms of *Escherichia coli. Adv Intern Med* 1988, 33:231–252.

33. Steffen R: Epidemiologic studies of traveler's diarrhea, severe gastrointestinal infections, and cholera. *Ref Infect Dis* 1986, 8(suppl 2):122–130.

34. Steffen R, Richernbach M, Wilhelm U, *et al.*: Health problems after travel to developing countries. *J Infect Dis* 1987, 156:84–91.

35. Kean BH, Schaeffner W, Brennan RW: The diarrhea of travelers: V. Prophylaxis with phthalylsulfathiazole and neomycin sulphate. *JAMA* 1962, 180:367–371.

36. Merson MH, Morris GK, Sack DA, *et al.*: Travelers' diarrhea in Mexico, a prospective study of physicians and family members attending a congress. *N Engl J Med* 1976, 294:1299.

37. Sack DA, Kaminsky DC, Sack RB, *et al.*: Enterotoxigenic *Escherichia coli* diarrhea of travelers: A prospective study of American Peace Corps volunteers. *Johns Hopkins Med J* 1977, 141:63.

38. Guerrant RL, Rouse JD, Hughes JM: Turista among members of the Yale Glee Club in Latin America. *Am J Trop Med Hyg* 1980, 29:895.

39. Taylor DN, Echeverria P: Etiology and epidemiology of traveler's diarrhea in Asia. *Rev Infect Dis* 1986, 8(suppl 2):131–135.

40. Griffin PM: *Escherichia coli* O157:H7 and other enterohemorrhagic *Escherichia coli. In* Blaser MJ, Ravdin JI, Smith PD, *et al.* (eds.): *Infections of the Gastrointestinal Tract.* New York: Raven Press; 1995:741.

41. Finegold SM, Baron EJ: *Bailey and Scott's Diagnostic Microbiology*, 7th ed. St. Louis: Mosby; 1986.

42. DuPont HL: Shigella species (bacillary dysentery). *In* Mandell GL, Bennett JE, Dolin R (eds.): *Principles and Practice of Infectious Diseases*, 4th ed. New York: Churchill Livingstone; 1995:2037.

43. Blaser MJ: *Campylobacter* and related species. *In* Mandell GL, Bennett JE, Dolin R (eds.): *Principles and Practice of Infectious Diseases*, 4th ed. New York: Churchill Livingstone; 1995:1949.

44. Blaser MJ: *Campylobacter jejuni. In* Blaser MJ, Ravdin JI, Smith PD, *et al.* (eds.): *Infections of the Gastrointestinal Tract.* New York: Raven Press; 1995:830.

45. Skirrow MB: *Campylobacter* and *Helicobacter*. *In* Greenwood D, Slack R, Peutherer J (eds.): *Medical Microbiology: A Guide to Microbial Infections: Pathogenesis, Immunity, Laboratory Diagnosis and Control*. Edinburgh: Churchill Livingstone; 1992:351–354.

46. Goldberg MB, Rubin RH: Nontyphoidal *Salmonella* infection. *In* Gorbach SL, Bartlett JG, Blacklow NR (eds.): *Infectious Diseases*. Philadelphia: W.B. Saunders; 1992:582.

47. Miller SI, Hohmann EL, Pegues DA: *Salmonella* (including *Salmonella typhi*). *In* Mandell GL, Bennett JE, Dolin R (eds.): *Principles and Practice of Infectious Diseases*, 4th ed. New York: Churchill Livingstone; 1995:201.

48. Hargrett-Bean NT, Pabin AT, Tauxe RV: Salmonella isolates from humans in the United States, 1984–1986. *MMWR* 1988, 37(SS-2):28.

49. Pegues DA, Hohmann EL, Miller SI: *Salmonella* including *S. typhi*. *In* Blaser MJ, Ravdin JI, Smith PD, *et al.* (eds.): *Infections of the Gastrointestinal Tract*. New York: Raven Press; 1995:791.

50. Goldberg MB, Miller SI, Rubin RH: Microbiologic aspects of salmonellae. *In* Gorbach SL, Bartlett JG, Blacklow NR (eds.): *Infectious Diseases*. Philadelphia: W.B. Saunders; 1992:1482.

51. Cover TL: *Yersinia enterocolitica* and *Yersinia pseudotuberculosis*. *In* Blaser MJ, Ravdin JI, Smith PD, *et al.* (eds.): *Infections of the Gastrointestinal Tract*. New York: Raven Press; 1995:812.

52. Tauxe RV, Hughes JM: Food-borne disease. *In* Mandell GL, Bennett JE, Dolin R (eds.): *Principles and Practice of Infectious Diseases*, 4th ed. New York: Churchill Livingstone; 1995:1012.

53. Snydman DR, Gorbach SL: Bacterial food poisoning (*Bacillus cereus, Clostridium perfringens, Vibrio parahemolyticus, Staphylococcus aureus, Yersinia enterocolitica*). *In* Evans AS, Feldman HA (eds.): *Bacterial Infections in Humans*. New York: Plenum; 1982:87–113.

54. Hatheway CL: *Clostridium botulinum*. *In* Gorbach SL, Bartlett JG, Blacklow NR (eds.): *Infectious Diseases*. Philadelphia: W.B. Saunders; 1992:1585.

55. Bartlett JG: Antibiotic-associated diarrhea. *In* Blaser MJ, Ravdin JI, Smith PD, *et al.* (eds.): *Infections of the Gastrointestinal Tract*. New York: Raven Press; 1995:896.

56. Kelly CP, LaMont JT: Treatment of *Clostridium difficile* diarrhea and colitis. *In* Wolfe MW (ed.): *Gastrointestinal Pharmacology*. Philadelphia: W.B. Saunders; 1993:199–212.

57. Kelly CP, Pothoulakis C, LaMont JT: *Clostridium difficile* colitis. *N Engl J Med* 1994, 330:257–262.

58. Lyerly DM, Wilkins TD: *Clostridium difficile*. *In* Blaser MJ, Ravdin JI, Smith PD, *et al.* (eds.): *Infections of the Gastrointestinal Tract*. New York: Raven Press; 1995:881.

59. Toskes PP, Donaldson R: Enteric bacterial flora and bacterial overgrowth syndrome. *In* Sleisenger MH, Fortran JS (eds.): *Gastrointestinal Disease*, 5th ed. Philadelphia: W.B. Saunders; 1995:1106–1118.

60. Toskes PP: Small intestine bacterial overgrowth, including blind loop syndrome. *In* Blaser MJ, Ravdin JI, Smith PD, *et al.* (eds.): *Infections of the Gastrointestinal Tract*. New York: Raven Press; 1995:343.

61. Toskes PP: Bacterial overgrowth of the gastrointestinal tract. *Adv Intern Med* 1993, 38:387–407.

62. Toskes PP: Bacterial overgrowth syndromes. *In* Haubrich WS, Schaffner F, Berk JE (eds.): *Bockus Gastroenterology*, 5th ed. Philadelphia: W.B. Saunders; 1995:1174–1182.

63. Toskes JP: Malabsorption. *In* Wyngaarden JB, Smith L, Bennett J (eds.): *Cecil Textbook of Medicine*, 19th ed. Philadelphia: W.B. Saunders; 1992:687–699.

64. Klipstein FA: Tropical sprue. *In* Bockus HL (ed.): *Gastroenterology*, 3rd ed. Philadelphia: W.B. Saunders; 1976:285–305.

65. Horsburgh CR Jr, Nelson AM: Mycobacterial disease of the gastrointestinal tract. *In* Blaser MJ, Ravdin JI, Smith PD, *et al.* (eds.): *Infections of the Gastrointestinal Tract*. New York: Raven Press; 1995:939.

66. Weber, *et al.*: Improved light microscopic detection of microsporidia spores in stool and duodenal aspirates. *N Engl J Med* 1992, 326:161–166.

67. Dobbins WO III: Whipple's disease. *In* Mandell GL, Bennett JE, Dolin R (eds.): *Principles and Practice of Infectious Diseases*, 4th ed. New York: Churchill Livingstone; 1995:1030.

68. Wilson KH, Blitchington R, Frothingham R, Wilson JA: Phylogeny of the Whipple's disease–associated bacterium. *Lancet* 1991, 338:474–475.

69. Relman DA: Whipple's disease. *In* Blaser MJ, Ravdin JI, Smith PD, *et al.* (eds.): *Infections of the Gastrointestinal Tract*. New York: Raven Press; 1995:922.

70. Silverstein FE, Tytgat GNJ: *Atlas of Gastrointestinal Endoscopy*. Philadelphia: W.B. Saunders; 1987.

71. Sartor RB: Microbial agents in the pathogenesis, differential diagnosis, and complications of inflammatory bowel disease. *In* Blaser MJ, Ravdin JI, Smith PD *et al.* (eds.): *Infections of the Gastrointestinal Tract*. New York: Raven Press; 1995:441.

SELECTED BIBLIOGRAPHY

Blaser MJ, Ravdin JI, Smith PD, *et al.* (eds.): *Infections of the Gastrointestinal Tract*. New York: Raven Press; 1995.

Guerrant RL: Lessons from diarrheal diseases: Demography to molecular pharmacology. *J Infect Dis* 1994, 169:1206–1218.

Guerrant RL: Principles and syndromes of enteric infection. *In* Mandell GL, Bennett JE, Dolin R (eds.): *Principles and Practice of Infectious Diseases*, 4th ed. New York: Churchill Livingstone; 1995:947.

Guerrant RL, Bobak DA: Bacterial and protozoal gastroenteritis. *N Engl J Med* 1991, 325:327–340.

CHAPTER 4

Helicobacter pylori Infection

David Y. Graham
Robert M. Genta

NORMAL GASTRIC HISTOLOGY

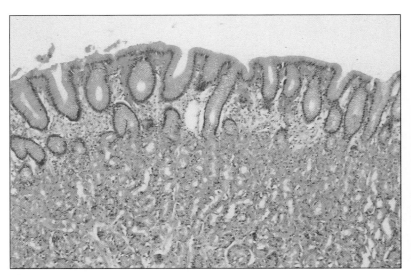

FIGURE 4-1 Low-power photomicrograph of normal gastric corpus. The gastric foveolae are much shorter than those in the antrum, reaching less than one fifth of the mucosal depth. The oxyntic glands are packed closely together. No lymphoid follicles are present.

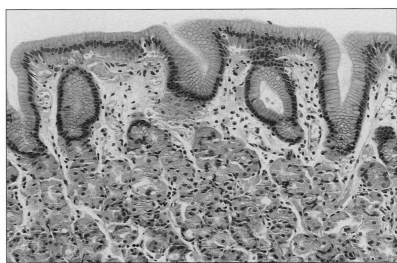

FIGURE 4-2 High-power photomicrograph of normal gastric corpus. The surface epithelium is similar to that of the antrum. Only a thin rim of lamina propria containing scattered plasma cells, lymphocytes, and eosinophils separates the surface epithelium from the underlying oxyntic glands.

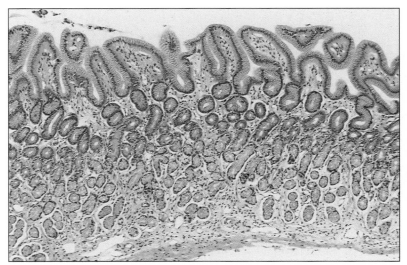

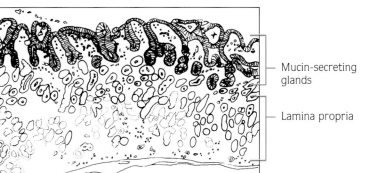

— Mucin-secreting glands

— Lamina propria

FIGURE 4-3 Low-power photomicrograph of normal gastric antrum. The foveolae are deep, and the surface may take a villous appearance. The mucin-secreting glands occupy the lower half of the mucosa. The lamina propria contains scattered plasma cells, lymphocytes, and rare eosinophils, but no neutrophils. Lymphoid follicles are not a feature of the normal antrum, but basally located aggregates of lymphocytes without germinal centers may be present.

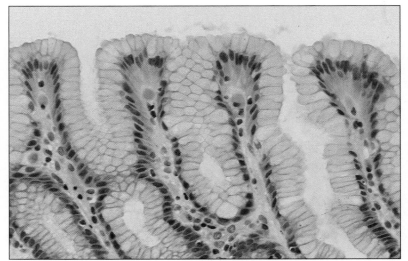

FIGURE 4-4 High-power photomicrograph of normal gastric antrum. The mucinous surface cells are aligned in an orderly arrangement along the basement membrane. The nuclei are small and basally located. An elongated mucin droplet, which stains positive with periodic acid–Schiff, is present in each cell.

SPECTRUM OF HISTOLOGIC INJURY IN *HELICOBACTER PYLORI* INFECTION

Histologic changes in the gastric mucosa induced by *Helicobacter pylori*

Acute and chronic inflammation
Surface epithelial damage
Lymphoid follicles
Mucosal atrophy ± intestinal metaplasia

FIGURE 4-5 Histopathologic changes in the gastric mucosa induced by *Helicobacter pylori* infection. The spectrum of histopathologic changes in the gastric mucosa always includes an acute and chronic inflammatory cellular response. Damage to the surface epithelium is typically seen as an alteration in the mucin content of the surface cells. The normal stomach is virtually devoid of lymphoid cells, but with infection, the chronic inflammatory cell response is associated with the development of lymphoid follicles, which may remain after cure of the infection. The most common pattern of histopathologic change seen in the United States is chronic gastritis without atrophy. With long-standing disease, a proportion of patients develop atrophic gastritis, often with intestinal metaplasia. Histologic evaluation of an *H. pylori*–infected gastric mucosa should reveal the presence of the organisms as well as inflammation and surface mucosal epithelial damage. The definitive diagnostic feature is the presence of *H. pylori* organisms.

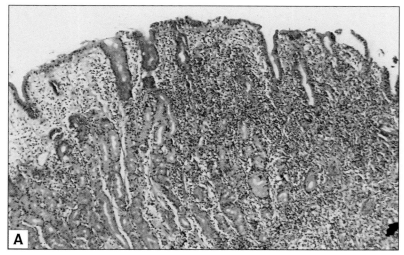

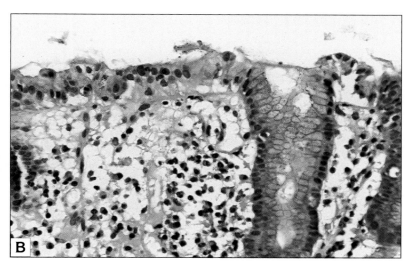

FIGURE 4-6 Histopathologic appearance of gastric mucosa in acute *Helicobacter pylori* infection. **A**, Dense patches of a mixed inflammatory infiltrate are scattered in the oxyntic mucosa. No bacteria are visible in these locations. **B**, On higher-power examination of the adjacent edematous and less-inflamed areas (on the left side of *panel 6A*), there are rare *H. pylori* closely attached to the epithelium and in the upper portion of a foveola.

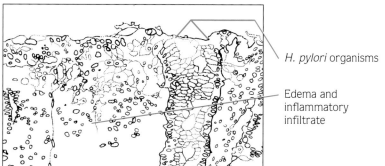

H. pylori organisms

Edema and inflammatory infiltrate

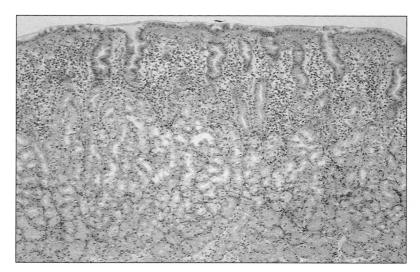

FIGURE 4-7 Classic chronic superficial gastritis. A dense band of lymphocytes and plasma cells separates the surface epithelium from the underlying oxyntic mucosa. Rare neutrophils infiltrate the lamina propria and the foveolar epithelium. This is the most common appearance of the gastric corpus with chronic *Helicobacter pylori* gastritis and represents the classic chronic superficial gastritis of the Whitehead classification.

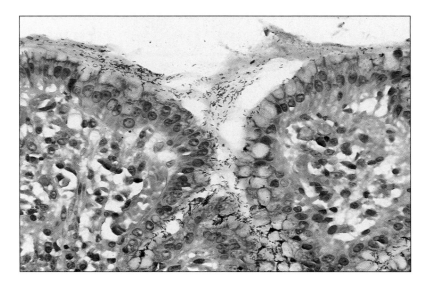

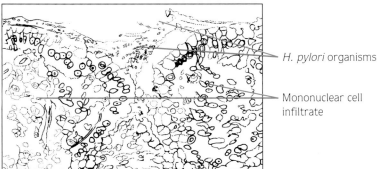

H. pylori organisms

Mononuclear cell infiltrate

FIGURE 4-8 Heavy *Helicobacter pylori* infection of the gastric antrum. Large numbers of bacteria are seen within the mucus and foveolae. The surface epithelium has lost its orderly arrangement, and the mucin component of the superficial cells is greatly reduced. The inflammatory infiltrate in the lamina propria is predominantly mononuclear.

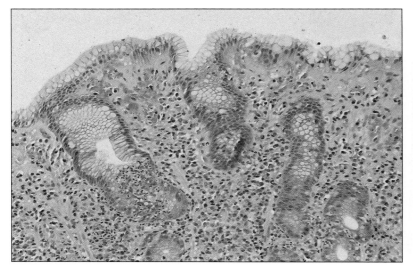

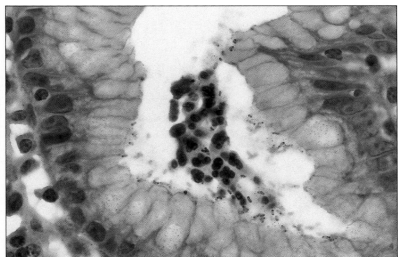

FIGURE 4-9 Predominantly neutrophilic inflammation in gastric pits infected with *Helicobacter pylori*. There is moderate edema of the superficial portion of the lamina propria.

FIGURE 4-10 *Helicobacter pylori* attached to the mucin cells and within the cytoplasm of neutrophils lying in the foveolar space.

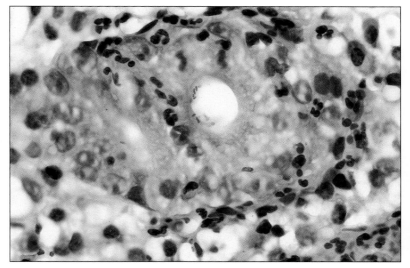

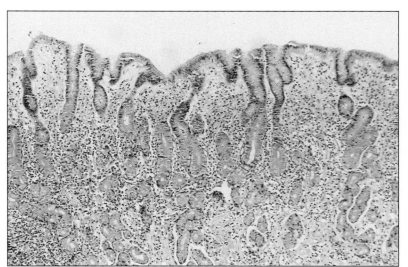

FIGURE 4-11 Antral gland with severe neutrophilic infiltration and few *Helicobacter pylori* within its lumen. Contrary to widespread belief, there is often little relationship between the location and intensity of the inflammatory infiltrate and the location and density of *H. pylori*.

FIGURE 4-12 Gastric atrophy. Only a few glands (*right*) show intestinal metaplasia; most of the other glands are long, tortuous, and sparse. There is little or no inflammatory infiltrate in the lamina propria. This condition is believed to be one of the late stages of *Helicobacter pylori* gastritis.

EPIDEMIOLOGY OF *HELICOBACTER PYLORI* INFECTION

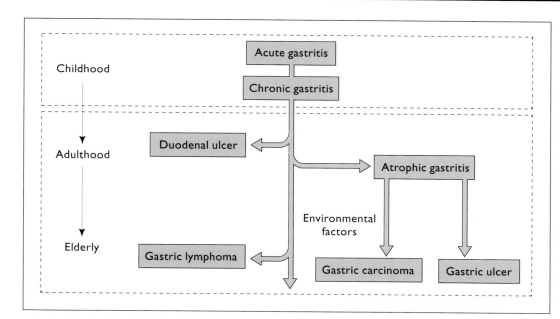

FIGURE 4-13 Time course of *Helicobacter pylori* infection and resultant diseases. *H. pylori* infection is typically acquired in childhood, and the pattern of acute and chronic inflammation is maintained throughout life. One in six infected persons develops peptic ulcer, with duodenal ulcer appearing at an earlier average age than gastric ulcer. Gastric adenocarcinoma is usually a very late event and may require environmental factors to bring about the transition from chronic atrophic gastritis to one with advanced stages of intestinal metaplasia. Gastric lymphoma can occur in any of the histologic types and is probably a chance occurrence related to the chronic stimulation of the chronic inflammatory reaction to the infection; in some cases, remission has been achieved with cure of the *H. pylori* infection. (*Adapted from* Graham [1].)

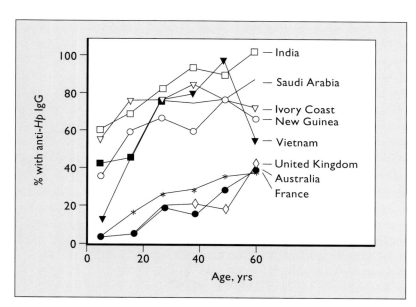

FIGURE 4-14 Prevalence of *Helicobacter pylori* (*Hp*) infection in different countries. In developed and developing countries, *H. pylori* is largely a childhood-acquired disease. In developing countries, 80% or more of the population is infected by age 20 years. In developed countries, there is an increased frequency with age, but this likely represents a cohort phenomenon, as the actual frequency of infection in any age has been falling. The major difference between populations in developed and developing nations is the rate of acquisition in childhood, which ranges from 0.5% to 5% per year in childhood, respectively for the two areas. In both developed and developing countries, the rate of acquisition in adults is lower, probably in the range of 0.5%. (*Adapted from* Graham *et al.* [2].)

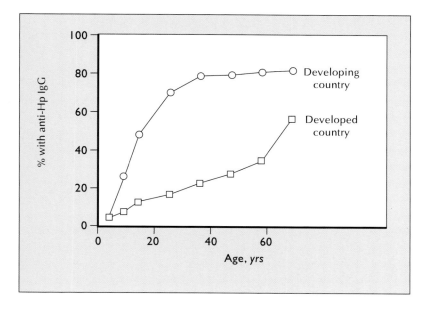

FIGURE 4-15 Differing prevalence of *Helicobacter pylori* (*Hp*) infection in developed versus developing countries. When prevalence rates for *H. pylori* infection in the different regions of the world are averaged, it shows the striking difference between developed and developing countries. This different epidemiologic pattern of *H. pylori* infection is due to the difference in rate of acquisition of the infection in childhood. (*Adapted from* Graham [1].)

Epidemiologic associations between gastritis and *Helicobacter pylori* infection

Factor	Gastritis	*H. pylori*
Age	✔	✔
Lower socioeconomic class	✔	✔
Duodenal ulcer	✔	✔
Gastric ulcer	✔	✔
Gastric cancer	✔	✔
Pernicious anemia	✔	—
Gender	—	—
Smoking or alcohol use	—	—
NSAID use	—	—

NSAID—nonsteroidal anti-inflammatory drug.

FIGURE 4-16 Comparison of epidemiologic associations in gastritis and *Helicobacter pylori* infection. The epidemiologic associations of gastritis and *H. pylori* infection are identical, with the exception of the lack of a clear role for *H. pylori* in pernicious anemia. By 1973, the epidemiology of gastritis had been fairly well defined, and the identification of *H. pylori* as a cause of gastritis allowed rapid progress and confirmed that most previous associations with gastritis could be transferred to *H. pylori*.

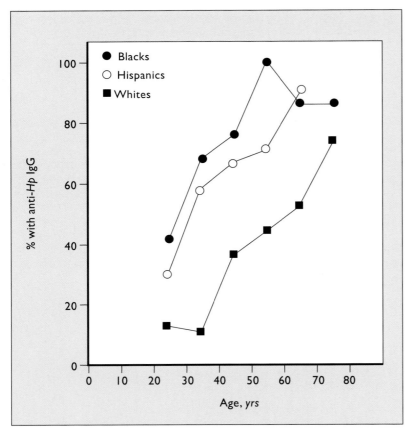

FIGURE 4-17 Prevalence of *Helicobacter pylori* (*Hp*) infection in the United States, by race (asymptomatic persons). In the United States, the prevalence of *H. pylori* infection in blacks and Hispanics is significantly greater than in age- and socioeconomic-status-matched whites. The difference in prevalence can be explained by the differences in socioeconomic status during childhood, with their related risks for acquisition of infection [3].

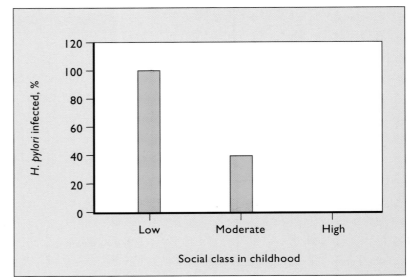

FIGURE 4-18 Influence of socioeconomic status in childhood on prevalence of *Helicobacter pylori* infection in black and Hispanic adults. A study examined the prevalence of *H. pylori* infection in black and Hispanic adults of current high socioeconomic status according to the socioeconomic class of the individuals' families during childhood. Socioeconomic class in childhood was an important variable for predicting current *H. pylori* status. For example, if a person has a high socioeconomic status today but had low socioeconomic status in childhood, the frequency of infection was 100% [4].

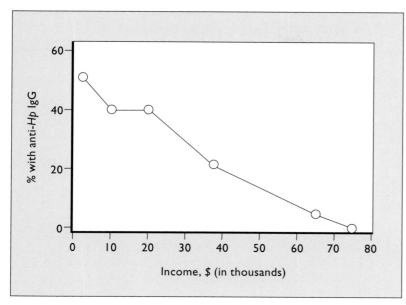

FIGURE 4-19 Effect of socioeconomic class on prevalence of *Helicobacter pylori* (*Hp*) infection in asymptomatic white Americans. Persons of high socioeconomic class are unlikely to be infected unless they were of low socioeconomic status in childhood (or were gastroenterologists who performed upper gastrointestinal endoscopy without the use of gloves) [5].

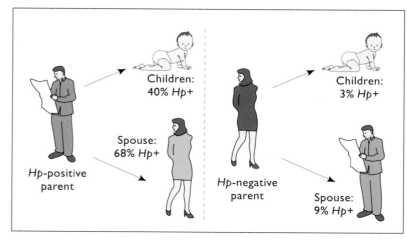

FIGURE 4-20 Transmission of *Helicobacter pylori* (*Hp*) infection in asymptomatic families. It has been shown repeatedly that *H. pylori* infection is transmitted within families with children. These studies have shown that if one parent is positive, either the mother or father, the frequency of infection of spouses and children is high. In contrast, if the parent is negative, infections in the spouse and children are uncommon [6].

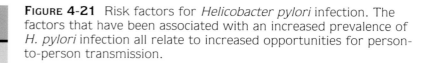

Risk factors for *Helicobacter pylori* infection

Low socioeconomic status
Birth in a developing country
Crowded living conditions
Sharing a bed as a child
Absence of hot water tap in home
Poor sanitary conditions

FIGURE 4-21 Risk factors for *Helicobacter pylori* infection. The factors that have been associated with an increased prevalence of *H. pylori* infection all relate to increased opportunities for person-to-person transmission.

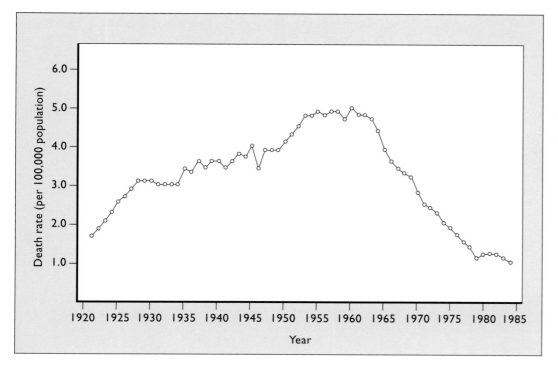

FIGURE 4-22 Duodenal ulcer mortality for men in the United States between 1920 and 1985. The rapid increase and then fall in both prevalence and mortality from duodenal ulcer suggests the involvement of an environmental factor. That factor is now known to be *Helicobacter pylori* infection. It is unclear whether other factors such as changes in diet or changes in prevalence of ulcerogenic strains also may be responsible in part. (*Adapted from* Kurata [7].)

DETECTION OF *HELICOBACTER PYLORI* INFECTION

Diagnostic tests for *Helicobacter pylori* infection

Noninvasive (indirect)
  Urea breath test
  IgG antibody detection
Invasive
  Rapid urease tests (CLOtest)
  Histology
  Culture

FIGURE 4-23 Diagnostic tests for *Helicobacter pylori* infection. Diagnostic methods for *H. pylori* infection basically can be grouped into those that do not require endoscopy (noninvasive) and those that do (invasive). The tests have in common high specificity and sensitivity but differ in cost and in usefulness for evaluating whether the infection has been cured. Invasive tests require gastric biopsy and therefore are more expensive. IgM and IgA serum antibodies have proved to be unreliable for initial diagnosis or follow-up, and the titers of IgG antibodies fall too slowly to be of use in confirming that infection has been cured. Hematoxylin-eosin staining of gastric mucosal biopsy specimens has a high rate of false-negative results, and thus special stains are recommended for the histologic evaluation of *H. pylori* status. Invasive tests provide definitive information about the presence or absence of the infection.

**When to test for *Helicobacter pylori*
(serology, breath test, both)**

History of ulcer or ulcer complication
Family history of gastric cancer in first-degree relative
Dyspepsia and suspect ulcer

FIGURE 4-24 Indications to test for *Helicobacter pylori* infection. The main reason to test for *H. pylori* infection is to identify persons who should be treated. Possibilities include patients with a past history of ulcer or an ulcer complication. Also, testing is indicated in persons with a family history of gastric cancer in a first-degree relative, because the presence of cancer in a first-degree relative increases the likelihood of cancer at least threefold. Finally, one might treat dyspeptic patients when an ulcer is suspected.

Use of diagnostic tests for *Helicobacter pylori* detection

Clinical setting	Diagnostic test
New, recurrent, or history of PUD	Serology/urea breath test
	Endoscopy with histology
Complicated PUD	Wait ≥ 4 wks, then endoscopy
Follow-up	(histology) or urea breath test
Patient undergoing endoscopy	Histology ± rapid urease test
Compliant patient with several treatment failures	Endoscopy, histology, culture, and susceptibility testing

PUD—peptic ulcer disease.

FIGURE 4-25 Approach to diagnostic tests in management of patients with suspected *Helicobacter pylori* infection. One approach to using the diagnostic tests for evaluation and follow-up of patients with suspected or proven *H. pylori* infection is shown. It is not necessary to reconfirm the presence of peptic ulcer disease in those with ulcer documented in the past. Endoscopy is generally indicated in those with complicated ulcer disease in order to plan the best strategy of management and to deal directly with the complication (*eg*, endoscopic hemostasis). To prevent recurrent symptoms, complications, need for visits, tests, and medications, the effect of therapy should be confirmed. The urea breath test is preferred, because it is noninvasive and significantly less expensive than endoscopy. In cases in which it has been difficult to obtain cure, endoscopy with culture and sensitivity testing is recommended.

When to determine *Helicobacter pylori* status

Before therapy
  Establish diagnosis to avoid treatment complications
    in uninfected persons
After treatment
  All persons with ulcers, especially those with ulcer
    complications
  If symptoms do not respond or recur

FIGURE 4-26 When to determine *Helicobacter pylori* status. In general, the potential side effects of antibiotics probably outweigh their benefits in treating patients who do not have an infection. Thus, prior to therapy, it is important to establish a diagnosis of infection in order to avoid treatment complications in the uninfected. Also, it is probably best to determine *H. pylori* status after therapy in all patients, but this step is definitely indicated in all those who have had ulcer complications and those in whom symptoms recur. All too frequently, patients are treated repeatedly, although their infection was cured with the first treatment.

Antibody tests for initial diagnosis of *Helicobacter pylori* infection

Used for initial diagnosis
Serum IgG antibody tests are sensitive, specific, and cost-effective (FDA-approved)
IgA and IgM tests are unapproved and poor
IgG titers decline slowly, limiting their use for follow-up
Saliva and urine tests are experimental

FDA—Food and Drug Administration.

FIGURE 4-27 Antibody tests for diagnosis of *Helicobacter pylori* infection. Antibody tests are particularly useful for the initial diagnosis of *H. pylori* infection. A number of Food and Drug Administration–approved tests are currently available. All of the tests are for serum IgG and are sensitive, specific, and cost-effective. There are no currently approved tests for IgA or IgM; both IgM and IgA have proved to be relatively poor predictors of the presence or absence of *H. pylori* infection and cannot be recommended. Saliva and urine tests for *H. pylori* are in development but are experimental, and overall their sensitivity and specificity have proved to be inferior to those of the serum IgG test.

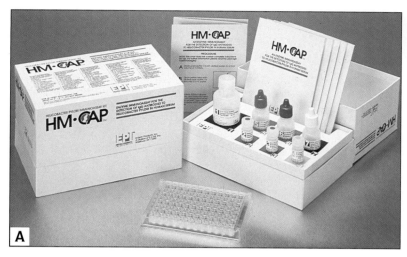

FIGURE 4-28 IgG antibody tests. **A** and **B**, IgG antibody tests are both sensitive and specific and convenient methods for the initial diagnosis of *Helicobacter pylori* infection. Examples of two commercially available tests are shown. Two rapid office-based tests are currently available (others are in development) and provide accurate results. Rapid tests that use whole blood are in development. Laboratory-based serologic tests also are based on detection of IgG antibody. Some laboratories offer IgA and IgM antibody tests, but these have poor sensitivity and specificity. Serologic tests have proved to be excellent for identifying the presence of *H. pylori* infection, but as the titer falls very slowly, they have not proved to be useful for follow-up of successful therapy. (*From* Graham [1]; with permission.)

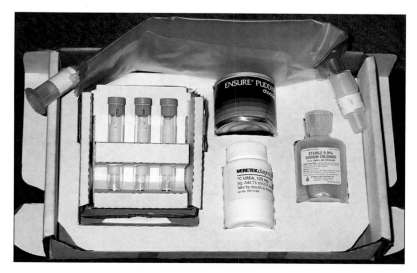

FIGURE 4-29 Components of the ^{13}C-urea breath test. After ingestion of urea labeled with the stable isotope of carbon-13, $^{13}CO_2$ is rapidly detected in the breath, signifying the presence of urease-containing bacteria in the stomach. (*Courtesy of* Meretek Diagnostics, Houston, TX.)

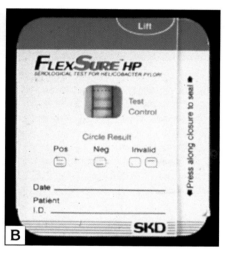

FIGURE 4-30 Mechanisms of the urea breath test. The basis of the urea breath test is hydrolysis of urea by the high urease activity of *Helicobacter pylori*. The ingestion of urea labeled with either the stable isotope ^{13}C or the radioactive ^{14}C results in the rapid appearance (within 5 minutes) of labeled CO_2 in the breath. The test is robust with specificity and sensitivities of approximately 95%. Its major advantage is that it measures the presence of active *H. pylori* infection, and it is the only noninvasive test to assess effectiveness of therapy. The ^{14}C test employs a very low dose of radioactivity, but approximately 25% is retained in the metabolic carbon pool, making it less attractive for repeated use or use in pregnant women or children.

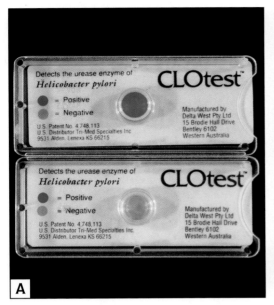

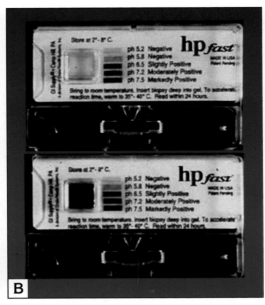

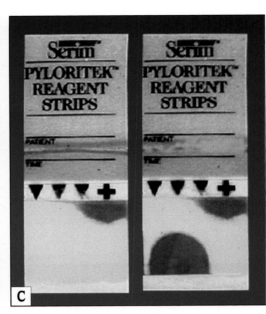

FIGURE 4-31 Rapid urease tests. Three commercially available rapid urease tests are shown. The rapid urease tests have a sensitivity and specificity of approximately 90% (95% confidence intervals for either false-positive or false-negative tests are 1%–13%). Both false-positive and false-negative tests occur, although false-negative tests outnumber false-positive ones. False-positive results are more common if one interprets the test in the afternoon or evening. **A** and **B**, The CLOtest (Delta West Pty. Ltd., Australia) (*panel 31A*) and hp*fast* (GI Supply, Camp Hill, PA) test (*panel 31B*) rely on a gastric biopsy specimen placed in a gel containing urea and a pH indicator. Production of ammonia increases pH and changes the color. The initial pH of the medium is lower for hp*fast* and theoretically excludes false-positive tests from other microorganisms with urease activity. **C**, The PyloriTek (Serim Research Corp., Elkhart, IN) test uses a membrane and pH indicator; both positive and negative results are shown. (*From* Graham [1]; with permission.)

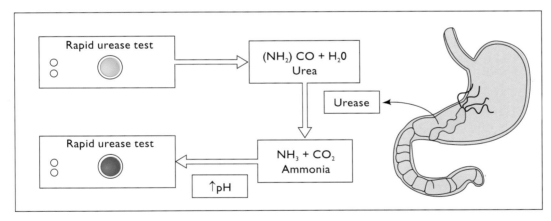

FIGURE 4-32 Mechanisms of rapid urease tests. The CLOtest and hp*fast* test rely on a gastric biopsy specimen placed in a gel containing urea and a pH indicator. Production of ammonia by *Helicobacter pylori* increases pH and changes the color from yellow to pink in the Clotest (yellow to blue in the hp*fast* test). The CLOtest is illustrated. (*Adapted from* Graham [1].)

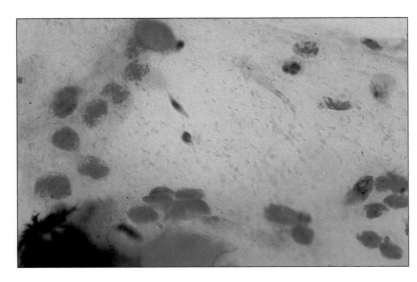

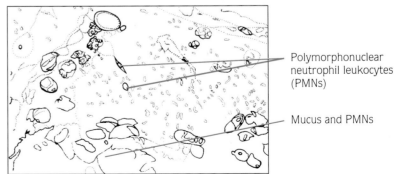

FIGURE 4-33 Gastric mucosal biopsy. A gastric mucosal biopsy specimen is rubbed on a glass slide and Gram-stained. Inflammatory cells and *Helicobacter pylori* are seen. This is a rapid but infrequently used technique to diagnose *H. pylori* infection. Most physicians rely on the combination of a rapid urease test and histology.

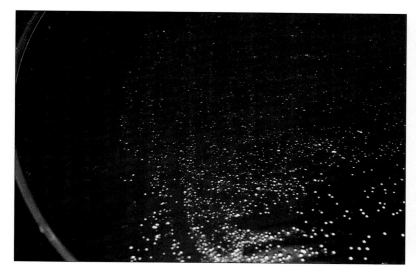

FIGURE 4-34 Culture of *Helicobacter pylori* on brain-heart infusion agar. The typical clear, glistening *H. pylori* colonies, approximately 1 mm in diameter, can be seen on freshly made brain-heart infusion agar with 7% horse blood. The rate of primary isolation is highest on this media. Culture is done at 37° C in 12% CO_2 with 100% humidity.

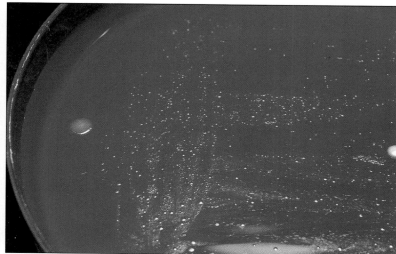

FIGURE 4-35 Culture of *Helicobacter pylori* on trypticase soy agar. *H. pylori* typically appears as approximately 1-mm, clear, glistening colonies when grown on commercially available trypticase soy agar with 5% sheep blood. Two contaminating yeast colonies are present on this plate, although the rate of contamination is low, possibly due to the hostile acid environment of the stomach.

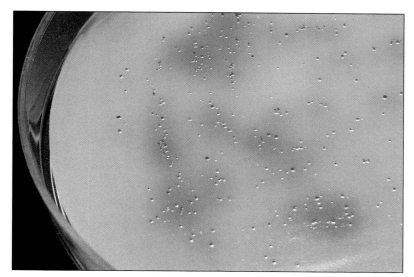

FIGURE 4-36 Typical *Helicobacter pylori* colonies on egg yolk emulsion agar containing triphenyleteroxolium chloride. The inclusion of an indicator may improve the identification [8].

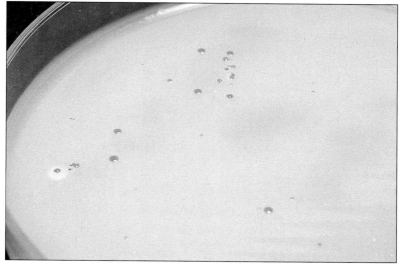

FIGURE 4-37 False-positive result on egg yolk emulsion agar. The colonies are those of a gram-positive coccus.

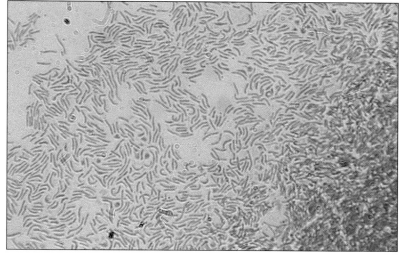

FIGURE 4-38 Gram stain of cultured *Helicobacter pylori* showing typical morphology.

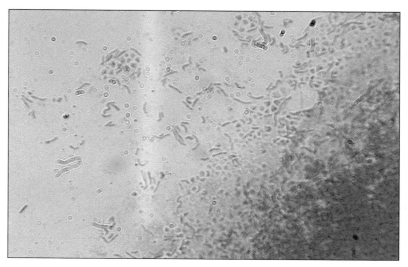

FIGURE 4-39 Gram stain of cultured *Helicobacter pylori* showing a mixture of coccoid and rod forms.

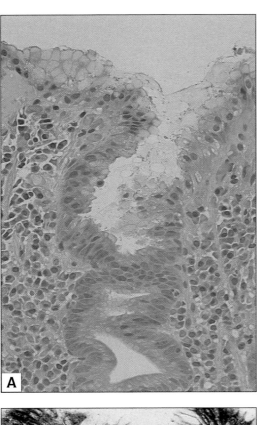

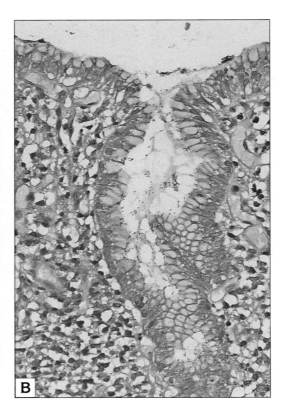

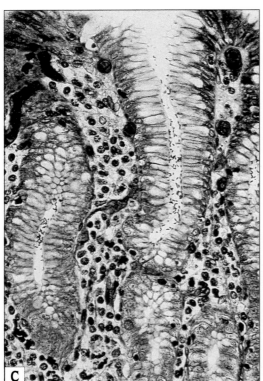

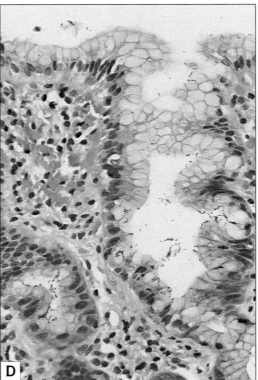

FIGURE 4-40 Histologic stains to detect *Helicobacter pylori* in biopsy specimens. Sections from the same biopsy specimen were stained with hematoxylin-eosin, Warthin-Starry, Giemsa, and Genta stains. *H. pylori* is rather difficult to detect with both the hematoxylin-eosin and modified Gram stains; in contrast, they are easily detected with both the Warthin-Starry and Giemsa stains. With the latter three stains, however, neither tissue morphology nor the nature of the inflammatory infiltrate can be evaluated. With the Genta stain [9], detection of *H. pylori* as well as the morphologic and inflammatory features of the gastric mucosa are easily appreciated. **A,** Hematoxylin-eosin stain. **B,** Warthin-Starry stain. **C,** Giemsa stain. **D,** Genta stain.

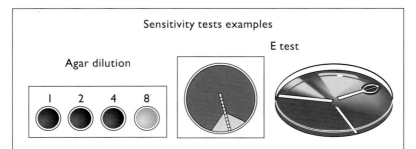

FIGURE 4-41 Antimicrobial sensitivity testing in *Helicobacter pylori* infection. Sensitivity testing is especially useful in identifying the best agent for patients who have failed previous therapy or who live in a region where either metronidazole or clarithromycin resistance is a problem. The E-test has proved to be simple and accurate for antimicrobial sensitivity testing of *H. pylori*. (*Adapted from* Graham [1].)

PATHOGENESIS OF *HELICOBACTER PYLORI*–INDUCED DUODENAL ULCER

A. Direct evidence implicating *Helicobacter pylori* in the pathogenesis of chronic gastritis

1. Voluntary ingestion of *H. pylori* results in gastritis.
2. Experimental animal challenge simulates human infection with resulting chronic gastritis.
3. Antimicrobial therapy that eradicates infection heals gastritis.

B. Indirect evidence implicating *Helicobacter pylori* in the pathogenesis of chronic gastritis

1. *H. pylori* only overlies gastric or gastric-type epithelium.
2. *H. pylori* infection is associated with only certain types of gastroduodenal inflammation, not all types.
3. There is universal systemic immune response to *H. pylori*.
4. Levels of *H. pylori*–specific antibodies decrease with therapy, concomitant with diminution in inflammation.
5. *H. pylori* is associated with epidemic gastritis and hypochlorhydria.

FIGURE 4-42 **A** and **B**, Evidence implicating *Helicobacter pylori* in the pathogenesis of chronic gastritis. Most frequently, chronic infection with *H. pylori* results in asymptomatic superficial gastritis. (*Adapted from* Blaser [10].)

Putative pathogenic mechanisms in *Helicobacter pylori* infection

Active motility enables bacteria to "swim" through mucus
Adherence to gastric mucosa
Multiply
Damage tissue
Internalization into epithelium (?)

Putative host immune response to *Helicobacter pylori* infection

Bacterial attachment stimulates proinflammatory cytokine secretion
   Interleukin-8, tumor necrosis factor-α
   Polymorphonuclear cell response
   Morphonuclear cell response
T and B cells are recruited, produce cytokines and antibodies
Inflammatory mediators may cause tissue damage (?)
Down-regulation of immune response to chronic infection

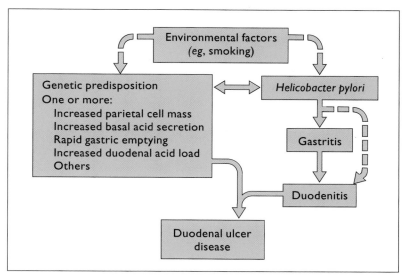

FIGURE 4-43 Pathogenesis of duodenal ulcer disease. The pathogenesis of peptic ulcer remains incompletely understood. Although some data suggest that specific clones of *Helicobacter pylori* are involved, other data suggest that host characteristics are extremely important. Approximately one in six infected persons develops peptic ulcer. The histologic pattern of gastritis is different in patients with duodenal ulcer than in those with gastric ulcer, gastric cancer, or asymptomatic gastritis. The pattern in duodenal ulcer is one of antral-predominant gastritis, sparing the gastric corpus and thus allowing acid secretion to remain high. *H. pylori* are found throughout the stomach but, for some reason, do not cause much inflammation in the gastric corpus. High acid secretion predating infection appears to be extremely common in those who develop duodenal ulcer disease, and it remains after the infection is cured. (*Adapted from* Graham [11].)

FIGURE 4-44 Putative pathogenic mechanisms in *Helicobacter pylori* infection. Following ingestion, the bacteria swim through the mucus, and some attach to the mucosa. They then multiply and cause tissue damage. There is increasing evidence that they are also internalized into the epithelium, where they are more accessible to the immune system. This internalization may in part be responsible for the systemic immune response seen as part of the infection.

FIGURE 4-45 Putative host immune response to *Helicobacter pylori* infection. The host launches a cellular and humoral immune response to the bacterial invasion. The presence of the bacteria and bacterial attachment to the mucosa stimulate the epithelial cells to produce a variety of chemokines. These subsequently attract inflammatory cells that produce cytokines and antibodies. It is thought that the inflammation may be the cause of tissue damage. The immune response is able to negate, reduce, or eliminate some of the factors responsible for the initial severe reaction, resulting in a down-regulation to the pattern of chronic infection. There are many examples of chronic mucosal infections in humans, with probably the best recognized being periodontal disease.

Determinants of outcome in *Helicobacter pylori* infection

Different exposures
Frequency, amount, strain
Cultural, social, diet, environmental
Genetic differences in susceptibility
To infection (twin study)
To specific disease (family studies)
Genetic differences in *H. pylori* strain
"Ulcer" strain, "cancer" strain, etc.

FIGURE 4-46 Determinants of outcome in *Helicobacter pylori* infection. In addition to genetic differences in bacterial virulence and genetic differences in host susceptibility, environmental cofactors may be critically important in the development of gastric cancer. Recent studies suggest that age of acquisition may not be important in that the infections typically occur in childhood.

Helicobacter pylori virulence factor genes

Urease	*ure*A-I
Flagella	*fla*A, *fla*B
Adhesin	*hpa*A
Neutrophil-activating protein	*nap*A
Superoxide dismutase	*sod*A
Vacuolating cytotoxin	*vac*A
Cytotoxin-associated gene	*cag*A
Catalase	*kat*A

FIGURE 4-47 *Helicobacter pylori* virulence factor genes. A large number of potential virulence factor genes have been identified. Urease, flagella, and adhesins all play a role in the initial infection. Urease seems unimportant or less important for maintenance of the infection. Whether the other gene products have critical roles in initiation or maintenance of infection remains unclear. (*From* Graham [1].)

*cag*A protein of *Helicobacter pylori*

128 K protein of unknown function
Product of the *cag*A gene
First gene found in only a proportion of isolates
Higher frequency in patients with ulcers (> 60%) than dyspepsia (~40%)
May be a marker for more virulent strains

FIGURE 4-48 CagA protein of *Helicobacter pylori*. CagA is a 128 K protein of unknown function. It is the first gene found in only a proportion of the *Helicobacter pylori* isolates. It appears in slightly higher frequency in patients with ulcers compared with those with asymptomatic gastritis. It is thought to be a possible marker for more virulent *H. pylori* strains.

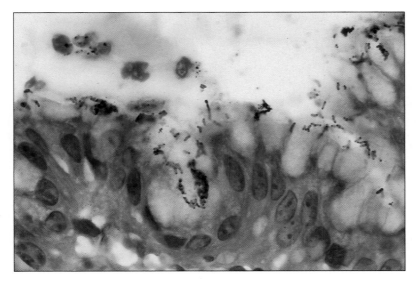

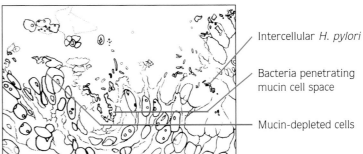

Intercellular *H. pylori*

Bacteria penetrating mucin cell space

Mucin-depleted cells

FIGURE 4-49 Histologic specimen showing epithelial damage inflicted on the surface epithelium by *Helicobacter pylori*. Some of the superficial cells are completely depleted of mucin. There is single-cell dropout, with clumps of bacteria apparently penetrating in the space previously occupied by a mucin cell. *H. pylori* can also be seen within intercellular spaces. Some authors consider this to represent the first step toward formation of erosions and ulcers.

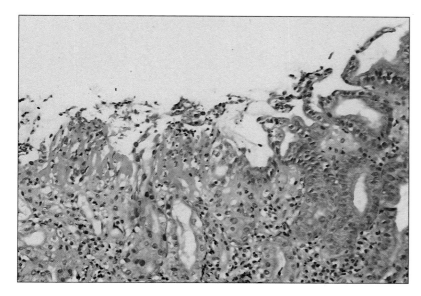

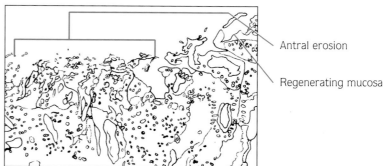

FIGURE 4-50 Histologic specimen showing antral erosion in *Helicobacter pylori* gastritis. The epithelium adjacent to the erosion shows prominent regenerative changes, with large dark nuclei and somewhat irregular architecture. Such changes (best described as *reactive atypia*) are completely reversed by eradication of *H. pylori* and should not be confused with dysplasia, a preneoplastic change believed to be irreversible.

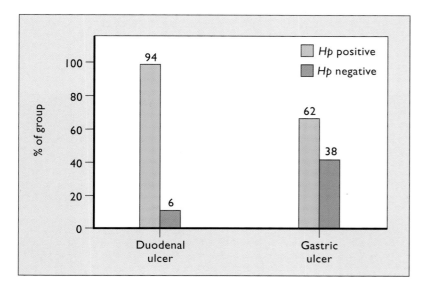

FIGURE 4-51 Frequency of *Helicobacter pylori* (*Hp*) infection in patients with duodenal versus gastric ulcer. The frequency of *H. pylori* infection was assessed in 302 consecutive patients with duodenal ulcer and 115 with gastric ulcer seen in one private practice. The majority of ulcers of both types were associated with *H. pylori* infection. The remainder were largely accounted for by use of nonsteroidal anti-inflammatory drugs [12,13].

DUODENAL ULCER

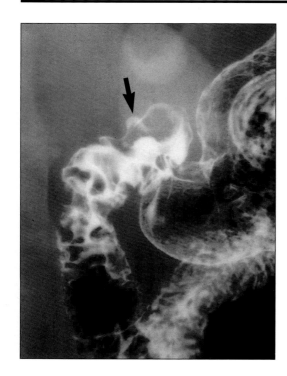

FIGURE 4-52 Barium upper gastrointestinal series showing marked deformity of the duodenal bulb with a typical ulcer crater (*arrow*) in the center. Barium contrast studies are less expensive than endoscopy but have much higher rates of false-positive and false-negative results. Endoscopy not only is able to identify the presence of gastroduodenal pathology but also has the added advantage of being able to obtain specimens for histology, rapid urease testing, and culture.

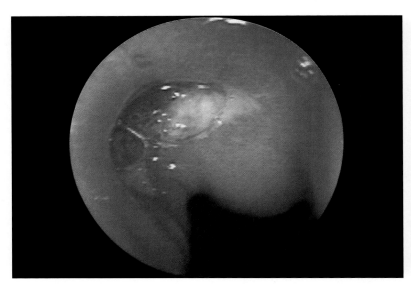

FIGURE 4-53 Endoscopic view showing deep, 1-cm duodenal ulcer prior to therapy. This is a typical ulcer at the apex of the bulb with deep excavation.

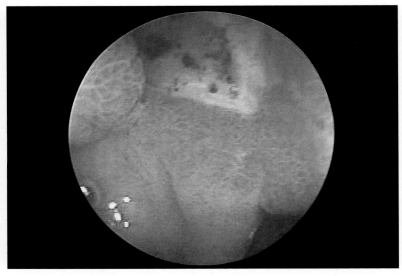

FIGURE 4-54 Close-up endoscopic view of the edge of a large duodenal ulcer. The almost featureless villous duodenal mucosa changes to one largely composed of gastric metaplasia. The ulcer base is stained by food or blood. The duodenum is deformed by the presence of both scar and edema.

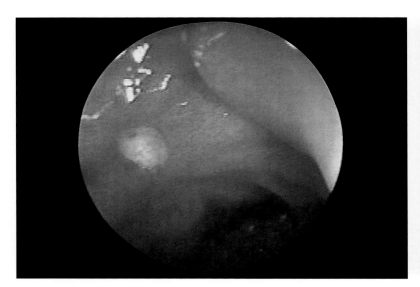

FIGURE 4-55 Endoscopic view of duodenal ulcer showing marked healing after 4 weeks of therapy with antisecretory drugs. Both the diameter and depth are greatly decreased, and the ulcer edges have become less distinct. The muscular spasm associated with the active inflammation has decreased, and so the duodenal wall is less deformed.

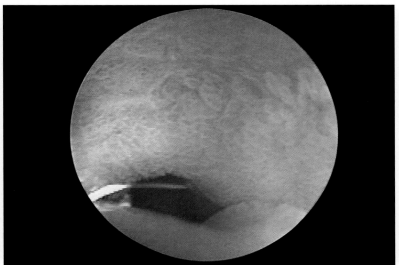

FIGURE 4-56 Close-up view of healed duodenal ulcer after successful therapy. The edge of the white thin scar is shown along with the large villi characteristic of a site of a healed ulcer.

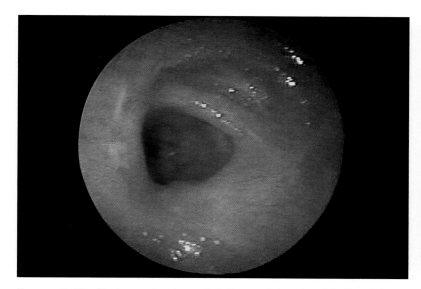

FIGURE 4-57 Endoscopic view of deformed duodenal bulb with several scars and a pseudodiverticulum. This type of deformity would in all likelihood be mistaken for a duodenal ulcer by a barium upper gastrointestinal tract series.

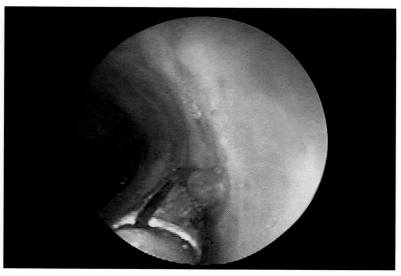

FIGURE 4-58 Endoscopic view of duodenal ulcer after a major upper gastrointestinal hemorrhage. A visible vessel is seen in the center of the ulcer. A heat probe, an endoscopic device for thermal hemostasis, is shown adjacent to the visible vessel in preparation for endoscopic hemostatic therapy.

GASTRIC ULCER

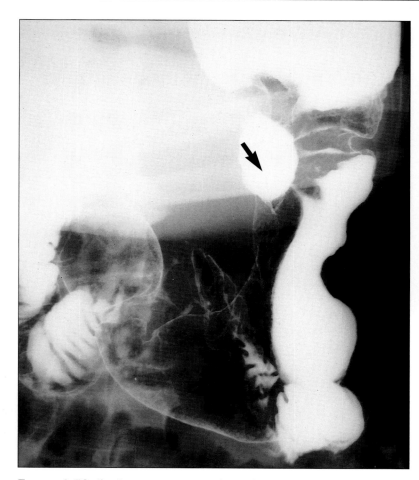

FIGURE 4-59 Barium upper gastrointestinal series showing a large deep gastric ulcer (*arrow*) with radiating folds high on the lesser curvature of the stomach. Most gastric ulcers are found on the lesser curvature near the angulus incisura.

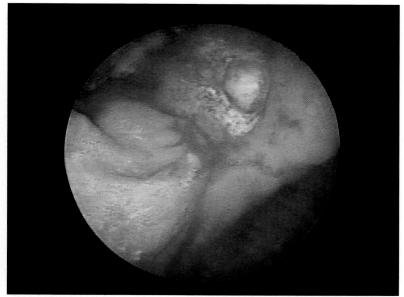

FIGURE 4-60 Retroflexed endoscopic view of the gastric angulus showing a gastric ulcer at the typical location for a benign gastric ulcer. The ulcer is sharply demarcated and appears punched out. This appearance is typical of an ulcer in which healing has not yet begun to outpace infection.

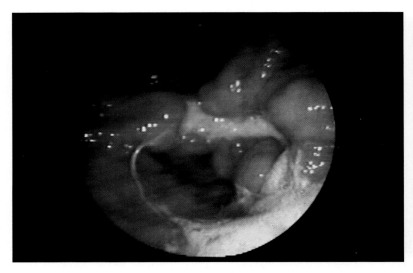

FIGURE 4-61 Endoscopic view of a very large gastric ulcer seen on the lesser curvature of the stomach with marked deformity of the stomach. On barium study, it would be difficult for the radiologist to determine whether such a large and irregular ulcer was benign or malignant. Endoscopy offers the opportunity to examine all the surfaces of the ulcer as well as to obtain tissue for histologic examination and cytology. This ulcer was benign.

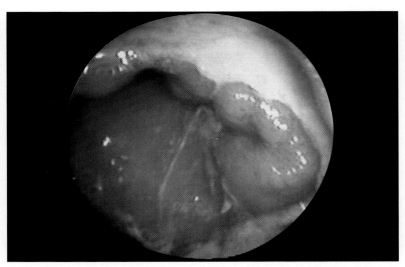

FIGURE 4-62 Close-up view of the edge of a large benign gastric ulcer. A close-up view of the edge of the gastric ulcer seen in Figure 4-61 shows the sharp edge undermined by the ulcer. This figure shows the typical sharp margins and white base of a gastric ulcer.

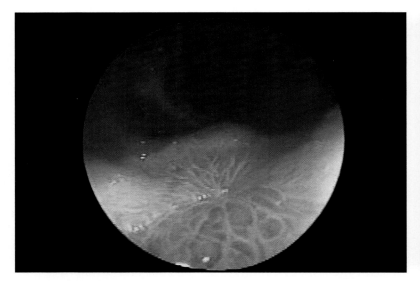

FIGURE 4-63 Close-up view of a healed gastric ulcer. At the site of a previous gastric ulcer, the gastric mucosa is intact but has not yet returned to the normal pattern. The mucosa is still red and inflamed, as would be expected of a recently formed scar anywhere in the body.

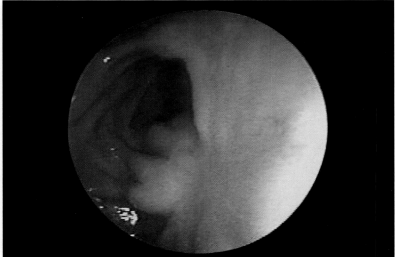

FIGURE 4-64 Endoscopic view showing marked deformity of the stomach due to the presence of a scar resulting from healed gastric ulcer. This deformity is permanent. One can see the radiating folds resulting from the large scar that underlies the mucosa at the site where the ulcer healed.

GASTRIC CANCER

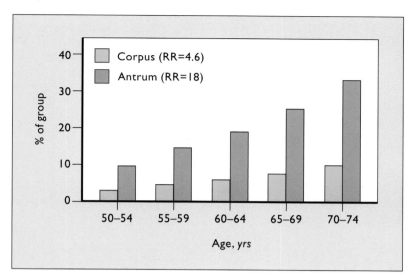

FIGURE 4-65 Risk of gastric cancer in persons with severe atrophic gastritis. The risk of developing gastric cancer over a 10-year period in a group of patients with severe atrophic gastritis ranged from approximately 2% to 30% and increased with patient age [14]. (RR—relative risk.)

Carcinogenicity of *Helicobacter pylori*: Conclusions of the WHO-IARC Working Group meeting, June 1994

H. pylori plays a causal role in chain of events leading to stomach cancer.
There is sufficient evidence in humans to indicate the carcinogenicity of infection with *H. pylori*.
H. pylori is a group 1 carcinogen.

WHO-IARC—World Health Organization International Agency for Research on Cancer.

FIGURE 4-66 Carcinogenicity of *Helicobacter pylori* infection: World Health Organization–International Agency for Research on Cancer Working Group meeting, June 1994. In June 1994, a Working Group of the International Agency for Research on Cancer of the World Health Organization concluded that there was sufficient evidence in humans for the carcinogenicity of *H. pylori* infection, and *H. pylori* was defined as a group 1, or definite, carcinogen [15].

Pathogenetic factors in gastric cancer

Histologic abnormality: underlying gastritis with atrophy
Intragastric synthesis of nitroso compounds
Facilitated by irritants (salt, carbohydrates, abrasive dusts)
Retarded by fresh fruits and vegetables (antioxidants ?)

FIGURE 4-67 Pathogenetic factors in gastric cancer. The histologic abnormality underlying gastric cancer is gastritis with atrophy. Correa proposed that one important factor in the pathogenesis is the intragastric synthesis of nitroso compounds [16]. There are clear epidemiologic data indicating that irritants enhance the frequency of gastric carcinoma and that fresh fruits and vegetables reduce the frequency, although the mechanisms are unknown. Direct trials of ascorbate supplementation have failed to reduce the risk of gastric cancer in high-risk populations.

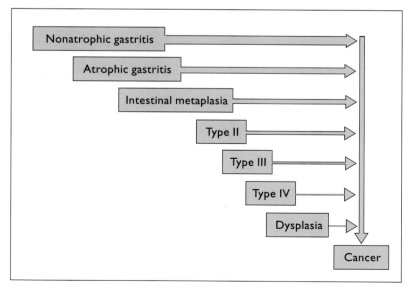

FIGURE 4-68 Time course of gastritis to cancer sequence. Although the pathogenesis of gastric carcinoma from *Helicobacter pylori* infection is unknown, the process is thought to begin with inflammation that leads to the development of metaplastic epithelium (intestinal metaplasia). In some individuals, this metaplasia subsequently leads to dysplasia and finally to gastric cancer. As with Barrett's esophagus, the step that promotes the change from an inflammatory response to metaplastic epithelium is unknown, and that step in the progression is unusual in the United States, because most individuals in developed countries maintain the pattern of nonatrophic gastritis. The width of the *arrows* in the figure represents the proportion of cases that move from one histologic type to another. The proportion of cases moving from nonatrophic to atrophic gastritis is small, and an even smaller proportion progresses on to one of the advanced stages of intestinal metaplasia. If the stage of advanced intestinal metaplasia is reached, it becomes more likely that the disease will progress toward dysplasia and cancer. (*Adapted from* Graham [1].)

Association between chronic gastritis and gastric cancer: Prospective case-control studies

Study	No.	No. with cancer	Hp+, %	OR	95% CI
Forman	22,000	29	69	2.8	1.0–8.0
Nomura	5908	109	94	6.0	2.1–17.3
Parsonnet	128,992	109	84	3.6	1.8–7.3

CI—confidence interval; OR—odds ratio.

FIGURE 4-69 Association between chronic gastritis and gastric carcinoma. Three recent nested case-control studies, which used serum collected and stored decades ago, have shown that gastric cancer is more common in people with *Helicobacter pylori* infection than in those without it. These studies provide a strong epidemiologic link between gastric carcinoma and *H. pylori* infection, and they complement and extend the previous, large number of studies showing the association between chronic gastritis and gastric carcinoma [17–19].

Increased risk of early gastric carcinoma with *Helicobacter pylori* infection

Group	No.	Hp+, %	OR	95% CI
Controls	213	74.6		
Gastric cancer	213	88.2*	2.6	1.35–4.37
Advanced	85	84.7	1.9	0.99–3.63
Early	128	93.0*	4.9	2.14–9.46
Histology				
Intestinal	125	90.4*	3.2	1.64–6.25
Diffuse	76	86.4*	2.2	1.01–4.29

*$P < 0.05$.

CI—confidence interval; OR—odds ratio.

FIGURE 4-70 Increased risk of early gastric carcinoma associated with *Helicobacter pylori* infection. Studies from Sapporo, Japan, have shown an increased risk of early gastric carcinoma associated with *H. pylori* infection. Such studies extend the findings of epidemiologic studies based on stored sera [20].

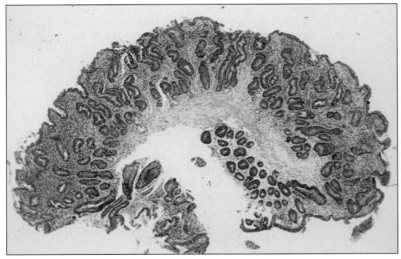

FIGURE 4-71 Histologic specimen showing atrophic gastritis with extensive intestinal metaplasia. Virtually the entire gastric mucosa is replaced by intestinal-type epithelium with goblet cells. The glands are sparse, long, and tortuous, and a moderately dense inflammatory infiltrate is present in the lamina propria. Intestinal metaplasia is believed to be the first step in the sequence leading to dysplasia and eventually carcinoma.

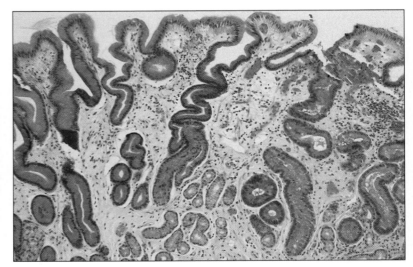

FIGURE 4-72 Atrophic gastritis with focal intestinal metaplasia. No inflammatory infiltrate is present. This is believed to represent the end stage of *Helicobacter pylori* gastritis. Patients with gastric atrophy usually have few or no detectable organisms, although many of them have circulating antibodies against *H. pylori* antigens.

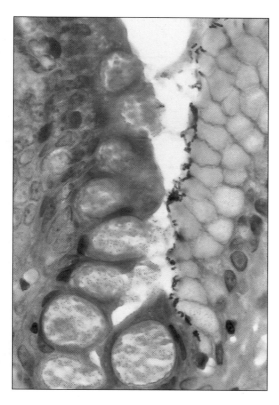

FIGURE 4-73 High-power microscopic view of intestinal metaplasia involving a gastric foveola. Intestinal metaplasia appears to create a hostile environment for *Helicobacter pylori*. Although there is heavy bacterial colonization in the *right* portion of this gastric foveola, no *H. pylori* are present in the *left* portion, which is entirely lined by intestinal-type epithelium. In some patients, however, *H. pylori* have been detected attached to areas of intestinal metaplasia.

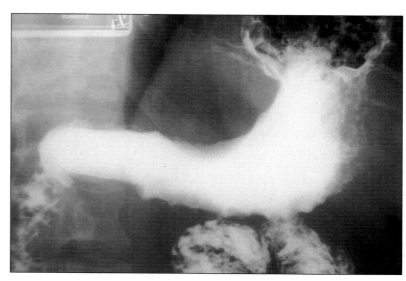

FIGURE 4-74 Barium upper gastrointestinal series showing a stiff gastric antrum with loss of normal mucosal features consistent with gastric carcinoma. Gastric carcinoma is one of the long-term consequences of chronic atrophic *Helicobacter pylori* gastritis.

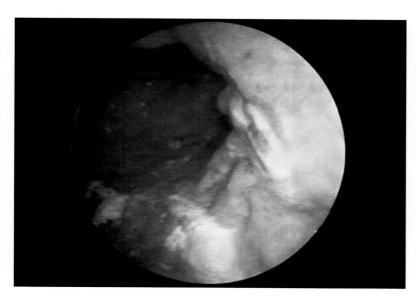

FIGURE 4-75 Endoscopic view of a large irregular ulcerated area seen on the posterior wall and lesser curvature of the stomach. Biopsy yielded gastric adenocarcinoma, a late complication of *Helicobacter pylori* infection.

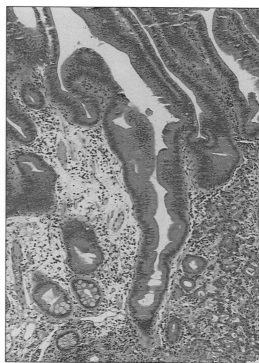

FIGURE 4-76 Histologic specimen showing dysplastic epithelium in a gastric villous adenoma. Between 5% and 40% of villous adenomas of the stomach contain foci of adenocarcinoma. In this photomicrograph, invasive carcinoma is seen in the lower right corner.

GASTRIC B-CELL LYMPHOMA

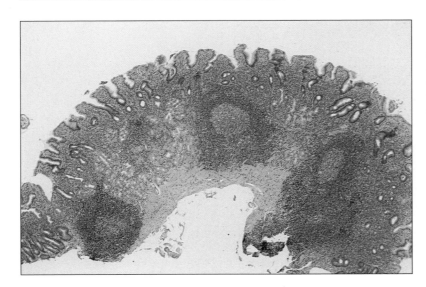

FIGURE 4-77 Low-power photomicrograph of antral biopsy specimen with three prominent lymphoid follicles. Lymphoid follicles are a constant inflammatory response in *Helicobacter pylori* gastritis. In some biopsy specimens, one may find several large and apparently confluent lymphoid follicles, which make the distinction from low-grade lymphomas arising from mucosa-associated lymphoid tissue difficult and sometimes impossible.

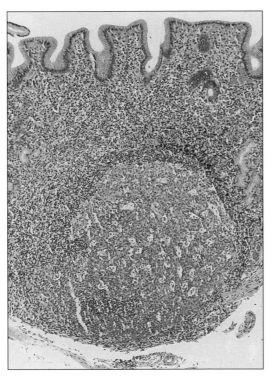

FIGURE 4-78 High-power view of a very large lymphoid follicle obliterating the entire lamina propria. In such cases, distinction from lymphoma requires extensive biopsy sampling, immunocytochemical stains, and gene-rearrangement studies.

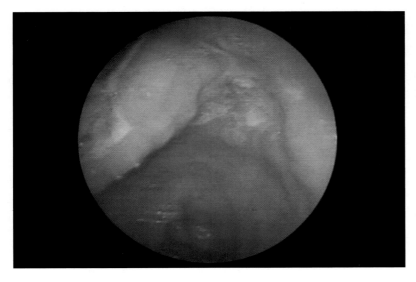

FIGURE 4-79 Endoscopic view of two irregularly shaped gastric ulcers seen at the angulus incisura. Biopsy showed well-differentiated gastric lymphoma. Biopsies of surrounding mucosa showed *Helicobacter pylori* infection. The lesions resolved with treatment of *H. pylori* infection. Primary gastric B-cell lymphoma is thought to be one consequence of the lymphocytic response to *H. pylori* infection.

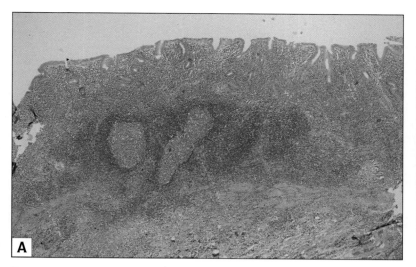

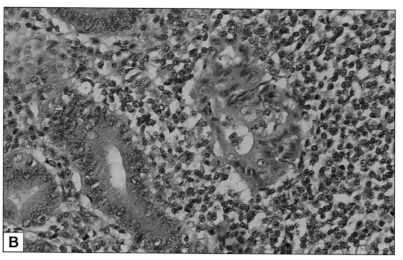

FIGURE 4-80 Histologic sections demonstrating mucosa-associated lymphoid tissue (MALT) lymphoma. **A,** Low-power photomicrograph of a MALT lymphoma. The lymphoid follicles are irregular in shape and distribution, and lymphocytes occupy the entire lamina propria displacing the antral glands.

B, A typical lymphoepithelial lesion, characteristic of MALT lymphomas but sometimes found around benign follicles in patients with *Helicobacter pylori* gastritis. Lymphocytes infiltrate the glandular epithelium, but the architecture of the gland is left largely intact.

THERAPY FOR *HELICOBACTER PYLORI* INFECTION

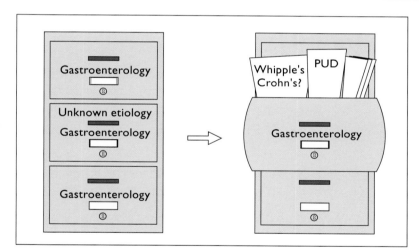

FIGURE 4-81 Conceptual reclassification of peptic ulcer disease (PUD). There recently has been a conceptual revolution relating to peptic ulcer disease. Peptic ulcer has been transformed from a digestive disease of unknown etiology to a bacterial infection. With this change comes recognition of a role for antimicrobial therapy.

NIH Consensus Conference guidelines on *Helicobacter pylori*
H. pylori plays an important role in ulcer pathogenesis. Antimicrobial treatment alters the natural history of ulcer disease. Antimicrobial therapy is indicated in all persons with peptic ulcer and *H. pylori* infection.
NIH—National Institutes of Health.

FIGURE 4-82 National Institutes of Health (NIH) Consensus Conference guidelines on *Helicobacter pylori*. The NIH Consensus Development Conference, in February 1994, laid down guidelines, including accepting *H. pylori* as having an important role in ulcer pathogenesis. In addition, these guidelines suggest that antimicrobial therapy alters the natural history of peptic ulcer disease and, therefore, should be given to all patients with peptic ulcer disease and *H. pylori* infection [21].

FIGURE 4-83 Effects of different antiulcer therapies on recurrence of duodenal ulcer within 1 year. The lack of ulcer recurrence after successful treatment of *Helicobacter pylori* (Hp) infection is a consistent finding worldwide [22]. (R$_x$—prescription.)

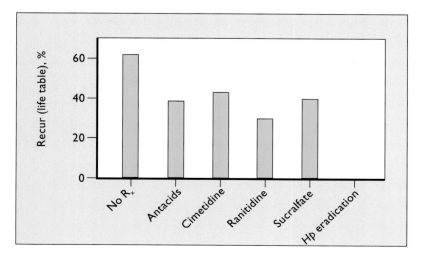

Antimicrobial treatments for *Helicobacter pylori* infection
Amoxicillin
Bismuth
Clarithromycin (macrolides)
Metronidazole
Tetracycline
Proton pump inhibitors

FIGURE 4-84 Antimicrobial treatments for *Helicobacter pylori* infection. All of these drugs have antimicrobial effectiveness, but none is useful as monotherapy.

Triple therapy for *Helicobacter pylori* infection*	
Tetracycline-HCl	500 mg four times a day
Metronidazole	250 mg three times a day
Bismuth subsalicylate	2 tablets four times a day
Tetracycline-HCl	500 mg four times a day
Clarithromycin	500 mg three times a day
Bismuth subsalicylate	2 tablets four times a day

*Duration × 14 days.

FIGURE 4-85 Triple therapy for *Helicobacter pylori* infection. Traditional triple therapy consists of tetracycline, metronidazole, and bismuth. Chlortetracycline and doxycycline yield inferior results. Seven days' therapy may be as efficacious as 14 days, although the ideal duration remains unsettled. The addition of an H_2 receptor antagonist or proton pump inhibitor may enhance effectiveness, although that question is also unsettled. When metronidazole resistance is suspected, one can substitute clarithromycin.

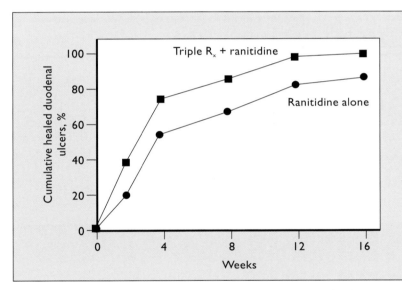

FIGURE 4-86 Rates of duodenal ulcer healing with triple therapy plus ranitidine versus ranitidine alone. Healing was significantly more rapid in patients who received triple therapy (bismuth subsalicylate, metronidazole, and tetracycline) plus ranitidine (*n*=53) than in those who received ranitidine alone (*n*=52). (R$_x$—prescription). (*Adapted from* Graham *et al*. [23].)

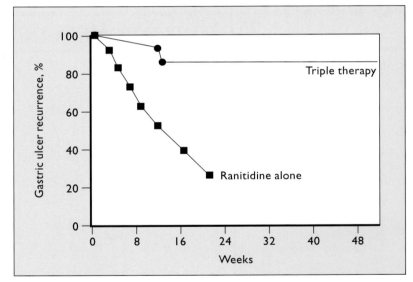

FIGURE 4-87 Rates of gastric ulcer recurrence for 1 year after successful ulcer healing with triple therapy plus ranitidine versus ranitidine alone. The recurrence rate of gastric ulcer was significantly greater in the ranitidine-alone group than in the triple-therapy/ranitidine group. (*Adapted from* Graham *et al*. [24].)

New twice-daily triple therapies for *Helicobacter pylori* infection*	
Metronidazole	500 mg twice a day
Omeprazole	20 mg twice a day
Clarithromycin	250 mg twice a day
Omeprazole	20 mg twice a day
Amoxicillin	1000 mg twice a day
Clarithromycin	500 mg twice a day

*Duration × 7 or 14 days.

FIGURE 4-88 New twice-daily triple therapies for *Helicobacter pylori* infection. The metronidazole-omeprazole-clarithromycin (MOC) combination has proved effective worldwide. The data suggest that 7 days' therapy may be sufficient. The therapy is effective in the face of metronidazole resistance but is markedly less effective when clarithromycin resistance is present. Side effects are uncommon. Omeprazole-amoxicillin-clarithromycin is slightly less effective than MOC and should be given for 14 days. Lansoprazole can be substituted for omeprazole in both regimens [25].

Dual therapies for *Helicobacter pylori* infection

Omeprazole	40 mg every morning × 14 days
Clarithromycin	500 mg three times a day × 14 days
Ranitidine–bismuth subcitrate	400 mg twice a day × 4 wks
Clarithromycin	500 mg three times a day × 14 days

FIGURE 4-89 Dual therapies for *Helicobacter pylori* infection. Two dual therapies have recently been approved by the Food and Drug Administration for use in *H. pylori* infection. The combination of clarithromycin, 500 mg three times a day, and omeprazole, 40 mg/day in the morning, and the ranitidine–bismuth subcitrate/clarithromycin combinations are both effective but may be less effective than the metronidazole-omeprazole-clarithromycin or omeprazole-amoxicillin-clarithromycin combinations.

Side effects of *Helicobacter pylori* therapies

Nausea (most common)
Diarrhea (usually mild)
Pseudomembranous colitis (very rare)
Rash (especially with amoxicillin)
Taste disturbance (especially with macrolides)
Black stool (with bismuth)
Candidal vaginitis (especially tetracycline)

FIGURE 4-90 Side effects of *Helicobacter pylori* therapies. The most common side effects are nausea and mild diarrhea. It is important to notify patients taking bismuths that they will probably develop black stool, so that they will not call the physician with the concern that they are bleeding. Vaginitis is a common accompaniment of *H. pylori* therapy in women.

FIGURE 4-91 Evaluation of the patient with ulcer. A new patient presenting with suspected ulcer or with a documented history or current finding of ulcer should be tested for the presence of *Helicobacter pylori* before antimicrobial therapy is prescribed. This step avoids the toxicity of antibiotic therapy in patients who are uninfected. Testing is done with a urea breath test (UBT) or serologic test for anti–*H. pylori* IgG antibodies. If patients present with "alarm" features, cancer should be suspected and investigated with endoscopy.

Alarm features

Advanced age
Long history
Weight loss
Significant anorexia
UGI bleeding/anemia
Significant vomiting
UGI series suggests "cancer"

UGI—upper gastrointestinal.

FIGURE 4-92 Alarm features suggesting cancer. Patients with suspected ulcer who present with any of a series of "alarm" features should be evaluated promptly for gastric cancer.

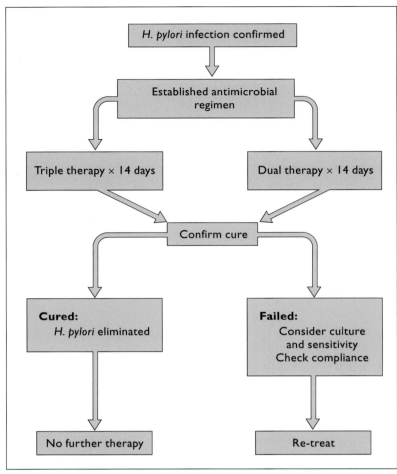

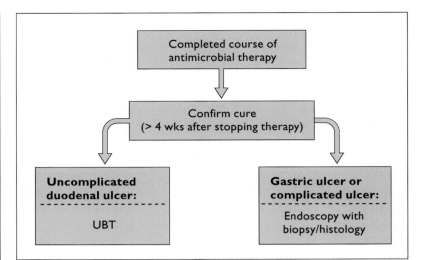

FIGURE 4-94 Follow-up of *Helicobacter pylori* treatment. Most, if not all, patients with peptic ulcer should be evaluated for the results of therapy. This step is mandatory in patients with a history of complicated peptic ulcer (*eg*, major hemorrhage) and desired in all others to prevent recurrence of symptoms, need to revisit physician, more tests, more drugs, and a risk of a major ulcer complication (~ 2%–3% per year). The effectiveness of therapy cannot be determined reliably until at least 4 weeks for an antibiotic- and proton pump inhibitor–free period have elapsed. The urea breath test (UBT) provides reliable information, but endoscopy with biopsy for histologic examination could also be done. A rapid urease test and/or culture can also be added. Serologic tests for anti–*H. pylori* IgG antibody are not useful because of the slow decline of antibody titers (months to years) after eradication of infection.

FIGURE 4-93 Strategy for antimicrobial treatment of *Helicobacter pylori* infection.

ACKNOWLEDGMENT

Parts of this chapter appeared in a previous publication: Graham DY: *An Update on Helicobacter pylori* [AGA educational slide/lecture program]. Alexandria, VA: American College of Gastroenterology; 1996. Reprinted with permission.

REFERENCES

1. Graham DY: *An Update on Helicobacter pylori* [AGA educational slide/lecture program]. Alexandria, VA: American College of Gastroenterology; 1996.

2. Graham DY, Adam E, Reddy GT, *et al.*: Seroepidemiology of *Helicobacter pylori* infection in India: Comparison of developing and developed countries. *Dig Dis Sci* 1991, 36:1084–1088.

3. Malaty HM, Evans DG, Evans DJ Jr, Graham DY: *Helicobacter pylori* in Hispanics: Comparison with blacks and whites of similar age and socioeconomic class. *Gastroenterology* 1992, 103:813–816.

4. Malaty HM, Graham DY: Importance of childhood socioeconomic status on the current prevalence of *Helicobacter pylori* infection. *Gut* 1994, 35:742–755.

5. Graham DY, Malaty HM, Evans DG, *et al.*: Epidemiology of *Helicobacter pylori* in an asymptomatic population in the United States: Effect of age, race, and socioeconomic status. *Gastroenterology* 1991, 100:1495–1501.

6. Malaty HM, Graham DY, Klein PD, *et al.*: Transmission of *Helicobacter pylori* infection. Studies in families of healthy individuals. *Scand J Gastroenterol* 1991, 26:927–932.

7. Kurata JH: Ulcer epidemiology: An overview and proposed research framework. *Gastroenterology* 1989, 96:569–580.

8. Westblom TU, Madan E, Midkiff BR: Egg yolk emulsion agar, a new medium for the cultivation of *Helicobacter pylori*. *J Clin Microbiol* 1991, 29:819–821.

9. Genta RM, Robason GO, Graham DY: Simultaneous visualization of *Helicobacter pylori* and gastric morphology: A new stain. *Hum Pathol* 1994, 25:221–226.

10. Blaser MJ: *Helicobacter pylori* and the pathogenesis of gastroduodenal inflammation. *J Infect Dis* 1990, 161:626–633.

11. Graham DY: *Campylobacter pylori* and peptic ulcer disease. *Gastroenterology* 1989, 96:615–625.

12. Borody TJ, George LL, Brandl S, *et al.*: *Helicobacter pylori*–negative duodenal ulcer. *Am J Gastroenterol* 1991, 86:1154–1157.

13. Borody TJ, Brandl S, Andrews P, *et al.*: *Helicobacter pylori*–negative gastric ulcer. *Am J Gastroenterol* 1992, 87:1403–1406.

14. Sipponen P, Kekki M, Haapakoski J, *et al.*: Gastric cancer risk in chronic atrophic gastritis: Statistical calculations of cross-sectional data. *Int J Cancer* 1985, 35:173–177.

15. IARC Monographs on the Evaluation of Carcinogenic Risks to Humans: Volume 61: Schistosomes, liver flukes and *Helicobacter pylori*. Lyon, France: International Agency for Research on Cancer; 1994.

16. Correa P: Clinical implications of recent developments in gastric cancer: Pathology and epidemiology. *Semin Oncol* 1985, 12:2–10.

17. Forman D, Newell DG, Fullerton F, *et al.*: Association between infection with *Helicobacter pylori* and risk of gastric cancer: Evidence from a prospective investigation. *BMJ* 1991, 302:1302–1305.

18. Nomura A, Stemmerman GN, Chyou P-H, *et al.*: *Helicobacter pylori* infection and gastric carcinoma in a population of Japanese-Americans in Hawaii. *N Engl J Med* 1991, 325:1132–1136.

19. Parsonnet J, Friedman GD, Vandersteen DP, *et al.*: *Helicobacter pylori* infection and risk of gastric carcinoma. *N Engl J Med* 1991, 325:1127–1131.

20. Asaka M, Kimura T, Kato M, *et al.*: Possible role of *Helicobacter pylori* infection in early gastric cancer development. *Cancer* 1994, 73:2691–2694.

21. NIH Consensus Development Panel: *Helicobacter pylori* in peptic ulcer disease. *JAMA* 1994, 272:65–69.

22. Hui WM, Lam SK, Lok AS, *et al.*: Maintenance therapy for duodenal ulcer: A randomized controlled comparison of seven forms of treatment. *Am J Med* 1992, 92:265–274.

23. Graham DY, Lew GM, Evans DG, *et al.*: Effect of triple therapy (antibiotics plus bismuth) on duodenal ulcer healing: A randomized controlled trial. *Ann Intern Med* 1991, 115:266–269.

24. Graham DY, Lew GM, Klein PD, *et al.*: Effect of treatment of *Helicobacter pylori* infection on the long-term recurrence of gastric or duodenal ulcer. A randomized, controlled study. *Ann Intern Med* 1992, 116:705–708.

25. Holtmann G, Talley NJ: Clinical approach to the *Helicobacter*-infected patient. *In* Blaser MJ, Smith PD, Ravdin JI, *et al.* (eds.): *Infections of the Gastrointestinal Tract*. New York: Raven Press; 1995:565–588.

SELECTED BIBLIOGRAPHY

Alpert LC, Graham DY, Evans DJ Jr, *et al.*: Diagnostic possibilities for *Campylobacter pylori* infection. *Eur J Gastroenterol Hepatol* 1989, 1:17–26.

Dixon MF: *Helicobacter pylori* and peptic ulceration: Histopathological aspects. *J Gastroenterol Hepatol* 1991, 6:125–130.

Genta RM, Hamner HW, Graham DY: Gastric lymphoid follicles in *Helicobacter pylori* infection: Frequency, distribution and response to triple therapy. *Hum Pathol* 1993, 24:577–583.

Genta RM, Robason GO, Graham DY: Simultaneous visualization of *Helicobacter pylori* and gastric morphology: A new stain. *Hum Pathol* 1994, 25:221–226.

Graham DY: *Helicobacter pylori*: Its epidemiology and its role in duodenal ulcer disease. *J Gastroenterol Hepatol* 1991, 6:105–113.

Tytgat GNJ, Lee A, Graham DY, *et al.*: The role of infectious agents in peptic ulcer disease. *Gastroenterol Int* 1993, 6:76–89.

CHAPTER 5

Viral Enteritis

Robert D. Shaw

Important agents of viral enteritis

Rotavirus
  Groups A, B, C
Caliciviruses
  Small round-structured viruses including Norwalk, Hawaii,
  Snow Mountain agents
Enteric adenovirus
Astrovirus

FIGURE 5-1 Important agents of viral enteritis. Rotaviruses are the leading cause of severe gastroenteritis in infants and young children worldwide. Small round-structured viruses (SRSVs), including the Norwalk virus, are known to be caliciviruses, which are a leading cause of epidemic outbreaks among adults. The SRSVs also include the agents previously known as Norwalk-like viruses.

ROTAVIRUS

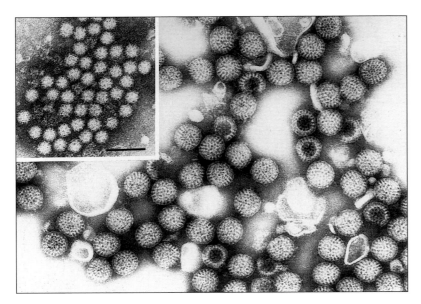

FIGURE 5-2 Human rotavirus particles in a stool filtrate prepared from an infant with gastroenteritis. Rotavirus was first identified as a human pathogen in 1973 by direct visualization with electron microscopy. This electron micrograph, first published in 1974, shows the classic double capsid particles thought to resemble wheels with spokes. This image explains the name of the virus, after the Latin *rota*, meaning wheel. (*From* Kapikiam [1]; with permission.)

Rotavirus gene coding assignments

Protein	Genomic segment	Protein MW	Function	Comments
VP4	4	86,775	Outer capsid	Hemagglutinin Cell-attachment
VP6	6	44,903	Inner capsid	Subgroup-specific antigen
VP7	9	37,198	Outer capsid	Surface glycoprotein serotype-specific

FIGURE 5-3 Rotavirus gene-coding assignments. The genome of rotaviruses consists of 11 segments of double-stranded RNA, which code for six structural and five nonstructural proteins. The genomic RNA can be easily extracted and separated by polyacrylamide gel electrophoresis. The RNA segments are numbered 1 to 11 according to their order of migration, RNA 1 being the slowest and 11 the fastest migrating RNA segment. Techniques for the cloning and sequencing of rotavirus genes have led to the rapid accumulation of information concerning the primary sequence of rotavirus proteins; however, the functions of some of these proteins are yet to be determined. Proteins VP4, VP6, and VP7 are three major components of the virus.

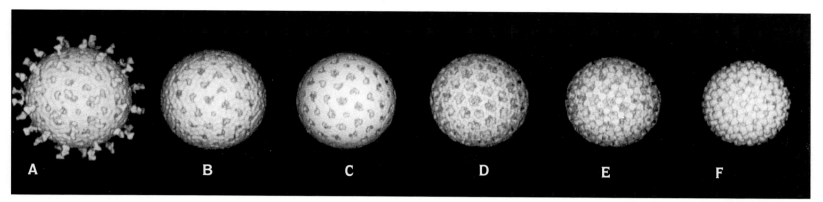

FIGURE 5-4 Three-dimensional structure of rhesus rotavirusvirus by cryoelectron microscopy and icosahedral image reconstruction. The surface-shaped representations were obtained by truncating the three-dimensional maps with spherical envelopes to reveal the internal structure. The six structures (from *left* to *right*) with their corresponding diameters are as follows: **A**, The virion outer capsid surface displays 60 spikes attributed to the VP4 hemagglutinin (1020 Å). **B**, The smoothly rippled outer capsid surface, attributed primarily to VP7, is perforated by 132 aqueous pores (790 Å). **C**, The space between the outer and inner capsids forms an open aqueous network that may provide pathways for the diffusion of ions and small regulatory molecules, as well as the extrusion of RNA (720 Å). **D**, The inner capsid has a "bristled" outer surface composed of 260 trimeric columns attributed to VP6 trimers (660 Å). **E**, The VP6 trimers merge with a smooth inner capsid shell, which is perforated by holes in register with those in the outer capsid (580 Å). **F**, A third protein shell (referred to as the *core*) is thought to be formed by VP1, VP2, and VP3 and encapsidates the double-stranded RNA segmented genome (530 Å). (*From* Yeager *et al.* [2]; with permission.)

A. Clinical importance of rotavirus proteins

VP4 and VP7, outer capsid
  Antibodies against these protect from disease
  Vaccine strategies maximize immunity to diverse types
  Epidemiology is based on diversity of these proteins

B. Clinical importance of rotavirus proteins

VP6, inner capsid
  Major structural protein (50% of viral mass)
  Target of major antibody response
  Most serology-based diagnostic tests detect antibodies to VP6

FIGURE 5-5 Clinical importance of rotavirus proteins. **A**, VP4 and VP7, outer capsid. **B**, VP6, inner capsid.

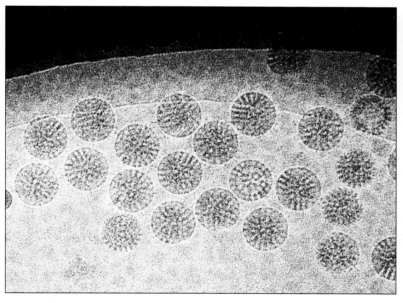

FIGURE 5-6 Modern electron microscopic image of rotavirus taken with the virus embedded in vitreous ice. The capsular structure of the virus is more clearly delineated by this technique. Extension of this technique was used to generate the computer-enhanced three-dimensional images in other figures. (*Courtesy of* M. Yeager, MD.)

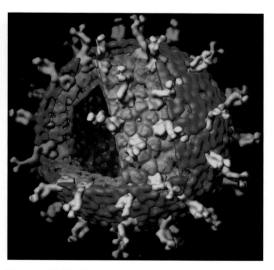

FIGURE 5-7 Computer-generated composite reconstruction of rotavirus showing surface views of the three nested capsid layers at 40 Å resolution. The outer capsid layer has been partially removed to reveal the interactions between VP4 spikes and VP6 in the inner capsid. The aqueous channels can be seen perforating VP7, VP6, and the core. (*Courtesy of* M. Yeager, MD.)

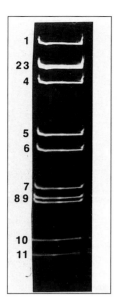

FIGURE 5-8 Polyacrylamide gel electrophoresis pattern of double-stranded (ds) RNA segments of a human rotavirus genome. Characteristic rates of mobility create a pattern called an *electropherotype*. In this representation, a typical size distribution pattern of 4–2–3–2 is seen. Each band contains a distinct dsRNA segment, and each codes for a single gene product (except for gene 9, which in some viruses codes for two variants of VP7). (*Courtesy of* H. Greenberg, MD.)

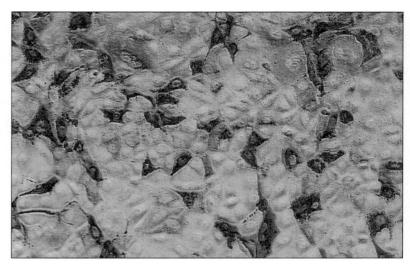

FIGURE 5-9 Rhesus rotavirus grown in tissue culture. Rotavirus research was expedited by the discovery that treatment of the viral particle with trypsin cleaved the outer capsid hemagglutinin VP4 and permitted growth in tissue culture. Virus is often grown on monolayer cultures of MA104 cells, a simian kidney cell line. This figure demonstrates rhesus rotavirus–infected MA104 cells (*darkly stained*) in which viral infection was permitted for 12 hours, at which time the monolayer was fixed and viral antigen detected with hyperimmune antiserum. Within 12 more hours' growth, the monolayer would have been completely destroyed by the lytic growth of the rotavirus. Tissue culture of this well-adapted rotavirus strain yields about 10^7 to 10^8 infectious viral particles/mL.

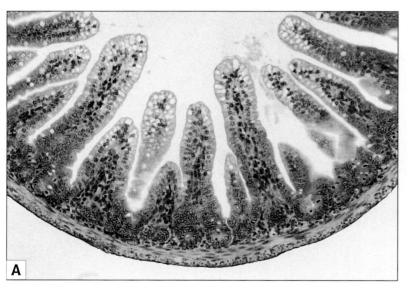

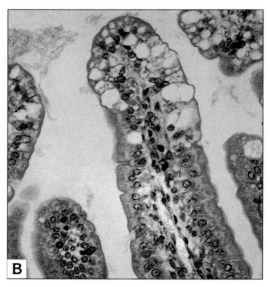

FIGURE 5-10 Histopathologic effects of rotavirus infection on murine intestinal epithelium. Rotavirus infection of the intestinal epithelium occurs in many mammalian and avian species in addition to humans. The characteristic lesions are similar in most species. In this figure, homologous infection of murine intestine is shown. **A** and **B**, The most striking abnormality in the murine intestine is vacuolation of the mature villus tip cells. (*Courtesy of* P. Offit, MD.)

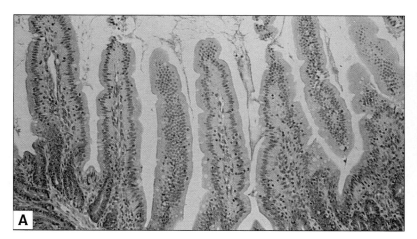

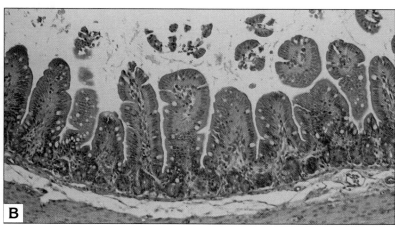

FIGURE 5-11 **A** and **B**, Histopathologic effects of rotavirus infection on rabbit ileum. Another typical finding of rotavirus infection is blunting and denuding of villi, which can be seen clearly if one compares the uninfected control ileum of a rabbit (*panel 11A*) with ileum 18 hours after infection (*panel 11B*). In addition to blunting, one may also see an increased mononuclear infiltrate in the mucosa. Polymorphonuclear leukocytes and epithelial ulceration is uncommon. (*Courtesy of* M. Conner, DVM.)

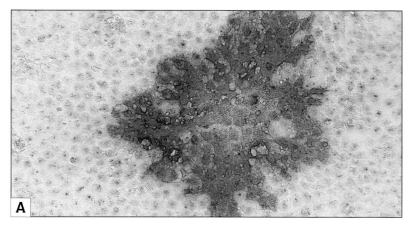

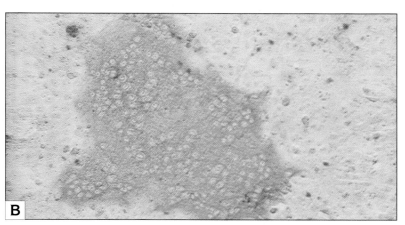

FIGURE 5-12 Tissue cultures of group B rotavirus, stained with immunochemical techniques. Human and animal rotaviruses may be classified in groups A to E. Group A infections are the leading cause of severe diarrhea in infants and young children. Group B and C infections occur less frequently and have different epidemiologic profiles. For instance, group B viruses have caused epidemic adult diarrheal disease in China. Group B viruses also display an ability to mediate cell fusion, a property not associated with other rotaviruses. **A**, A group B rotavirus infected a monolayer of simian kidney cells (MA104) and was detected by immunochemical means using a monoclonal antibody specific for group B VP6 protein. Fusion of monolayer cells has resulted in the formation of a giant cell syncytium. **B**, Group B rotavirus has infected African green monkey kidney cells and was detected by hyperimmune serum directed at the human group B virus that caused disease in China. (*Courtesy of* E. Mackow, PhD.)

Clinical and epidemiologic features of rotavirus enteritis, by subgroup

	Group A	Group B	Group C
Epidemiology	Common cause of endemic diarrhea in infants and young children Winter peak in temperate zones	Outbreaks in adults and older children reported from China	Sporadic episodes in young children
Signs/symptoms	Dehydrating diarrhea for several days Vomiting and fever usual	Severe watery diarrhea for 3–5 days	Similar to group A
Diagnosis	Immunoassay, EM, PAGE, rt-PCR	EM, PAGE, rt-PCR	EM, PAGE, rt-PCR

EM—electron microscopy; PAGE—polyacrylamide gel electrophoresis; rt-PCR—reverse transcriptase and polymerase chain reaction genomic amplification.

FIGURE 5-13 Clinical and epidemiologic features of rotavirus enteritis, by subgroup. Rotaviruses are categorized into groups as determined by group antigens located on viral protein VP6. These groups cause human disease but are genetically quite distinct [3].

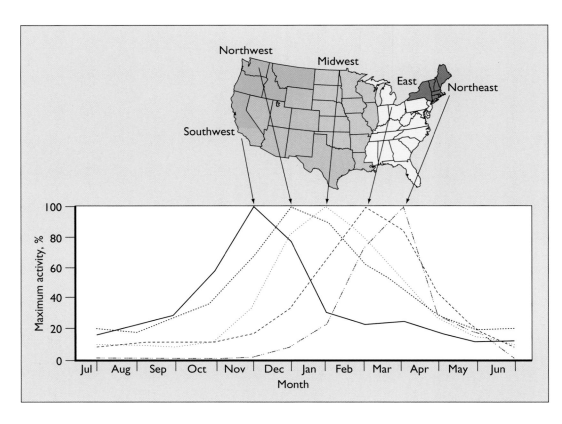

FIGURE 5-14 Regional rotavirus activity by month in the United States between 1984 and 1988. Data were collected in a 5-year retrospective survey of sentinel laboratories in the United States, covering the period 1984 to 1988. Results showed that rotavirus infections occur as epidemics predominantly in the winter months. The earliest outbreaks of each season tend to be in the western states in the fall months, with a wave-like progression across the continent toward the northeast, where the peak incidence of outbreaks is in the late winter and early spring.(*Adapted from* LeBaron *et al.* [4].)

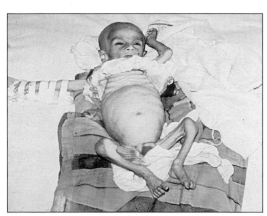

FIGURE 5-15 Acute rotavirus gastroenteritis in a child. Viral gastroenteritis occurs worldwide, but mortality is unusual in developed regions with ready access to medical care. In many areas of Asia, Africa, and Latin America, this illness is an important cause of mortality in children under the age of 2 years. Rotavirus is the most frequent cause of severe gastroenteritis in this population. The severity of the illness is accentuated by preexisting malnutrition. This photograph is typical of such a child suffering acute rotavirus gastroenteritis. (*Courtesy of* H. Greenberg, MD)

Clinical features of group A rotavirus gastroenteritis in children

Symptoms	Frequency, %
Diarrhea	98
Diarrhea > 10 × daily	28
Vomiting	87
Vomiting > 5 × daily	51
Fever	84
Abdominal pain	18
Gross blood in stool	1
Hospitalization	39

FIGURE 5-16 Clinical features of group A rotavirus gastroenteritis in children. Rotavirus-induced gastroenteritis in infants and young children most commonly presents with watery diarrhea, fever, vomiting, and occasional dehydration. There is no blood or mucus in the stools; leukocytes may be detected in the feces of a small percentage of patients. (*Adapted from* Uhnoo *et al.* [5].)

Clinical features of rotavirus gastroenteritis in adults

Symptoms	Adults, *n*
Diarrhea	14
Abdominal cramps	11
Vomiting	4
Upper respiratory symptoms	3
Fever	2
Nausea	1

FIGURE 5-17 Clinical features of rotavirus gastroenteritis in adults. Rotaviruses are less commonly a cause of severe diarrhea in adults than in infants and young children. Outbreaks of rotavirus gastroenteritis in adults have been reported in nursing home and hospital settings. Adult contacts of children with symptomatic rotavirus infection usually develop asymptomatic infection and shed rotavirus in their feces. In this prospective family study, of the 11 patients having abdominal cramps, three of these subjects had no diarrhea. The three patients with upper respiratory tract symptoms had no gastrointestinal symptoms. (*Adapted from* Wenman *et al.* [6].)

Appearance of rotavirus-specific immune markers after acute gastrointestinal infection in infants			
	Serum	**Stool**	**Duodenal fluid**
IgM	6 days	—	6 days
IgG	1 mo	2 wks	1 mo
IgA	4 mos	2 wks	4 mos

FIGURE 5-18 Appearance of rotavirus-specific immune markers after acute gastrointestinal infection in infants. Humoral immune response to rotavirus infection in humans is characterized by the appearance in serum and duodenal fluid of rotavirus-specific IgM followed by IgG and IgA. There are few data on the virus-specific cellular immune response to rotavirus infection in humans. Infants and young children mount a rotavirus-specific Th-cell response in blood lymphocytes after acute rotavirus gastroenteritis.

Composition of oral rehydration solutions		
	WHO-ORS, g/L H₂0	**Reduced-osmolarity ORS, g/L H₂0**
Sodium	90	60
Potassium	20	20
Chloride	80	50
Citrate	10	10
Glucose	111	84
Osmolarity	311	224

ORS—oral rehydration solution; WHO—World Health Organization.

FIGURE 5-19 Composition of oral rehydration solutions (ORS). Oral rehydration therapy with the standard World Health Organization (WHO) rehydration formula effectively prevents dehydration during rotavirus diarrhea. The WHO-ORS consists of NaCl, 3.5 g/L of water; $NaHCO_3$, 2.5; KCl, 1.5; and glucose, 20. Recently, use of reduced-osmolarity oral rehydration salt solutions has been shown to have a beneficial effect on the clinical course of acute diarrhea. Rice-based and amino acid-containing ORS formulations are not generally recommended because they have no clinical advantage over WHO-ORS for children with acute noncholera diarrhea [7].

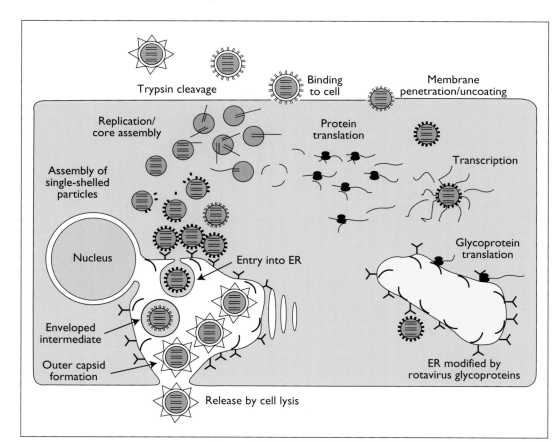

FIGURE 5-20 Life cycle of rotavirus. Numerous steps have been identified as potential targets for disease-preventing vaccines. It is known that antibodies may prevent trypsin cleavage, which is required for membrane penetration; prevent binding to the cell surface; or prevent viral uncoating and release of the viral genomic material in the cytoplasm. Many of the specific mechanisms that accomplish transcription, translation, and assembly are not yet known in detail. (ER—endoplasmic reticulum.) (*Adapted from* Dormitzer and Greenberg [8].)

CALICIVIRUSES (INCLUDING NORWALK VIRUS)

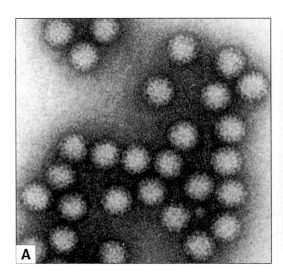
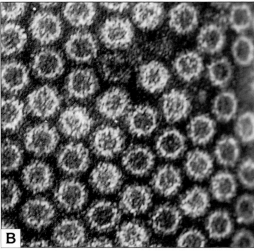

A

B

FIGURE 5-21 **A** and **B**, Negative-stained transmission electron micrographs of Norwalk virus. This virus is a member of the viral family Caliciviridae, so named because of the cuplike surface depression seen by electron microscopy, which give it the appearance of a chalice. (*From* Estes and Hardy [9]; with permission.)

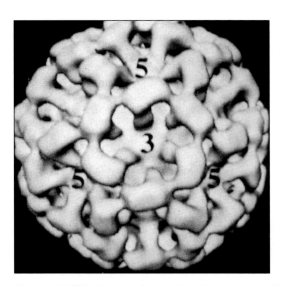

Figure 5-22 Three-dimensional structure of recombinant Norwalk virus particles viewed along the isosahedral threefold axis. This is a complete reconstruction of a recombinant Norwalk virus–like particle. The Norwalk genome, which has been cloned, can be expressed in laboratory systems, yielding large amounts of Norwalk virus protein, which self-assemble into the structure shown in this figure. This particle contains 90 dimeric copies of the single structural protein. (*Courtesy of* B.V.V. Prasad; *from* Estes and Hardy [9]; with permission.)

Clinical and epidemiologic features of calicivirus infections	
Epidemiology	Epidemics of vomiting and diarrhea in older children and adults
	Occurs in families, communities, nursing homes, cruise ships
	Often associated with shellfish, other food, water
Signs/symptoms	Vomiting, diarrhea, fever, myalgia, headache
	Lasts 24–48 hours
Diagnosis	Immunoassay, immune electron microscopy, rt-PCR

rt-PCR—reverse transcription and polymerase chain reaction genomic amplification.

FIGURE 5-23 Clinical and epidemiologic features of calicivirus infections. This group of viruses is responsible for a large number of previously undiagnosed outbreaks. The diversity and prevalence of these agents is becoming better known with more widespread use of new molecular tools for diagnosis and epidemiologic studies.

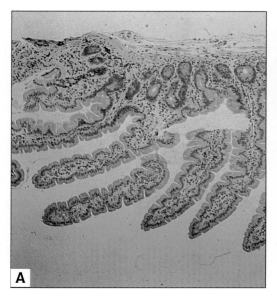
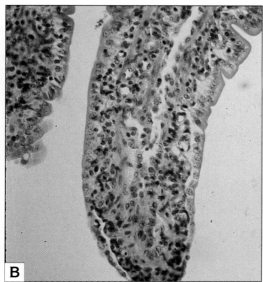
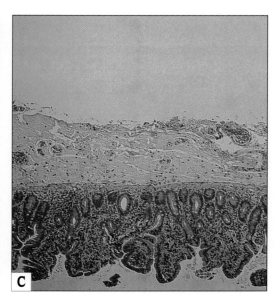

FIGURE 5-24 Intestinal histopathology of acute Norwalk virus infection. **A,** Normal intestinal (duodenal) villi prior to infection. **B,** Acute Norwalk virus infection showing a disorganized epithelium on broad flattened villi. The virus selectively infects the surface epithelial cells. **C,** Acute infection at higher magnification showing vacuolization of epithelial cells and mononuclear inflammatory cell infiltration. These abnormalities return to normal within 2 weeks. Brush border enzymatic activity may lead to mild malabsorption of lactose and fat during this period. (*From* Agus *et al.* [10]; with permission.)

ENTERIC ADENOVIRUSES

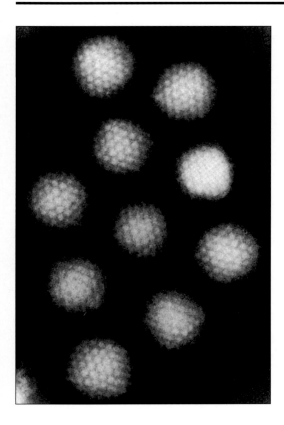

FIGURE 5-25 Negative-stained electron micrograph of enteric adenovirus type 40. Enteric adenoviruses, like rotaviruses and caliciviruses, lack a lipid envelope. The repeating protein structure gives a characteristic appearance by electron microscopy. Measuring 65 to 80 nm in diameter, these particles are approximately the same size as rotavirus (70 nm) but larger than caliciviruses (~ 30 nm). The genomic material of adenoviruses is DNA, unlike rotavirus of caliciviruses, which contain RNA. (Bar=50 nm) (*Courtesy of* W.D. Cubitt; *from* Hermann and Blacklow [11]; with permission.)

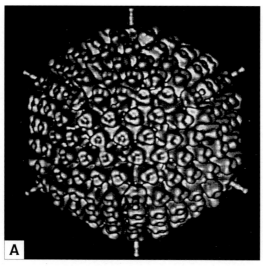

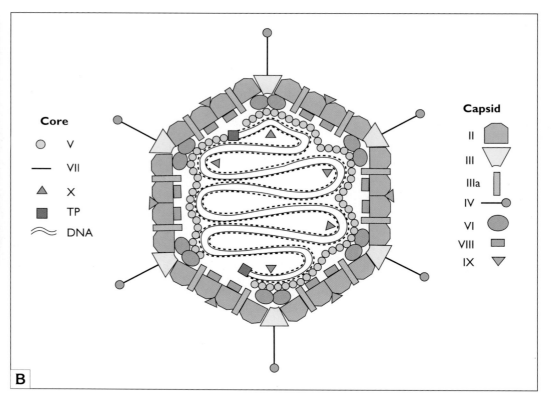

FIGURE 5-26 Models of the adenovirus virion. **A,** A three-dimensional image reconstruction of the intact adenovirus particle viewed along an icosahedral threefold axis. **B,** Diagrammatic cross-section of the adenovirus particle based on current understanding of its polypeptide components and DNA. No real section of the icosahedral virion would contain all components. Virion constituents are designated by their polypeptide numbers with the exception of the terminal protein (TP). (*From* Stewart *et al.* [12]; with permission.)

Clinical and epidemiologic features of enteric adenovirus infections	
Epidemiology	Endemic diarrhea in infants and young children
Signs/symptoms	Diarrhea for 5–12 days Vomiting and fever
Diagnosis	Immunoassay, electron microscopy with PAGE, rt-PCR

PAGE—polyacrylamide gel electrophoresis; rt-PCR reverse transcription and polymerase chain reaction genomic amplification.

FIGURE 5-27 Clinical and epidemiologic features of enteric adenovirus infections. The clinical syndromes caused by enteric adenovirus infection and rotavirus infection of young children are quite similar. Adenovirus causes less severe dehydration.

ASTROVIRUSES

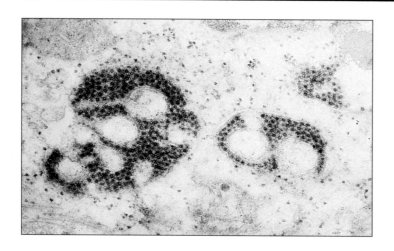

FIGURE 5-28 Astrovirus in tissue culture. Astroviruses have been noted to be important human pathogens, causing a gastroenteritis syndrome. Recent progress in the cultivation of these viruses *in vitro* will facilitate research into important areas of viral structure and function, including neutralization. The virus can be seen in this figure replicating within LLCMK2 cells. (*Courtesy of* L. Oshiro, MD, and S. Matsui, MD.)

Clinical features of astrovirus gastroenteritis

Age predilection	Usually affects children Reported in nursing homes
Signs/symptoms	Watery diarrhea, usually for 2–3 days, sometimes longer
Diagnosis	Immunoassay, electron microscopy, rt-PCR

rt-PCR—reverse transcription and polymerase chain reaction genomic amplification.

FIGURE 5-29 Clinical features of astrovirus infections. Astrovirus has only recently been characterized as a human pathogen. The characterization of a typical clinical syndrome and the importance of this agent as a cause of viral gastroenteritis will emerge more fully in the future.

Epidemiologic features of astrovirus infections

Worldwide distribution
Primarily affects children
  Outbreaks in elderly and immunocompromised patients also
Antibody acquisition in childhood
Antibody prevalence 75% by age 10 yrs
  Antibody to serotypes 1–5 in US gamma globulin pools
  Serotype 1 predominance in Oxford region of United Kingdom
Fecal–oral transmission (person-to-person, contaminated food/water, fomites[?])
Peak incidence in winter in northern temperate regions

FIGURE 5-30 Epidemiologic features of astrovirus infections. (*Adapted from* Matsui [13].)

REFERENCES

1. Kapikiam AZ: Acute viral gastroenteritis. *Prev Med* 1974, 3:535–542.

2. Yeager M, Dryden KA, Olson NH, *et al.*: Three-dimensional structure of rhesus rotavirus by cryoelectron microscopy and image reconstruction. *J Cell Biol* 1990, 110:2133–2144.

3. Blacklow NR, Greenberg HB: Viral gastroenteritis. *N Engl J Med* 1991, 325(4):252–264.

4. LeBaron CW, Lew J, Glass RI, et al.: Annual rotavirus epidemic patterns in North America: Results of a 5-year retrospective survey of 88 centers in Canada, Mexico, and the United States. Rotavirus Study Group. *JAMA* 1990, 264:983.

5. Uhnoo I, Olding SE, Kreuger A: Clinical features of acute gastroenteritis associated with rotavirus, enteric adenoviruses, and bacteria. *Arch Dis Child* 1986, 61:732–738.

6. Wenman WM, Hinde D, Feltham S, Gurwith M: Rotavirus infection in adults: Results of a prospective family study. *N Engl J Med* 1979, 301:303–306.

7. Multicentre evaluation of reduced-osmolarity oral rehydration salts solution: International Study Group on reduced-osmolarity ORS solutions. *Lancet* 1995, 345:282.

8. Dormitzer P, Greenberg HB: Rotavirus gastroenteritis: Basic facts and prospects for prevention and treatment. *In* Root RK, Sande MA (eds.): *Viral Infections*. New York: Churchill Livingstone, 1993.

9. Estes MK, Hardy ME: Norwalk virus and other enteric caliciviruses. *In* Blaser MJ, Ravdin JI, Smith PD, *et al.* (eds.): *Infections of the Gastrointestinal Tract*. New York: Raven Press; 1995:1009–1035.

10. Agus SG, Dolin R, Wyatt RG, *et al.*: Acute infectious nonbacterial gastroenteritis: Intestinal histopathology: Histologic and enzymatic alterations during illness produced by the Norwalk agent in man. *Ann Intern Med* 1973, 79:18–25.

11. Hermann JE, Blacklow NR: Enteric adenoviruses. *In* Blaser MJ, Ravdin JI, Smith PD, *et al.* (eds.): *Infections of the Gastrointestinal Tract*. New York: Raven Press; 1995:1047–1055.

12. Stewart PL, Burnett RM, Cyrklaff M, Fuller SD: Image reconstruction reveals the complex molecular organization of adenovirus. *Cell* 1991, 67:145–154.

13. Matsui SM: Astroviruses. *In* Blaser MJ, Ravdin JI, Smith PD, *et al.* (eds.): *Infections of the Gastrointestinal Tract*. New York: Raven Press; 1995:1035–1047.

SELECTED BIBLIOGRAPHY

Bellamy AR, Both GW: Molecular biology of rotaviruses. *Adv Virus Res* 1990, 38(1):1–43.

Blacklow NR, Greenberg HB: Viral gastroenteritis. *N Engl J Med* 1991, 325:252–264.

Fields BN, Knipe DM, Howley PM (eds.): *Fields Virology*, 3rd ed. Philadelphia: Lippincott-Raven; 1996.

Herrmann JE, Taylor DN, Echeverria P, Blacklow NR: Astroviruses as a cause of gastroenteritis in children. *N Engl J Med* 1991, 324:1757–1760.

Yeager M, Dryden KA, Olson NH, *et al.*: Three-dimensional structure of rhesus rotavirus by cryoelectron microscopy and image reconstruction. *J Cell Biol* 1990, 110:2133–2144.

CHAPTER 6

Parasitic Enteritis

Rosemary Soave

Common clinical syndromes caused by parasitic infections in the gastrointestinal tract

Diarrhea
1. Bloody diarrhea (dysentery)
   Entamoeba histolytica
   Balantidium coli
   Trichuris trichiura
   Schistosoma spp
   Strongyloides stercoralis
2. Watery diarrhea
   Giardia lamblia
   Cryptosporidium parvum
   Cyclospora spp
     (*Cyanobacterium*-like bodies)
   Isospora belli
   Microsporidium spp

Abdominal pain (± diarrhea)
Ascaris lumbricoides
Strongyloides stercoralis
Hookworm
Schistosoma spp
Taenia spp

Failure to thrive (weight-for-height deficit)
1. Parasitic infections frequently
   with diarrhea
     Giardia lamblia
     Trichuris trichiura
     Entamoeba histolytica
     Cryptosporidium parvum
     Isospora belli
2. Parasitic infections frequently
   without diarrhea
     Ascaris lumbricoides
     Strongyloides stercoralis
     Hookworm
     Taenia spp

Gastrointestinal blood loss/anemia
Hookworm (*Necator, Ancylostoma*)

FIGURE 6-1 Common clinical syndromes caused by parasitic infections in the gastrointestinal tract. (*Adapted from* Oberhelman and Krogstad [1].)

PROTOZOA

Giardia lamblia

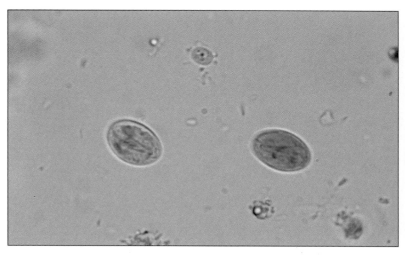

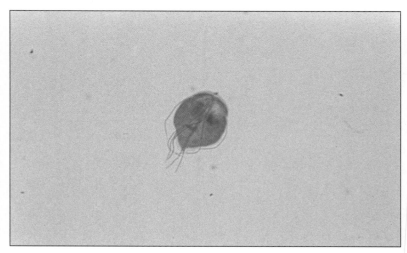

FIGURE 6-2 *Giardia lamblia* cysts. *G. lamblia* (also called *G. intestinalis* or *duodenalis*) cysts are oval, thin-walled, and approximately 8 to 14 × 7 to 10 μm. In the infective form of the protozoan, cysts are formed in the large intestine and pass into the environment in the feces. (Iodine stain.) (*Courtesy of* M. Scaglia, MD.)

FIGURE 6-3 *Giardia lamblia* trophozoite. Trophozoites are pear-shaped, bilaterally symmetrical bodies and measure 9 to 21 × 5 to 15 μm. Characteristic structures include four pairs of flagella and two nuclei in the area of the sucking disc. Trophozoites move by oscillating about the long axis, producing motion said to resemble a falling leaf. (Giemsa stain.) (*Courtesy of* M. Scaglia, MD.)

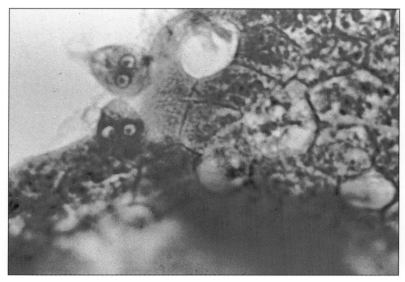

FIGURE 6-4 Peroral biopsy specimen showing *Giardia lamblia* trophozoites attached to the duodenal epithelium. (*Courtesy of* D. Heyneman, MD; *from* Zaiman [2]; with permission.)

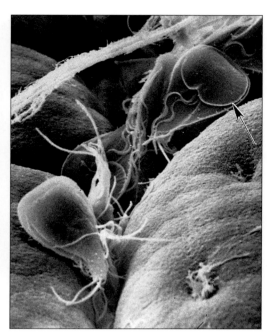

FIGURE 6-5
Scanning electron micrograph of *Giardia lamblia* trophozoites in a crevice over human jejunal villus. On the ventral surface of the organism, note the slightly concave attachment disc (*arrow*). The irregular dorsal surface of the *Giardia* is seen in the organism to the lower left. (× 2000.) (*Courtesy of* R. Owen, MD; *from* Pennsylvania *et al.* [3]; with permission.)

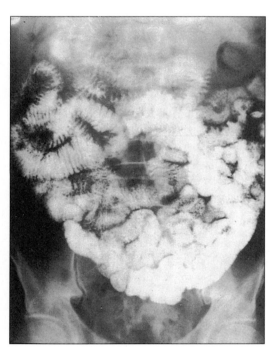

FIGURE 6-6 Barium follow-through radiograph in a man with chronic giardiasis and hypogammaglobulinemia, showing diffuse lymphoid nodular hyperplasia throughout the small intestine. Immunodeficiency states, particularly hypogammaglobulinemia and malnutrition, are apparently associated with increased susceptibility to giardiasis. (*From* Farthing [4]; with permission.)

Treatment of giardiasis

Drug	Adults	Children
Metronidazole	250 mg three times a day × 5–7 days	5 mg/kg three times a day × 7 days
Quinacrine	100 mg three times a day × 5–7 days	2 mg/kg three times a day × 7 days
Furazolidone	100 mg four times a day × 7–10 days	2 mg/kg four times a day × 10 days
Tinidazole	2 g × 1 dose	—
Paromomycin	25–30 mg/kg/d in 3 doses × 5–10 days	—

FIGURE 6-7 Treatment of giardiasis. The most commonly used agent to treat giardiasis is the nitroimidazole, metronidazole, despite its never having received a Food and Drug Administration indication for this use. Although quinacrine is considered the drug of choice by many practitioners, it is no longer being produced in the United States and is available only through the Centers for Disease Control and Prevention. The nitrofurantoin, furazolidone, is often used for children because it is available in a suspension form. Tinidazole is not licensed in the United States. Despite lower efficacy rates, paromomycin is often recommended for pregnant women with giardiasis because it is not absorbed from the gastrointestinal tract and thus may have negligible effects on the fetus; none of the other anti-*Giardia* agents are known to be safe for use in pregnant women. (*Adapted from* Hill [5].)

Entamoeba histolytica

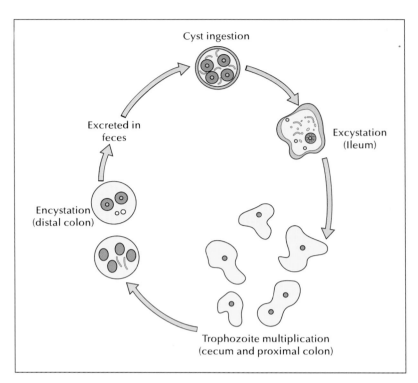

FIGURE 6-8 Life cycle of *Entamoeba histolytica*. Infection is initiated when the host ingests food or water contaminated with *E. histolytica* cysts. In the small intestine, excystation of the cysts results in liberation of the trophozoites, the tissue-invasive form of the parasite. Trophozoites multiply in the cecum and proximal colon. The low water content of the distal colon induces encystation, *ie*, transformation of trophozoites into cystic forms, with resultant expulsion of cysts into the environment.

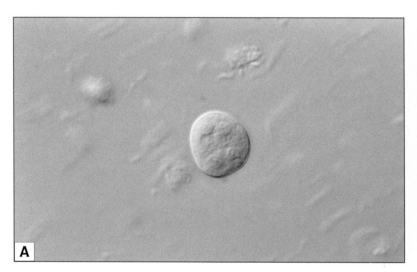

A

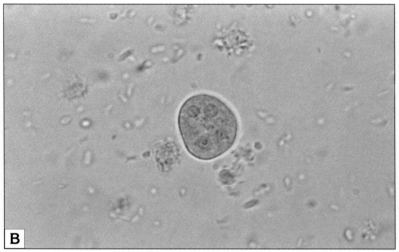

B

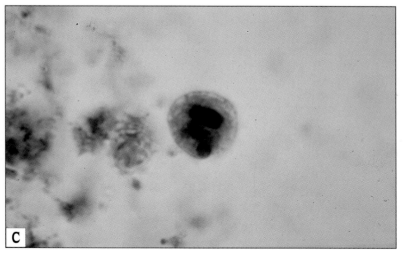

C

FIGURE 6-9 *Entamoeba histolytica* cysts. **A–C**, The environmentally resistant *E. histolytica* cyst is spherical or ovoid and 10 to 20 µm in diameter. Characteristic features include a hyaline wall (*panel 9A*), which is strongly refractive in unstained preparations, up to four nuclei (*panels 9A–C*), and rod-shaped chromatoid bodies seen best on stained preparations (*panel 9C*). (*Panel 9A*, Nomarski interference-contrast microscopy; *panel 9B*, iodine stain; *panel 9C*, hematoxylin stain.) (Panels 9A and 9B *courtesy of* M. Scaglia, MD.)

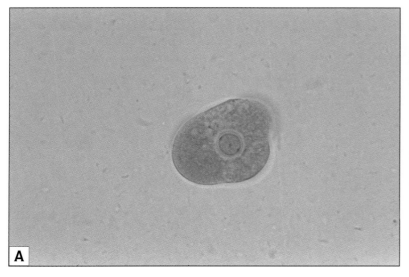

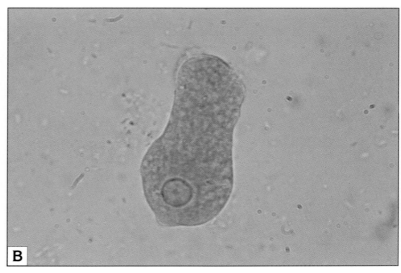

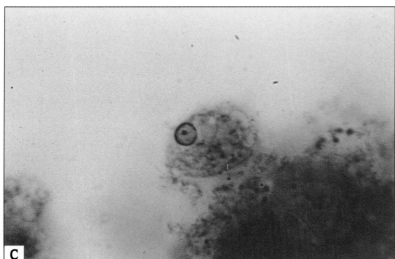

FIGURE 6-10 *Entamoeba histolytica* trophozoites. **A–C,** The trophozoites vary in diameter from 12 to 60 µm. Details of the eccentric nucleus, including the peripheral chromatin and prominent karyosome, are best seen on stained preparations (*panel 10C*). Trophozoites have directed motility that is mediated by pseudopodia, cytoplasmic protrusions that impart a torpedo-like shape (*panel 10B*). Motility can be enhanced in freshly passed fecal specimens by warming the slide. Trophozoites inhabit the large intestine where they feed on red blood cells, invade mucosa to form ulcers, and may disseminate through the bloodstream to other organs. (*Panels 10A and 10B*, iodine stain; *panel 10C*, trichrome stain.) (Panels 10A and 10B *courtesy of* M. Scaglia, MD; panel 10C *courtesy of* J.S. Tatz, MD; *from* Zaiman [2]; with permission.)

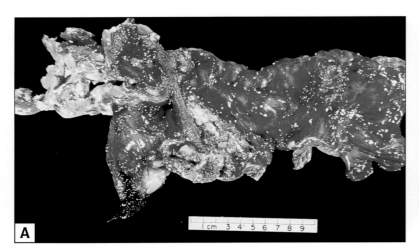

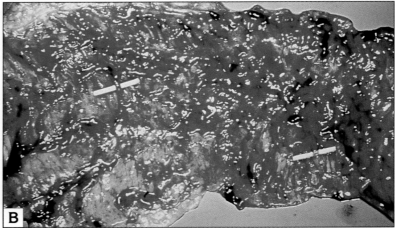

FIGURE 6-11 Gross anatomical findings of amebiasis at postmortem examination. The patient, a man aged 28 years, died unexpectedly after being diagnosed with rectal carcinoma metastatic to liver. **A,** Intestinal examination revealed ulceration of the entire cecum with appendiceal perforation and a 7-cm abscess. **B,** The distal 10 cm of colon was covered with ulcerations with heaped-up margins. (*continued*)

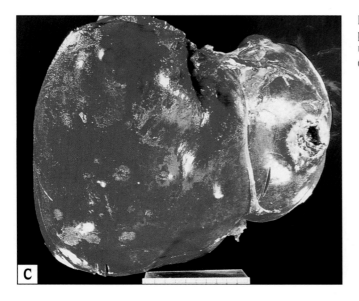

FIGURE 6-11 (*continued*) **C.** Seventy percent of the liver was replaced with pus-filled abscess cavities ranging from 1 to 14 cm in diameter. Intestinal ulcers and hepatic pus contained numerous *E. histolytica* trophozoites. No carcinoma was found. (*Courtesy of* W.D. Johnson, MD.)

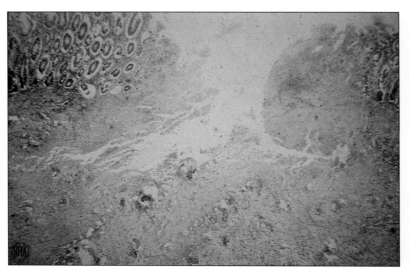

FIGURE 6-12 Colonic biopsy specimen from a patient with amebic dysentery. The specimen shows a flask-shaped ulcer with necrosis and an inflammatory exudate. This pathologic finding indicates amebic invasion into the submucosa. (Periodic acid–Schiff stain.)

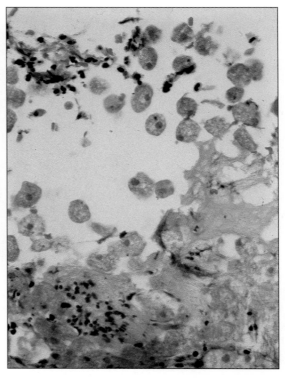

FIGURE 6-13 Numerous *Entamoeba histolytica* trophozoites in a colonic biopsy specimen from a patient with amebic colitis. The presence of intracytoplasmic red cells is indicative of intense phagocytic activity. (Hematoxylin-eosin stain.) (*From* the collection of B.H. Kean, MD.)

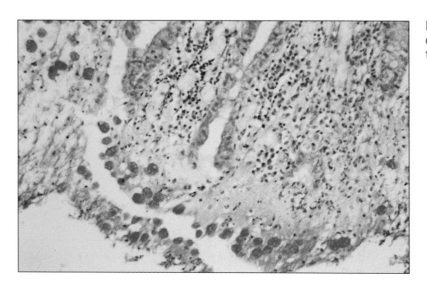

FIGURE 6-14 Rectal biopsy specimen from a patient with amebic colitis revealing numerous organisms. (Best carmine stain.) (*From* the collection of B.H. Kean, MD.)

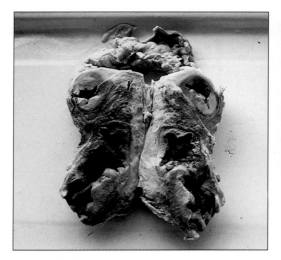

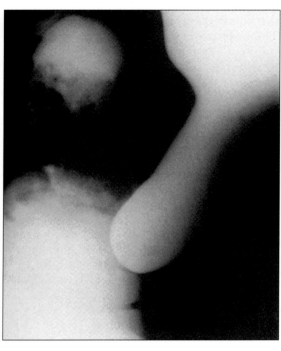

FIGURE 6-16 Barium enema examination revealing ameboma. Ameboma is an unusual presentation of amebic intestinal infection, occurring in < 1% of patients with invasive intestinal disease. This patient, a Filipino man aged 26 years, presented with asymptomatic left lower quadrant mass. The appearance on radiographs mimics a carcinoma, presenting as an "apple core–like" lesion. (*Courtesy of* the Department of Radiology, UCSD Medical Center; *from* Reed and Ravdin [6], with permission.)

FIGURE 6-15 Gross specimen of a cecal ameboma with bowel stricture. This chronic granulomatous lesion is a rare complication of amebic infection that is clinically indistinguishable from rectal carcinoma. (*From* the collection of B.H. Kean, MD.)

Nonpathogenic amebae

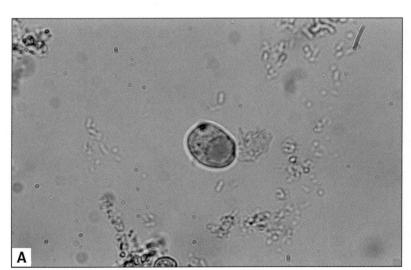

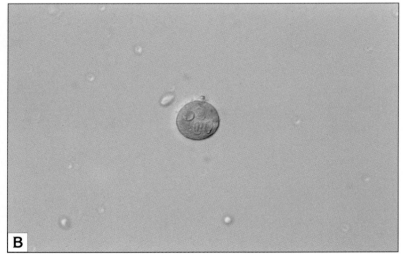

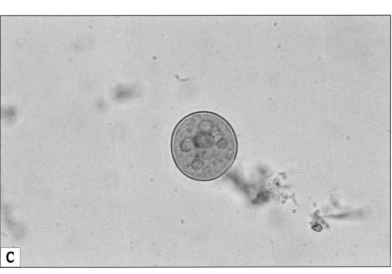

FIGURE 6-17 Nonpathogenic, commensal amebas in human feces. **A–C,** *Iodamoeba bütschlii* (*panel 17A*), *Entamoeba hartmanni* (*panel 17B*), and *Entamoeba coli* (*panel 17C*) are examples of nonpathogenic, commensal amebas that are often found in fecal specimens. Cysts (as shown) and/or trophozoites may be present. Although treatment for these commensal organisms is not recommended, they must be distinguished from pathogenic *E. histolytica*, which does require prompt treatment. (All, iodine stain.) (*Courtesy of* M. Scaglia, MD.)

Blastocystis hominis

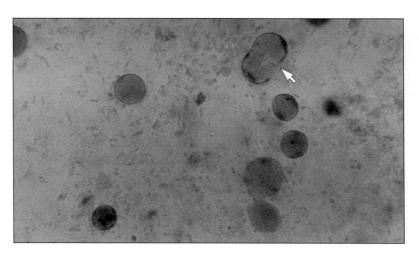

FIGURE 6-18 *Blastocystis hominis* on fecal smear. This organism, previously considered a yeast, has now been reclassified as a protozoan. The clinical significance of finding this frequently detected organism in fecal specimens is controversial. As shown on the fecal smear, organisms are generally round, approximately 6 to 40 μm, and they reproduce by binary fission (*arrow*). (Trichrome stain.)

Cryptosporidium

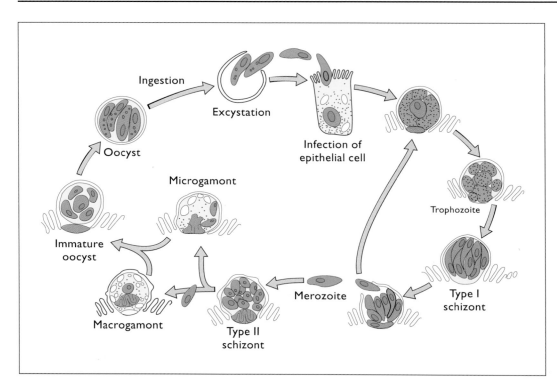

FIGURE 6-19 Monoxenous life cycle of *Cryptosporidium.* On excystation, infective sporozoites implant on intestinal epithelium and develop into trophozoites. Asexual multiplication results in the formation of merozoites enclosed within a schizont. On their release, merozoites either may reinfect the intestinal epithelium and reinitiate merogony, or they may initiate the sexual phase, which includes gametogony, fertilization, and oocyst formation. The newly formed oocyst is immediately infective to the same host.

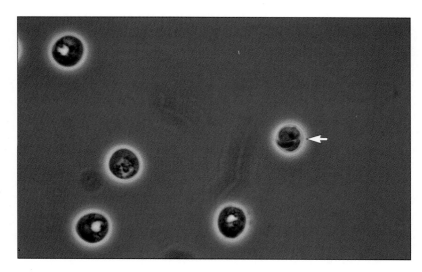

FIGURE 6-20 Suspension of *Cryptosporidium* oocysts purified from infected human feces. Oocysts are approximately 4 μm in diameter and contain four infective sporozoites; two are visible in the oocyst on the right (*arrow*). (Phase-contrast microscopy, × 1000.)

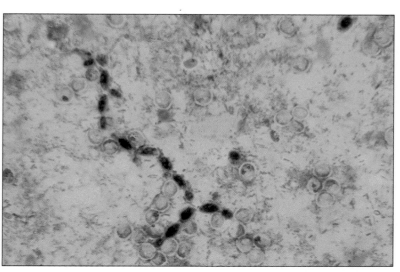

FIGURE 6-21 Four comma-shaped, motile, infective sporozoites released from a *Cryptosporidium* oocyst. Excystation is stimulated by trypsin, bile acids, and warm temperatures. (Phase-contrast microscopy, × 630.)

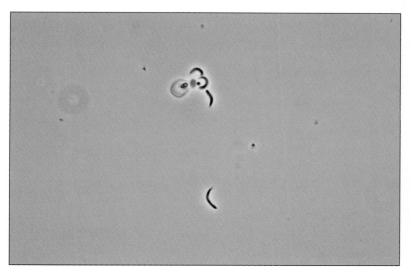

FIGURE 6-22 Modified Kinyoun-stained fecal smear from an immunocompetent traveler returning from Mexico shows cryptosporidia. Acid-fast (*red*) cryptosporidia can be easily distinguished from yeasts (*green*) with this stain. (× 630.)

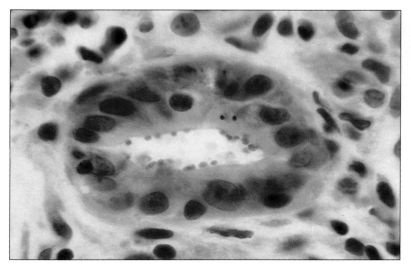

FIGURE 6-23 Colonic biopsy specimen from an AIDS patient with severe, chronic watery diarrhea. Numerous cryptosporidia are seen adhering to the epithelial surface. (Giemsa stain; × 630.)

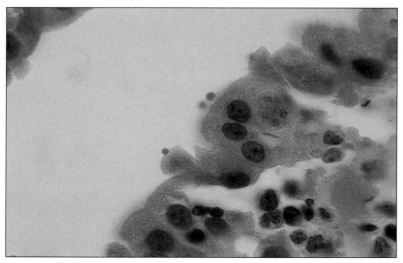

FIGURE 6-24 Section of a gallbladder removed from a patient with cryptosporidial enteritis. Round, blue-staining cryptosporidia are attached to the gallbladder epithelium. The tissue is edematous, inflamed, and necrotic in parts. Tissue autolysis with loss of organisms often makes diagnosis of biliary cryptosporidiosis difficult. (Giemsa stain; × 400.)

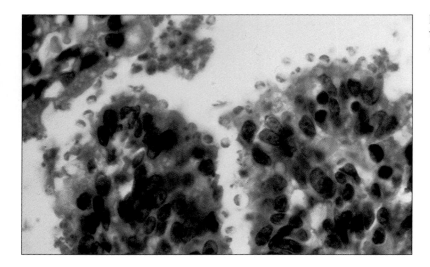

FIGURE 6-25 Multiple cryptosporidial organisms infecting the surface epithelium of the ileum of a *rnu/rnu* athymic rat. (*From* Gardner *et al.* [7]; with permission.)

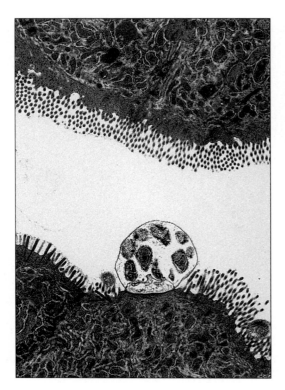

FIGURE 6-26
Electron micrograph of a cryptosporidial schizont attached to the brush border of small intestinal epithelium from a patients with AIDS. (× 10,000.)

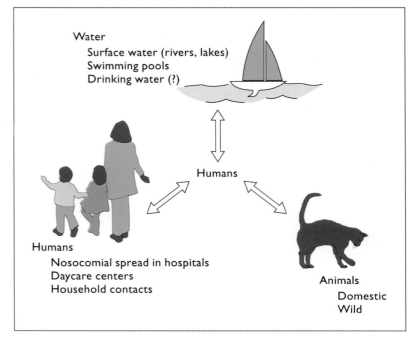

Water
    Surface water (rivers, lakes)
    Swimming pools
    Drinking water (?)

Humans

Humans
    Nosocomial spread in hospitals
    Daycare centers
    Household contacts

Animals
    Domestic
    Wild

FIGURE 6-27 Transmission patterns of *Cryptosporidium*. Initially, transmission of *Cryptosporidium* was thought to be primarily zoonotic, from animals to humans. Recent, well-documented water-borne and nosocomial outbreaks of infection indicate that zoonotic transmission of *Cryptosporidium*, though important, is not as common as spread via contaminated water and from person-to-person contact. In addition to spreading infection to other persons, humans also may be responsible for contaminating water (swimming pool and wave-pool outbreaks) and for spread of infection to animals. Chlorination of pools is ineffective for killing *Cryptosporidium*. Transmission of *Cryptosporidium* via drinking water in a nonepidemic situation has not as yet been demonstrated. A recent outbreak of cryptosporidiosis in Maine traced to consumption of contaminated apple cider was the first documentation of food-borne transmission.

Water-borne outbreaks of cryptosporidiosis

Location	Cases, *n*	Source
San Antonio, TX (1984)	346	Artesian well
Albuquerque, NM (1986)	78	Surface water
Carrollton, GA (1987)	13,000	Municipal water
Los Angeles, CA (1988)	44	Swimming pool
Medford and Talent, OR (1992)	5000	Municipal water
Milwaukee, WI (1993)	403,000	Municipal water
Dane County, WI (1993)	85	Swimming pools
Cape May, NJ (1994)	135	Lake

FIGURE 6-28 Water-borne outbreaks of cryptosporidiosis. During the period 1981 to 1992, 345 water-borne outbreaks resulting in 85,061 cases of illness and seven deaths were reported in the United States. An etiologic agent was identified in more than half of the outbreaks. *Giardia lamblia* or *Cryptosporidium parvum* was identified as the etiologic agent in 53% of the outbreaks in which an etiology was established. In 1993, contamination of the drinking water system with *Cryptosporidium* in Milwaukee, Wisconsin, is estimated to have resulted in more than 400,000 cases of watery diarrhea, 4000 hospitalizations, and approximately 100 deaths. This contamination is the largest water-borne outbreak to have been reported in the United States since 1920, when record keeping began.

Isospora belli

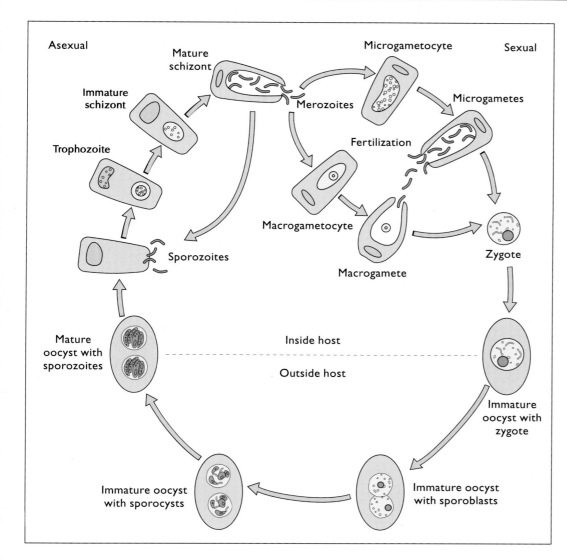

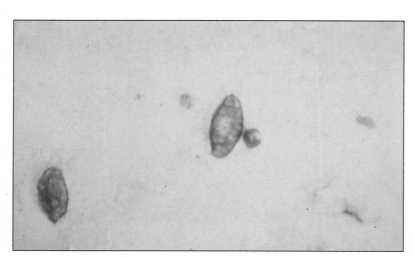

FIGURE 6-29 Life cycle of *Isospora belli*. Ingested oocysts release their sporozoites in the duodenum and small intestine. Sporozoites invade the epithelial cells and multiply asexually (schizogony or merogony) to produce merozoites. The latter either reinfect the intestine or undergo sexual differentiation to form micro- and macrogametocytes. Fertilization results in formation of oocysts, which are expelled into the environment where they mature and become infective. Oocysts are very resistant and may persist in the environment for long periods. (*Adapted from* Sun [8].)

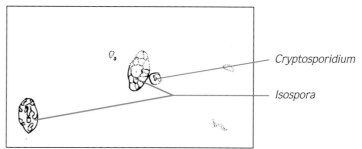

FIGURE 6-30 Fecal smear from an AIDS patient who was dually infected with *Cryptosporidium* and *Isospora*. (Modified Kinyoun acid-fast stain; × 450.) (*Courtesy of* M. Boncy.)

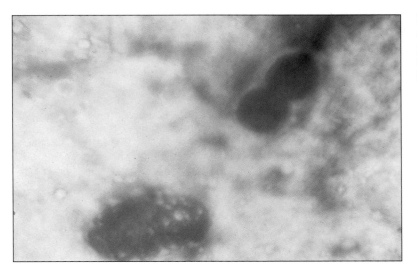

FIGURE 6-31 An immature (*bottom*) and a fully sporulated, mature (*top*) *Isospora belli* oocyst in the feces of an infected AIDS patient. The mature, infective oocyst contains two sporocysts, each of which, in turn, contains four sporozoites. (Modified Kinyoun stain; × 650.) (*Courtesy of* M. Boncy.)

Cyclospora

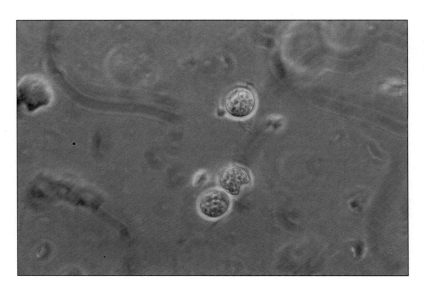

FIGURE 6-32 Fecal wet mount showing *Cyclospora* oocysts from an immunocompetent host with watery diarrhea. Morulae and refractile globules can be seen within the spherical cysts. (Phase-contrast microscopy; × 630.)

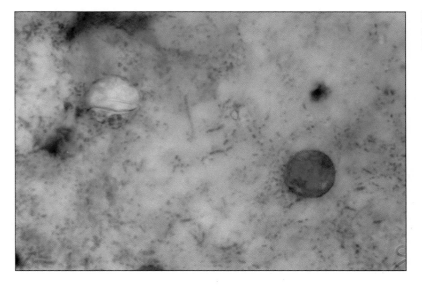

FIGURE 6-33 Fecal smear showing acid-fast and unstained *Cyclospora* oocysts. Variability in staining is typical for this organism. (Modified Kinyoun stain; × 1000.)

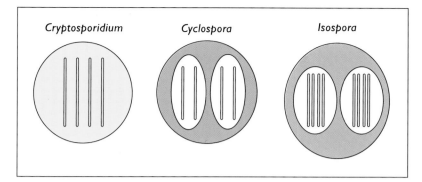

FIGURE 6-34 Comparative morphology of coccidian organisms. *Cryptosporidium*, *Cyclospora*, and *Isospora* are taxonomically related coccidians that differ by the number of sporocysts per oocyst and sporozoites per sporocyst. *Cryptosporidium* oocysts contain four sporozoites. *Isospora* oocysts have two sporocysts, each of which harbors four sporozoites. *Cyclospora* oocysts contain two sporozoites in each of two sporocysts.

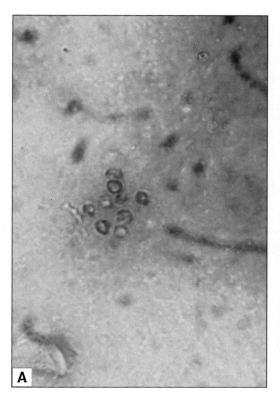

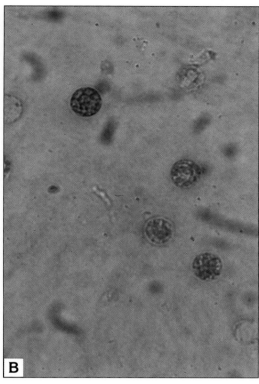

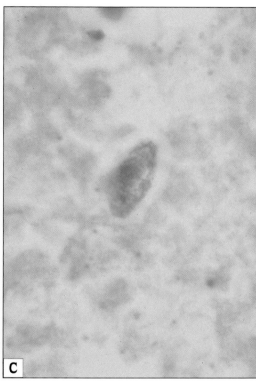

FIGURE 6-35 Comparative staining patterns of coccidians on fecal smears. **A–C,** *Cryptosporidium* (*panel 35A*), *Cyclospora* (*panel 35B*), and *Isospora* (*panel 35C*) are easily detected with acid-fast–stained smears of fecal specimens. The three organisms can be differentiated by their morphologic features: *Cryptosporidium* are 4 μm, round, and sometimes crescent-shaped; *Cyclospora* are 8 μm and round; and *Isospora* are elliptical, 23 to 33 μm long × 10 to 19 μm wide. Enteritis caused by the three organisms is clinically indistinguishable. (Modified Kinyoun stain; × 630.)

Microsporidium

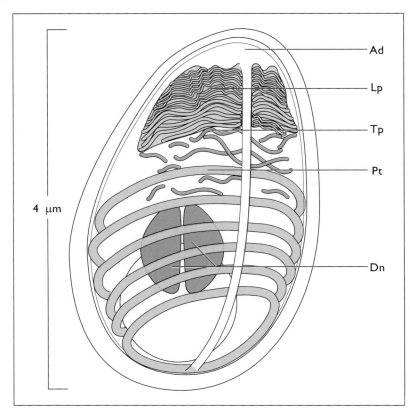

FIGURE 6-36 Diagram of the internal structure of a microsporidian spore. The spore coat has an outer electron-dense exospore and an inner, thicker, electron-lucent endospore. The extrusion apparatus (anchoring disk [Ad], polar tubule [Pt], lamellar polaroplast [Lp], and tubular polaroplast [Tp]) dominates the spore contents and is diagnostic of microsporidia. The number of polar tubule coils varies among species. (Dn—diplokaryon nuclei.) (*Adapted from* Cali and Owen [9].)

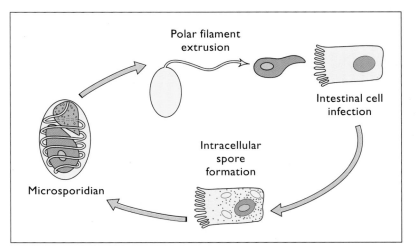

FIGURE 6-37 Life cycle of a microsporidia. Infection occurs when an ingested spore everts its polar tube and uses it like a syringe to inject the spore contents into an intestinal cell. New spores are formed intracellularly and released when the cell is sloughed.

Microsporidia species that infect humans, with clinical manifestations

	HIV-infected	Non–HIV-infected
Encephalitozoon		
E. cuniculi	Disseminated infection	Seizures
E. hellem	Keratoconjunctivitis, disseminated infection	—
E. intestinalis*	Enteritis, disseminated infection	—
Enterocytozoon bieneusi	Enteritis, cholangitis, respiratory infection (rare)	Enteritis[†]
Pleistophora spp	Myositis	Myositis
Nosema spp	—	Keratitis,[‡] disseminated infection
Microsporidium		
M. africanum	—	Corneal ulcer
M. ceylonensis	—	Corneal ulcer

*Formerly *Septata intestinalis*.

[†]Two cases, one immunocompetent.

[‡]Two cases, both immunocompetent.

FIGURE 6-38 Microsporidia species that infect humans with clinical manifestations. Microsporidia refers to members of the phylum Microspora, order Microsporidia. There are more than 1000 species within approximately 100 genera in this phylum. Four genera have been implicated in human infection. Species associated with human infection but not fitting these four genera have been grouped under the genus *Microsporidium*. Hundreds of cases of microsporidiosis involving HIV-infected patients have been reported. Of the 10 non–HIV-related cases of microsporidiosis that have been reported, only three were known to occur in immunocompetent individuals. (*Adapted from* Davis and Soave [10].)

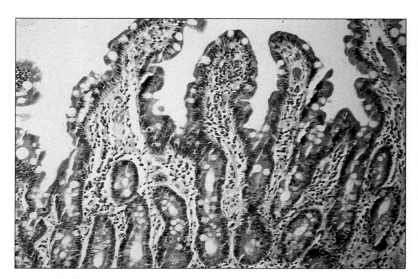

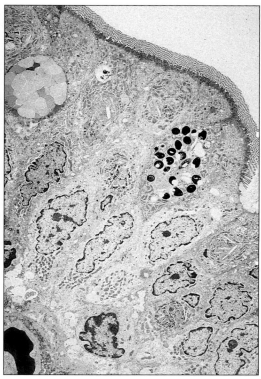

FIGURE 6-40
Electron micrograph showing *Enterocytozoon bieneusi* spores inside a small intestinal epithelial cell. (*Courtesy of* J.M. Orenstein, MD.)

FIGURE 6-39 Small intestinal biopsy specimen from an AIDS patient with chronic diarrhea due to *Enterocytozoon bieneusi*. Villi are blunted or bulbous shaped; cells in infected areas have vacuolated cytoplasm. Degenerating and necrotic cells are present in heavily infected areas. (Hematoxylin-eosin stain.)

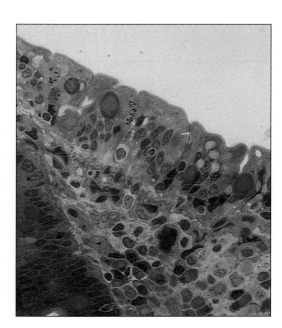

FIGURE 6-41
Duodenal biopsy specimen from a patient with AIDS, showing lightly stained oval parasites (*Enterocytozoon bieneusi*). Clusters of densely stained spores and intraepithelial lymphocytes are also apparent. (Methylene blue-azure II, basic fuchsin stain; × 640.) (*From* Orenstein [11]; with permission.)

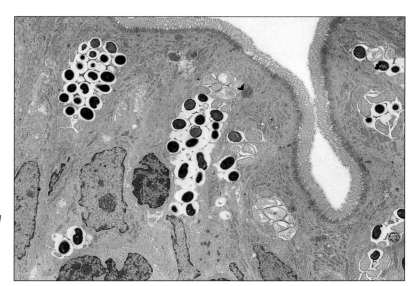

FIGURE 6-42 Transmission electron micrograph of a duodenal biopsy specimen from a patient with AIDS and *Encephalitozoon intestinalis* (previously called *Septata intestinalis*) infection. Septated vacuoles containing developing spores are especially concentrated in the apical cytoplasm of these duodenal enterocytes. (× 3330.) (*From* Orenstein *et al.* [12]; with permission.)

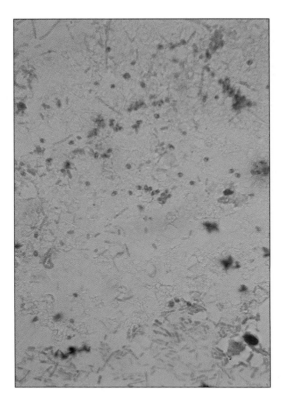

FIGURE 6-43
Fecal smear of microsporidian spores, stained with a modified trichrome stain. The chromotrope-based stain (modified trichrome) is useful in identifying the small (0.1 μm) microsporidian spores in fecal smears. The pink, beltlike stripe is a characteristic finding.

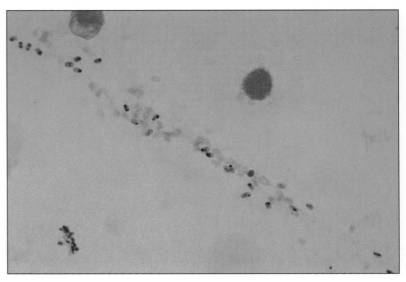

FIGURE 6-44 *Encephalitozoon hellem* spores in a Gram-Weigert–stained bronchoalveolar lavage specimen from an AIDS patient. The patient suffered cough, shortness of breath, and pulmonary infiltrates. *E. hellem* is a newly recognized microsporidian species that has been detected exclusively in AIDS patients. It is associated with pneumonia, keratoconjunctivitis, and renal disease but appears to spare the intestine.

NEMATODES

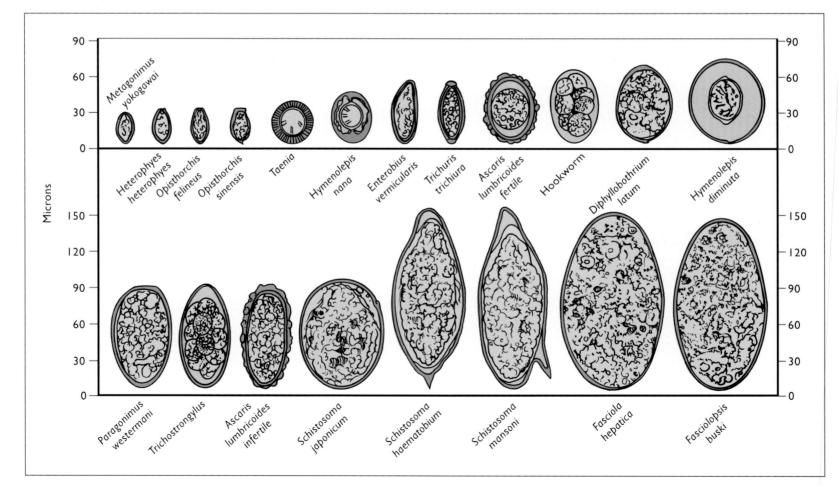

FIGURE 6-45 Relative sizes of helminth eggs. Diagnosis of helminthic infection most commonly depends on careful examination of stool or urine for eggs. (*Adapted from* Brooke and Melvin [13].)

Enterobius vermicularis

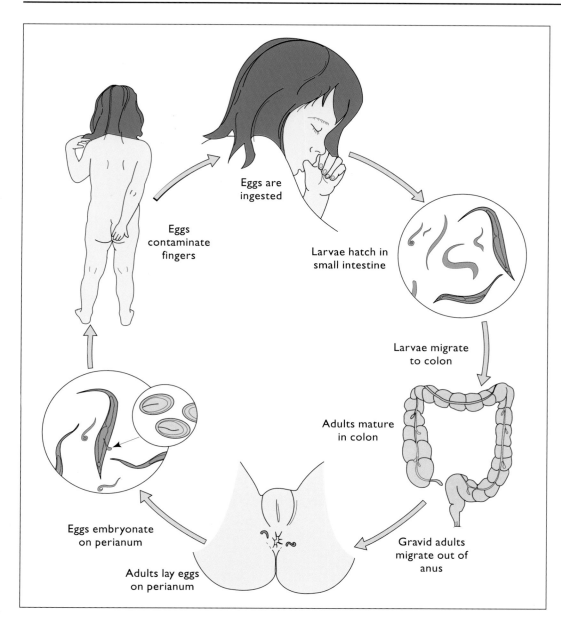

FIGURE 6-46 Life cycle of *Enterobius vermicularis*. Ingested pinworm eggs hatch into larvae in the small intestine and then migrate to the colon, where they mature into adult worms. At night, female worms migrate through the anus, onto the perianal skin, where they expel their eggs and then die. Anal itching predisposes to finger contamination with eggs, which are then easily ingested. (*Adapted from* Katz *et al.* [14].)

Eggs are
ingested

Eggs
contaminate
fingers

Larvae hatch in
small intestine

Larvae migrate
to colon

Adults mature
in colon

Eggs embryonate
on perianum

Adults lay eggs
on perianum

Gravid adults
migrate out of
anus

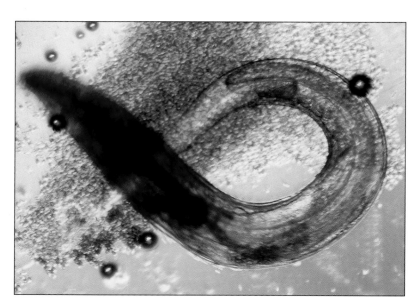

FIGURE 6-47 Pinworm spewing its eggs. *Enterobius vermicularis* is prevalent throughout the world but occurs more commonly in temperate climates. There are an estimated 42 million cases in the United States. The name is derived from the long, sharply pointed tail of the female worm. Gravid females contain an average of 11,000 ova, which they deposit in the perianal and perineal areas during their nightly migrations. Resultant anal pruritus is the most common symptom of this infection. (*From* the collection of B.H. Kean, MD.)

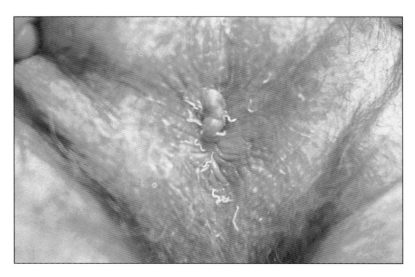

FIGURE 6-48 Multiple adult pinworms on perianal skin. (*Courtesy of* F. Ciferri; *from* Zaiman [2]; with permission.)

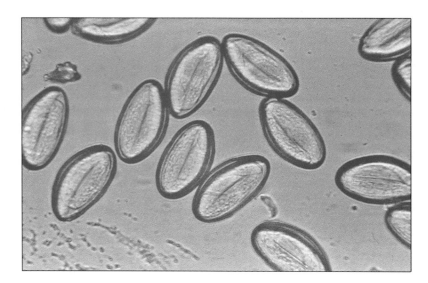

FIGURE 6-49 Clear adhesive tape applied to the perianal area of a child reveals numerous football-shaped *Enterobius* ova. Scratching the perianal area leads to hand contamination with infective ova and reinfection of the host. (*Courtesy of* E.D. Wagner, MD; *from* Zaiman [2]; with permission.)

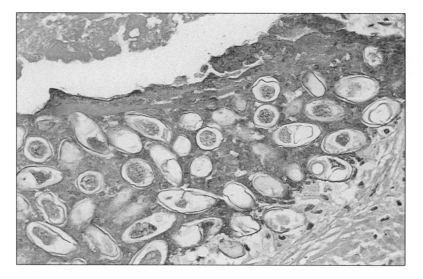

FIGURE 6-50 *Enterobius* eggs in an ovary. Rarely, female worms migrate into the vagina and gain entrance to the peritoneal cavity via the female reproductive system. Granuloma capsules form around the ova and may be responsible for chronic pelvic peritonitis. (*From* the collection of B.H. Kean, MD.)

Trichuris trichiura

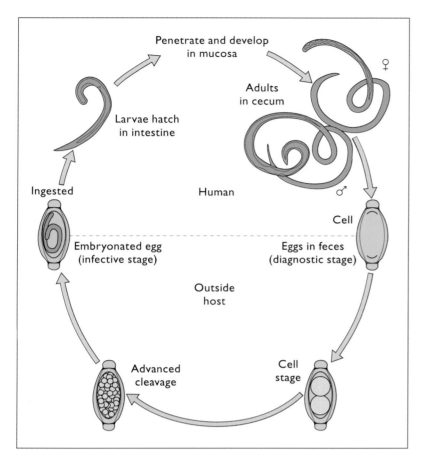

Penetrate and develop
in mucosa

Larvae hatch
in intestine

Adults
in cecum

Ingested

Human

♀

♂

Cell

Embryonated egg
(infective stage)

Eggs in feces
(diagnostic stage)

Outside
host

Advanced
cleavage

Cell
stage

FIGURE 6-51 Life cycle of *Trichuris trichiura* (whipworm). Infection occurs after ingestion of embryonated eggs. After 10 to 30 days in the small intestine, the larvae migrate to the large intestine (primarily cecum and appendix). They embed their anterior end into the mucosa and "whip" the free posterior end in the intestinal lumen. The mature adults lay eggs, which pass from feces into the soil, and mature if temperature and humidity are favorable.

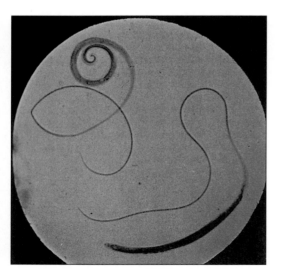

FIGURE 6-52 Adult *Trichuris* worms. (*From* Gopinath and Keystone [15]; with permission.)

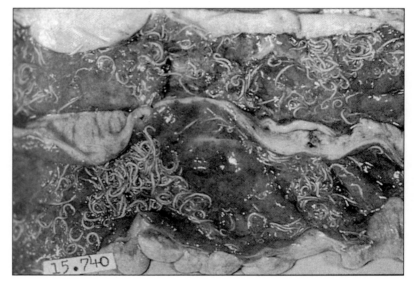

FIGURE 6-53 *Trichuris trichiura* in resected colon. (*From* Gopinath and Keystone [15]; with permission.)

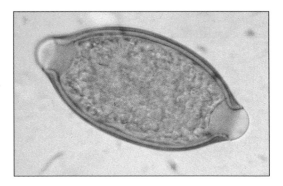

FIGURE 6-54 *Trichuris* eggs. Female worms in the human cecum shed between 3000 and 20,000 eggs per day. Embryonation occurs after the egg passes out into the environment and requires tropical temperatures. On average, an infective egg survives for less than 1 year. (*Courtesy of* M. Scaglia, MD.)

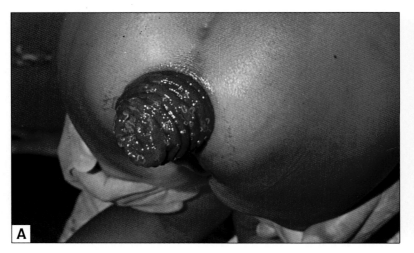

A

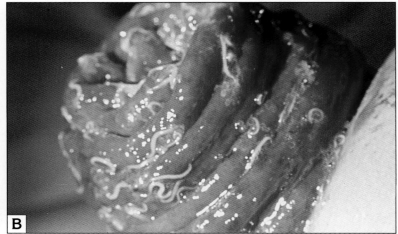

B

FIGURE 6-55 Prolapsed anus due to the presence of whipworm (*Trichuris trichiura*). **A**, Prolapsed rectum in a child. **B**, Close-up view of the adult whipworms on the prolapsed rectal mucosa. (*Courtesy of* F. Beltran; *from* Zaiman [2], with permission.)

Ascaris lumbricoides

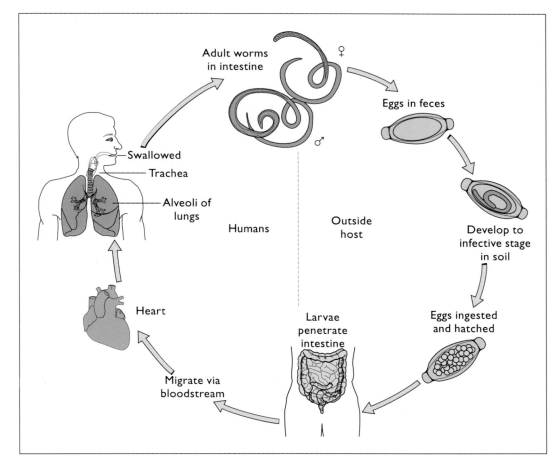

Adult worms in intestine

♀

♂

Eggs in feces

Swallowed

Trachea

Alveoli of lungs

Humans

Outside host

Develop to infective stage in soil

Heart

Larvae penetrate intestine

Eggs ingested and hatched

Migrate via bloodstream

FIGURE 6-56 Life cycle of *Ascaris*. Embryonated *Ascaris* eggs are ingested by humans. Larvae form in the small intestine and enter the liver via the enterohepatic circulation. From the liver they travel to the heart and lungs, out the alveolar spaces, up the trachea, and then are swallowed. Mature adult worms form in the small intestine, and they pass unembryonated eggs into the environment via the feces. Embryonation occurs in the soil within 2 to 4 weeks. Ingestion of the eggs completes the life cycle. (*Adapted from* Garcia [16].)

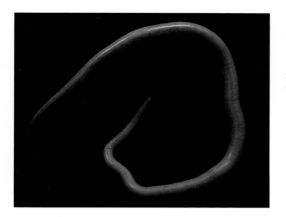

FIGURE 6-57 Adult *Ascaris lumbricoides* worm. Female worms may be as thick as a pencil and range from 20 to 35 cm in length, whereas males are slender and usually < 30 cm long. Ascariasis is the most common helminthic infection worldwide, with an estimated prevalence of 1 billion. Because virtually 100% of individuals living in areas of inadequate sanitation are infected, and each individual may be carrying hundreds of worms, the worm burden for our planet is staggering. (*From* the collection of B.H. Kean, MD.)

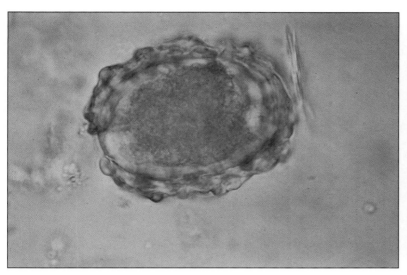

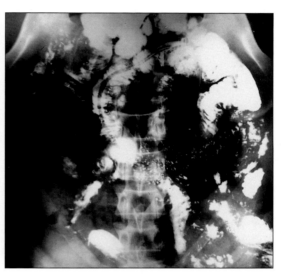

FIGURE 6-58 Fertilized *Ascaris lumbricoides* egg. The fertilized egg measures 45 to 75 µm × 35 to 50 µm. Mature female worms are estimated to produce an average of 200,000 eggs daily. Fertilized eggs become infective within approximately 2 weeks in a moist, warm soil, where they can then survive for months to years.

FIGURE 6-59 Barium radiograph showing intestinal ascariasis. *Ascaris* intestinal infection may be diagnosed radiographically. A radiolucent worm is shown in the barium-filled intestine of this patient; contrast material can also be seen in the worm's digestive tract. Adult worms that reside in the bowel do not generally cause symptoms, unless they migrate into the ampulla of vater, bile ducts, gallbladder, or pancreas. They may also perforate the intestine or occlude the appendix. (*From* the collection of B.H. Kean, MD.)

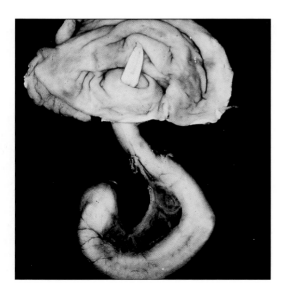

FIGURE 6-60 Gross specimen showing *Ascaris* occluding the appendix of a patient who presented with severe abdominal pain. Mebendazole is used to treat intestinal infections. Piperazine may help to relieve obstructions in the bile ducts or intestine by narcotizing the worms. (*From* the collection of B.H. Kean, MD.)

Hookworm

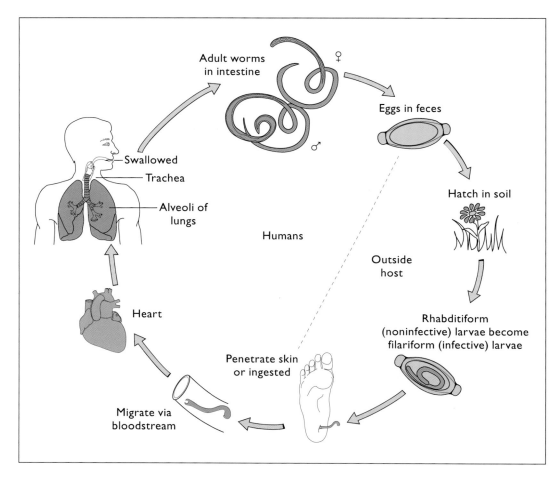

FIGURE **6-61** Hookworm life cycle. Hookworm filariform larvae enter the human body via the skin. They are transported to the small intestine via the heart and lungs in a fashion similar to *Ascaris* larvae. Adults mature in the intestine and pass unembryonated eggs into the soil where filariform larvae develop. (*Adapted from* Garcia [16].)

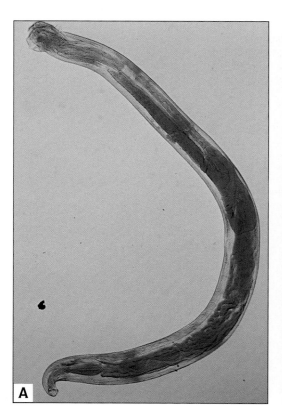

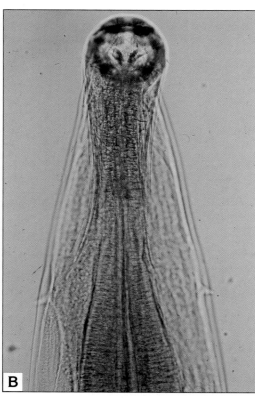

FIGURE **6-62** The New World hookworm, *Necator americanus*. **A**, *Necator* ranges from 5 to 9 mm for males to 1 cm for females. **B**, The sharply bent head is hooked-shaped, and the buccal capsule has a pair of cutting plates that help anchor it to the intestinal mucosa where it sucks blood from the host. (*From* the collection of B.H. Kean, MD.)

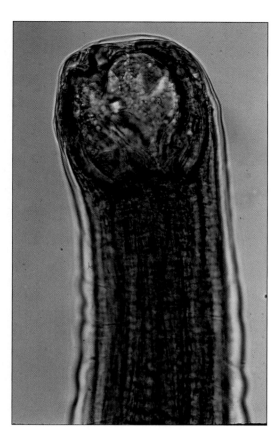

FIGURE 6-63 The Old World hookworm, *Ancyclostoma duodenale.* *A. duodenale* is slightly larger than *Necator* and has a set of teeth with which it attaches to the mucosa of the upper small intestine. The average daily blood loss for *Necator* infections is 0.03 mL, whereas it is 0.2 mL for *Ancyclostoma.* (*From* the collection of B.H. Kean, MD.)

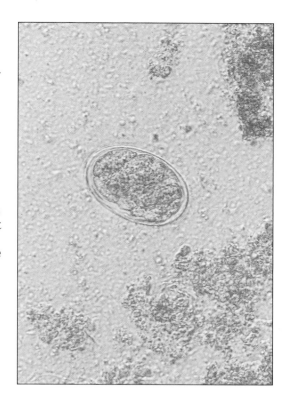

FIGURE 6-64 Fecal smear showing a single hookworm ova. Hookworm infection is diagnosed by detection of ova in feces. Adult worms lay an average of 7000 eggs daily, which are expelled to the environment in feces. Moist, shady, warm soil provides optimal conditions for eggs to survive and hatch into infective larvae. Contact with contaminated soil for 5 to 10 minutes allows the larvae to penetrate the human host's skin. (*From* the collection of B.H. Kean, MD.)

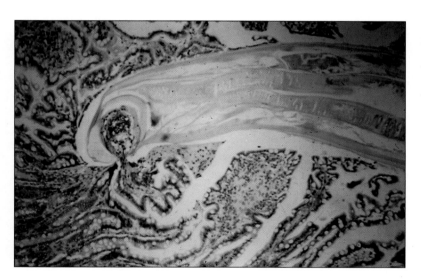

FIGURE 6-65 Tissue section showing a hookworm attached to the small intestinal mucosa, where it deprives the host of nutrients. Iron-deficiency anemia, chronic protein-calorie malnutrition, and weight loss are the most common manifestations of hookworm infection, but abdominal pain and diarrhea may also occur. (*From* the collection of B.H. Kean, MD.)

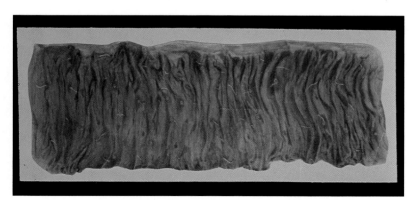

FIGURE 6-66 Resected specimen of small intestine showing numerous hookworms attached. (*From* the collection of B.H. Kean, MD.)

Strongyloides stercoralis

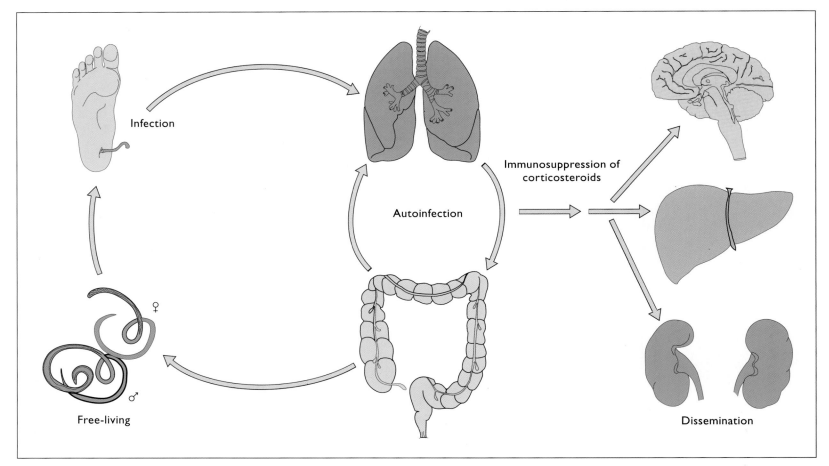

FIGURE 6-67 Life cycle of *Strongyloides stercoralis*. The *Strongyloides* life cycle is complex and not completely understood. It resembles that of the hookworms in that larvae migrate via the bloodstream to the lungs and eventually to the small intestine. The administration of corticosteroids may disrupt the usual cycle of autoinfection, resulting in disseminated infection. (*Adapted from* Genta [17].)

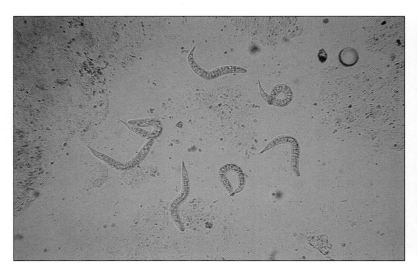

FIGURE 6-68 Fecal smear showing *Strongyloides stercoralis* larvae. Larvae demonstrated in feces or duodenal fluid are the basis for diagnosis of infection. Rhabditiform larvae exit in the feces, and transform either into free-living adult nematodes or filariform larvae, which must penetrate the skin of their host in order to complete their life cycle.

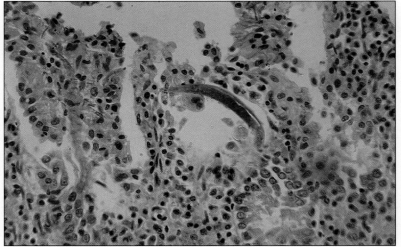

FIGURE 6-69 *Strongyloides stercoralis* in a tissue section from the small intestine of a renal transplant patient with abdominal pain and diarrhea. With heavy infections, there may be severe intestinal damage, but this is unusual. Peripheral eosinophilia of 50% to 75% may be seen, especially in immunocompetent hosts. Immunocompromised patients or those with chronic illness often have much less eosinophilia.

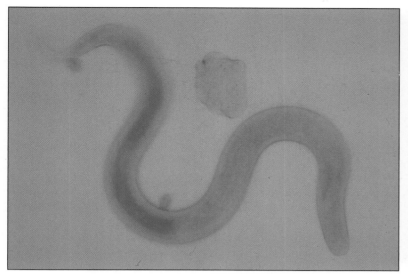

FIGURE 6-70 *Strongyloides* larva in bronchoalveolar lavage fluid of a bone marrow transplant patient who presented with bilateral pulmonary infiltrates. Autoinfection is probably the mechanism that allows for persistent infection in those individuals from an endemic area. Parasite and host are able to survive without problems until the host is immunosuppressed, at which time the larvae then begin to proliferate and disseminate to multiple organs. Mortality is very high in the hyperinfection syndrome. (Iodine stain.)

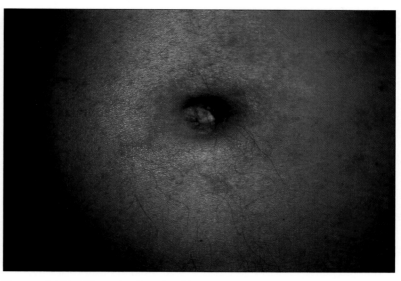

FIGURE 6-71 "Thumbprint sign" in a bone-marrow transplant patient with *Strongyloides* hyperinfection syndrome. This petechial, periumbilical rash is thought to be a consequence of larval migration.

CESTODES
Diphyllobothrium latum

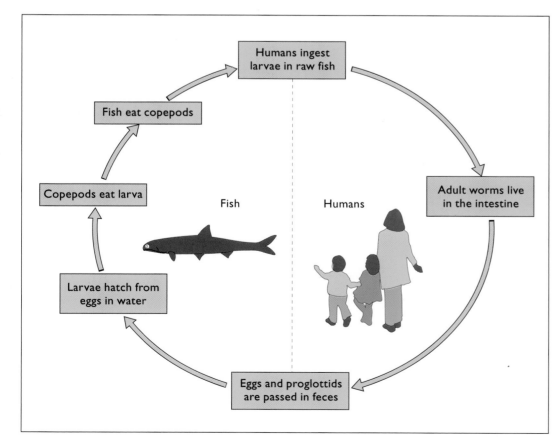

FIGURE 6-72 Life cycle of *Diphyllobothrium latum*. Humans become infected with the adult worm by eating raw, poorly cooked, or pickled freshwater fish (pike, perch, trout, salmon, whitefish). The worm matures in the human gastrointestinal tract and may reach a length of 10 meters with up to 3000 proglottids. Eggs and proglottids are passed with feces into freshwater. The eggs hatch, and ciliated, coracidium larvae are ingested by the intermediate host, the copepod. The second intermediate host, larger fish ingest the larval stage and in turn are eaten by humans, thus initiating infection with the adult worm.

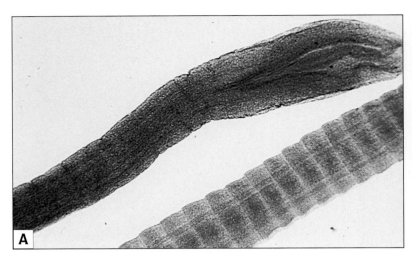

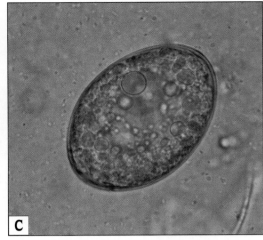

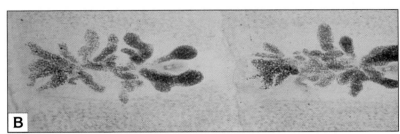

FIGURE 6-73 *Diphyllobothrium latum* morphology. **A**, Scolex. **B**, Proglottid. **C**, Egg. The fish tapeworm of humans has a worldwide distribution. Infected persons are usually asymptomatic but may have diarrhea or abdominal pain. Prolonged infection results in vitamin B$_{12}$ deficiency. (Panels 73A and 73B *from* the collection of B.H. Kean, MD; panel 73C *courtesy of* M. Scaglia, MD.)

Taenia saginata

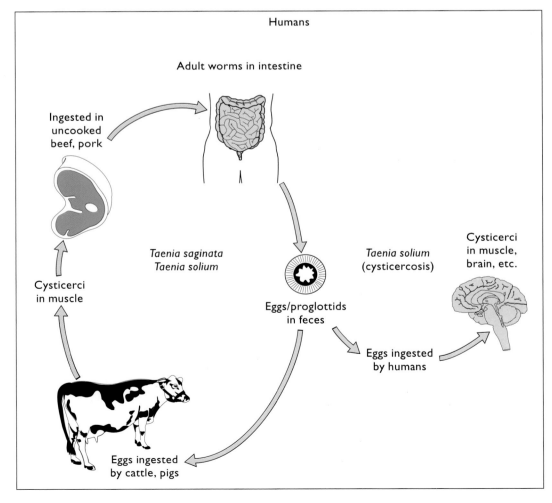

FIGURE 6-74 Life cycle of *Taenia saginata* (beef tapeworm) and *Taenia solium* (pork tapeworm). The life cycles of these two cestodes involve alternate larval and adult stages in two hosts: intermediate and definitive. Adult worms attach to the intestine by means of the scolex and absorb nutrients from the host. A ribbonlike chain of segments called *proglottids* form, each of which contains male and female sexual organs and produce ova. Proglottids or ova are passed in the feces sporadically; multiple examinations may be required for diagnosis. Intermediate hosts (cattle, pigs) ingest the eggs and develop larval cysts in their tissues. Cysts are eaten by the definitive host in uncooked meat; they mature into tapeworms in the digestive tract. Humans may also ingest *T. solium* eggs, which may travel to brain or muscle to form cysticeri (cysts). (*Modified from* Garcia [16].)

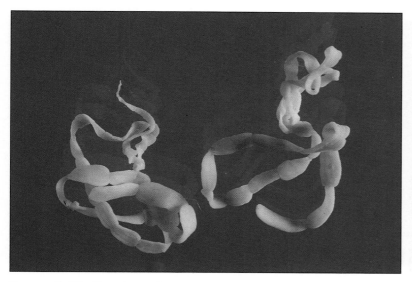

FIGURE 6-75 *Taenia saginata* proglottids. (*Courtesy of* M. Scaglia, MD.)

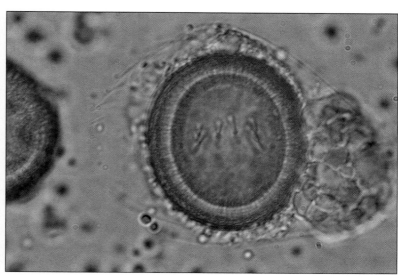

FIGURE 6-76 *Taenia saginata* egg. (*Courtesy of* M. Scaglia, MD.)

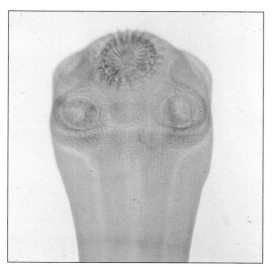

FIGURE 6-77 *Taenia solium* scolex. (*Courtesy of* M. Scaglia, MD.)

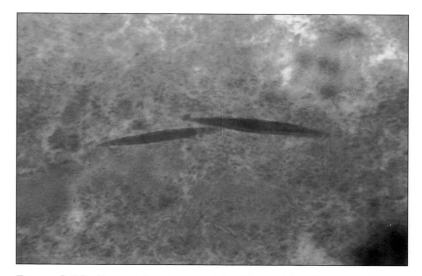

FIGURE 6-78 Charcot-Leyden crystals. Charcot-Leyden crystals stain purple-red with trichrome and may be found in either stool or sputum specimens. They are formed from the breakdown products of eosinophils, but their presence does not correlate with peripheral blood eosinophilia. They are not specific for infection with any particular organism but are seen in specimens from patients with either protozoan or helminthic infections.

REFERENCES

1. Oberhelman RA, Krogstad DJ: Use of the parasitology laboratory in the diagnosis of gastrointestinal infections. *In* Blaser MJ, Ravdin JI, Smith PD, *et al.* (eds.): *Infections of the Gastrointestinal Tract.* New York: Raven Press; 1995:1279–1291.

2. Zaiman H: *A Pictorial Presentation of Parasites.* Valley City, ND: Herman Zaiman.

3. Pennsylvania LL, Owen R, Fogel R, *et al.*: Giardiasis and traveler's diarrhea [clinical conference]. *Gastroenterology* 1980, 78:1602–1614.

4. Farthing MJG: *Giardia lamblia. In* Gorbach SL, Bartlett JG, Blacklow NR (eds.): *Infectious Diseases.* Philadelphia: W.B. Saunders; 1992:1959–1967.

5. Hill DR: Giardiasis: Issues in management and treatment. *Infect Dis Clin North Am* 1993, 7:503–525.

6. Reed SL, Ravdin JI: Amebiasis. *In* Blaser MJ, Ravdin JI, Smith PD, *et al.* (eds.): *Infections of the Gastrointestinal Tract.* New York: Raven Press; 1995:1065–1081.

7. Gardner AL, *et al.*: Intestinal cryptosporidiosis: Pathophysiologic alterations and specific cellular and humoral immune responses in rnu/+ and *rnu/rnu* (athymic) rats. *Am J Trop Med Hyg* 1991, 44:49–62.

8. Sun T: *Color Atlas and Textbook of Diagnostic Parasitology.* New York: Igaku-Shoin; 1988.

9. Cali A, Owen R: Microsporidiosis. *In* Balow A (ed.): *The Laboratory Diagnosis of Infectious Diseases: Principles and Practice,* 4th ed. New York: Springer-Verlag; 1988:929–950.

10. Davis L, Soave R: *Cryptosporidium, Isopora, Dientamoeba. In* Gorbach SL, Bartlett JG, Blacklow NR (eds.): *Infectious Diseases*, 2nd ed. Philadelphia: W.B. Saunders; 1996.

11. Orenstein JM, Tenner M, Cali A, Kotler DP: A microsporidian previously undescribed in humans, infecting enterocytes and macrophages, and associated with diarrhea in an acquired immunodeficiency syndrome patient. *Hum Pathol* 1990, 21:475–481.

12. Orenstein JM, Chiang J, Steinberg W, *et al.*: Intestinal microsporidiosis as a cause of diarrhea in human immunodeficiency virus-infected patients: A report of 20 cases. *Hum Pathol* 1992, 23:722–728.

13. Brooke MM, Melvin DM: Morphology and Diagnostic Stages of Intestinal Parasites of Man. Atlanta: Centers for Disease Control and Prevention; 1972. [DHEW publication no. (PHS) 72-H116.]

14. Katz M, Despommier DD, Gwadz RW: *Parasitic Diseases*. New York: Springer-Verlag; 1989.

15. Gopinath R, Keystone JS: Ascariasis, trichuriaris, and enterobiasis. *In* Blaser MJ, Ravdin JI, Smith PD, *et al.* (eds.): *Infections of the Gastrointestinal Tract*. New York: Raven Press; 1995:1167–1179.

16. Garcia LS: Laboratory methods for diagnosis of parasitic infections. *In* Finegold SM, Baron EJ (eds.): *Diagnostic Microbiology*, 7th ed. St. Louis: C.V. Mosby Co.; 1986.

17. Genta RM: *Strongyloides stercoralis. In* Blaser MJ, Ravdin JI, Smith PD, *et al.* (eds.): *Infections of the Gastrointestinal Tract*. New York: Raven Press; 1995:1197–1209.

Selected Bibliography

Mannheimer SB, Soave R: Protozoal infections in patients with AIDS. *Infect Dis Clin North Am* 1994, 8:483–498.

Markell EK, Voge M, John DT: *Medical Parasitology*, 7th ed. Philadelphia: W.B. Saunders Co; 1992.

Ravdin JL (ed.): *Amebiasis: Human Infections by Entamoeba histolytica*. New York: Churchill Livingstone; 1988.

Rondanelli EG, Scaglia M (eds.): *Atlas of Human Protozoa*. Milan: Masson; 1993.

Schantz P: The dangers of eating raw fish. *N Engl J Med* 1989, 320:1143–1145.

Wolfe MS: Giardiasis. *Clin Microbiol Rev* 1992, 5:93–100.

CHAPTER 7

Fungal Enteritis

Helen Buckley

Mycoses of the gastrointestinal tract	
Organism	**Tissue form**
Candida albicans	Yeasts, pseudohyphae, septate hyphae
Histoplasma capsulatum	Intracellular yeast cells within the cells of the reticuloendothelial system
Aspergillus fumigatus	Septate hyphae, dichotomous branching
Mucorales	Branching nonseptate hyphae
Paracoccidioides brasiliensis	Multibudding yeast cells

FIGURE 7-1 Mycoses of the gastrointestinal tract. Fungal pathogens infect the gastrointestinal tract via two routes: direct transmucosal inoculation (*eg*, *Candida*) and dissemination from extrasystemic primary infection (*eg*, pulmonary infection with *Histoplasma capsulatum*).

CANDIDIASIS

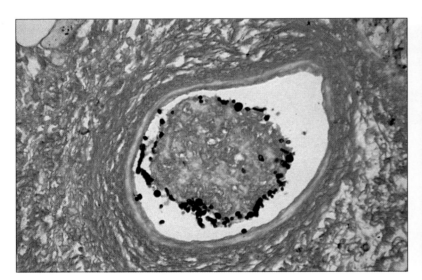

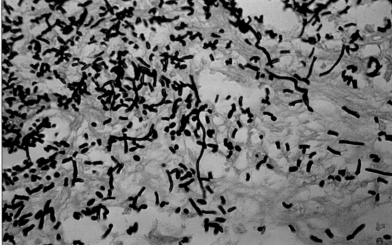

FIGURE 7-2 Mesenteric artery embolus seen in a severely neutropenic patient who had hematogenously disseminated candidiasis involving the liver and spleen. Note the presence of yeast cells and hyphae of candida within the embolus. Candidiasis represents a spectrum of infections caused by *Candida* species. The disease manifestations are protean and range from mucosal and superficial, to acute life threatening, to chronic disease. *Candida albicans* is part of the gastrointestinal flora of humans, and disease caused by this species is usually endogenous in origin. Other candidal species, such as *C. tropicalis*, *C. parapsilosis*, *C. lusitania*, *C. krusei*, *C. guilliermondii*, and *C. glabrata*, are generally thought to be exogenously acquired. Many factors will determine the development of these protean clinical manifestations and include local, physiological, and iatrogenic ones. Candida blood infections are common in university hospitals and most likely as a result of medical progress. (Gomori methenamine silver stain; × 100.) (Courtesy of M. Rinaldi, PhD.)

FIGURE 7-3 Gastric tissue section demonstrating disseminated candidiasis. This case of fatal disseminated *Candida* infection occurred in a leukemia patient. The organism is seen in gastric tissue, demonstrating budding yeasts, pseudohyphae of varying lengths, and true hyphae. Most cases of life-threatening candidal infections are seen in the immunosuppressed, and esophageal lesions are a great source of morbidity in patients with AIDS and those undergoing chemotherapy. (Gomori methenamine silver stain; × 400.) (*Courtesy of* M. Rinaldi, PhD.)

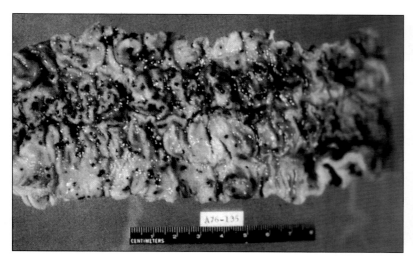

FIGURE 7-4 Gross specimen of small intestine showing numerous shallow mucosal lesions due to *Candida* infection. The patient had acute leukemia and developed fatal disseminated candidiasis. Autopsy data indicate that the small bowel is affected in approximately 20% of patients with multiple sites of gastrointestinal candidiasis, usually in neutropenic hosts. (*From* Washburn and Bennett [1]; with permission.)

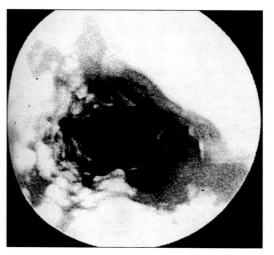

FIGURE 7-5 Endoscopic appearance of *Candida* esophagitis. Endoscopy shows the characteristic raised white plaques of *Candida* opposite and esophageal ulcer due to cytomegalovirus in a patient with AIDS and esophagitis due to both *Candida* and cytomegalovirus. (*Courtesy of* D.T. Dieterich, MD; *from* Polis [2]; with permission.)

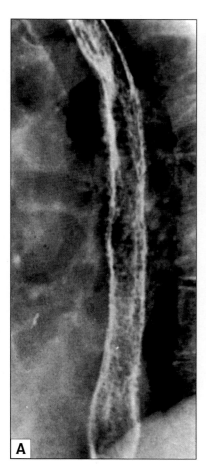
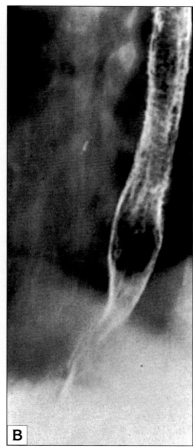

FIGURE 7-6 Barium contrast esophagograms of *Candida* esophagitis. **A** and **B**, Esophagograms show a markedly irregular esophagus due to multiple plaques in a patient with AIDS and severe odynophagia. (*From* Polis [2]; with permission.)

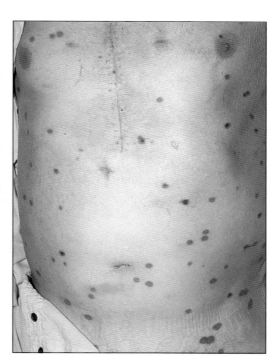

FIGURE 7-7 Multiple skin lesions in disseminated candidiasis. Disseminated disease is often manifested by multiple skin lesions. A neutropenic chemotherapy patient developed fever, myalgias, and a purpuric rash. The source of this hematogenously disseminated infection was a contaminated vascular catheter. (*Courtesy of* G.J. Raugi, MD.)

HISTOPLASMOSIS

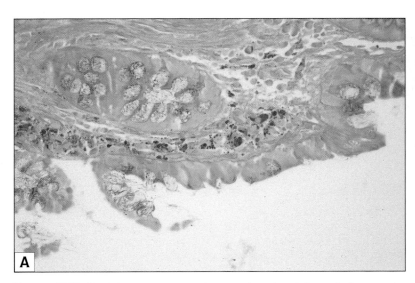

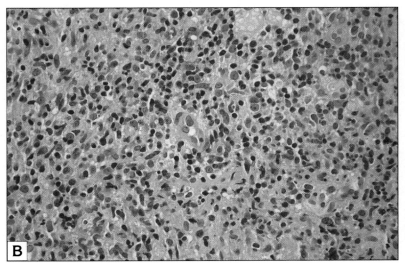

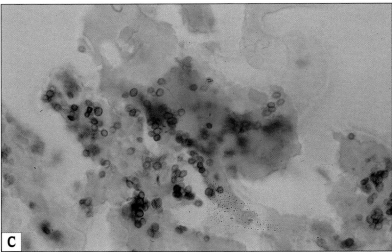

FIGURE 7-8 Gastric mucosa specimens showing intracellular yeast cells in disseminated histoplasmosis. The specimens are from the autopsy of a patient with AIDS who developed disseminated histoplasmosis. *Histoplasma capulatum* is a mold that lives in soil and accumulates in the presence of feces from blackbirds, chickens, or bats. The organism is acquired by inhalation, and most cases are subclinical, not requiring hospitalization. This is a dimorphic organism, the infective form being the mold phase, and once inhaled, it converts to the yeast phase within the alveolar macrophages. **A,** *Histoplasma capsulatum* in the gastric mucosa. The yeasts stained with periodic acid–Schiff. (× 100.) **B,** On hematoxylin-eosin staining, the gastric mucosa show an inflammatory reaction consisting of lymphocytes and occasional eosinophils. Intracellular small budding yeasts of *H. capsulatum* are often missed in routine hematoxylin-eosin stains. (× 400.) **C,** Silver stain readily demonstrating the yeast phase of *Histoplasma* in the gastric mucosa. Note that the cells of *Histoplasma* are relatively uniform in size. (× 1000.) (*Courtesy of* M. Rinaldi, PhD.)

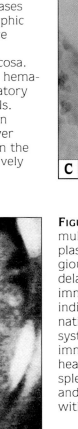

FIGURE 7-9 Abdominal computed tomography scan showing multiple calcified granulomas in the spleen due to resolved histoplasmosis. Histoplasmosis mimics tuberculosis but is not contagious. After inhalation of the mold form, the individual develops delayed-type hypersensitivity, which remains positive for life in immunocompetent hosts. However, in the immunosuppressed individual, the calcifications in the lung breakdown and dissemination can occur, notably to the organs of the reticuloendothelial system. In immunocompetent hosts, the onset of cell-mediated immunity causes the granulomas in the lung and distant sites to heal uneventfully, leaving these marble-sized calcifications. Such splenic calcifications are very common in highly endemic areas and are diagnostic of remote histoplasmosis. (*From* Lee *et al.* [3]; with permission.)

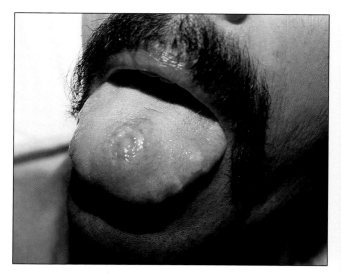

FIGURE 7-10 Oral ulcer of disseminated histoplasmosis in a patient with AIDS. (*Courtesy of* E.J. Bottone, PhD.)

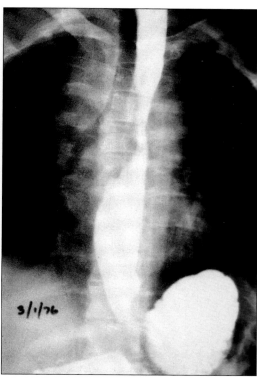

FIGURE 7-11 Esophagogram showing esophageal histoplasmosis lesions. The patient had dysphagia resulting from esophageal compression by massive mediastinal lymphadenopathy. (*From* Washburn and Bennett [1]; with permission.)

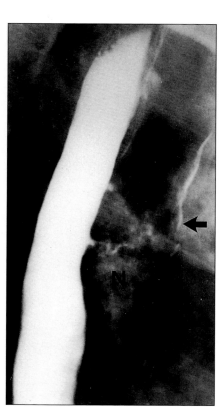

FIGURE 7-12 Barium esophagogram showing tracheoesophageal fistula due to histoplasmosis. This man aged 54 years noted a sensation of air passing from one portion of his chest to another when he lay on his left side. A single-contrast esophagogram shows a pinpoint fistula filled with barium extending from the esophageal lumen through an enlarged, mediastinal, calcified lymph node (*N*) into the trachea (*arrow*). (*From* Morgan and Koehler [4]; with permission.)

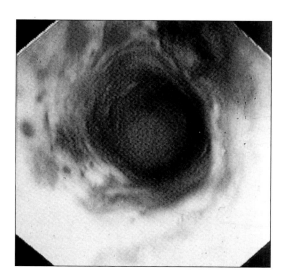

FIGURE 7-13 Endoscopic view of histoplasmosis esophagitis in an AIDS patient. Endoscopy with brushing can be used for diagnosing histoplasma esophagitis that involves ulcerations and mass lesions. (*From* Young *et al.* [5]; with permission.)

Sources of exposure to *Histoplasma capsulatum*	
Microfocus	**Activities**
Caves	Spelunking (bat droppings)
Chicken coops	Cleaning, demolition, use of bird droppings in garden
Bird roosts	Excavation, camping
Bamboo canebreaks	Cutting cane, recreation
Schoolyards	Routine activities, cleaning
Prison grounds	Routine activities, cleaning
Decayed wood piles	Transporting or burning wood
Dead trees	Recreational, cutting wood
Contaminated chimneys	Cleaning, demolition (bats)
Old buildings	Demolition, remodeling, cleaning
Laboratories	Research projects, epidemiologic studies at contaminated microfoci

FIGURE 7-14 Sources of exposure to *Histoplasma capsulatum.* Histoplasmosis is endemic in the United States in the Ohio and Mississippi River valleys. (*Modified from* Wheat [6].)

MUCORMYCOSIS

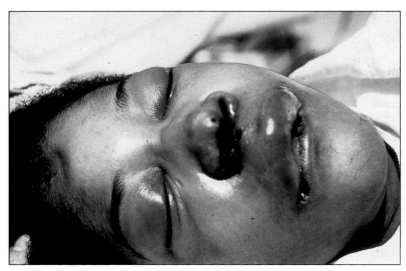

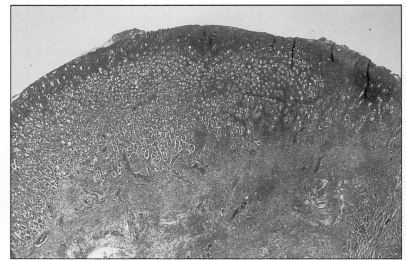

FIGURE 7-15 Rhinocerebral mucormycosis in a diabetic patient. Mucormycosis is a rapidly fatal disease caused by members of the order Mucorales. These organisms are ubiquitous, have nonseptate hyphae and usually produce their vegetative spores in sporangia. The disease is seen in patients in acidosis caused by diabetes or other metabolic conditions or in severely immunosuppressed patients. The organism is inhaled, and the disease is usually first manifested as a rhinocerebral disease. It is rapidly fatal and is marked by the invasion of blood vessels. Intravenous drug abuse is a predisposing factor in patients with brain abscesses. The control of the underlying condition in the patient is imperative in controlling dissemination of this infection. (*Courtesy of* J.T. Herdegen, MD, and R. Bone, MD.)

FIGURE 7-16 Hemorrhagic necrosis of the gastric mucosa in disseminated *Rhizopus* infection. Tissue is usually hemorrhagic in disseminated mucormycosis. This specimen is from an autopsy of a severely immunocompromised patient who died of disseminated disease caused by *Rhizopus.* (Hematoxylin-eosin stain; × 50.) (*Courtesy of* W. Merz, PhD.)

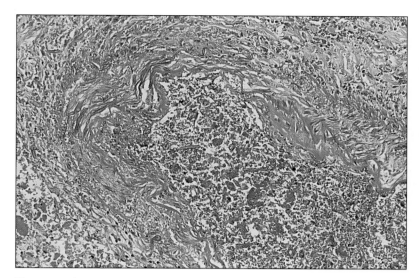

FIGURE 7-17 Blood vessel invasion in mucormycosis. The pathology of this disease is characterized by blood vessel invasions. The hematoxylin-eosin–stained section, from the same case as Figure 7-16, shows blood vessel invasion with thrombosis by fungal elements. (× 200.) (*Courtesy of* W. Merz, PhD.)

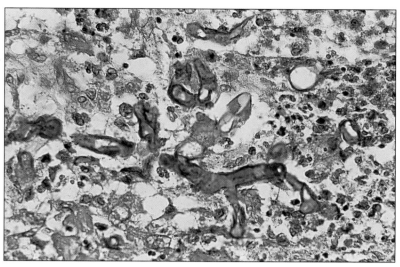

FIGURE 7-18 Periodic acid–Schiff-staining of a tissue section shows large nonseptate hyphae with 90° angle branching typical of *Rhizopus*. Note the ribbon appearance of the hyphae, which occurs because the hyphae fold when cut. (× 400.) (*Courtesy of* W. Merz, PhD.)

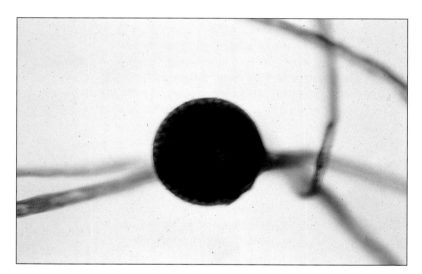

FIGURE 7-19 Microscopic findings of *Mucor* organisms grown in culture. In culture and in nature, nonseptate hyphae are seen with spores produced in sporangia. The organism must be seen in tissue for diagnosis, because these organisms are common contaminants in the laboratory. (Lactophenol mount; × 400.)

ASPERGILLOSIS

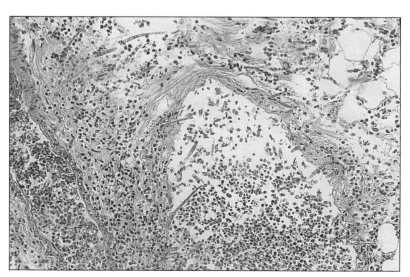

FIGURE 7-20 Vascular invasion of gastric mucosa by *Aspergillus*. Aspergillosis represents illness caused by *Aspergillus* species. These organisms are ubiquitous in nature but, when their spores are inhaled, they can affect the lung in three ways: 1) they are a very common cause of uncomplicated allergy; 2) they can cause fungus balls within necrotic tissue present in the lung of patients with preexisting lung disease; and 3) in the immunocompromised patient, they can invade lung tissue and disseminate throughout the body. In the immunosuppressed host, organisms can be seen invading blood vessels and causing infarction and hemorrhage. As seen in this bone marrow transplant patient who developed pulmonary disease that disseminated to all organs, one of the characteristics of disseminated aspergillosis is penetration of blood vessel walls. This patient was severely immunosuppressed. Bone marrow transplant patients are very susceptible to this complication. (Hematoxylin-eosin stain; × 100.)

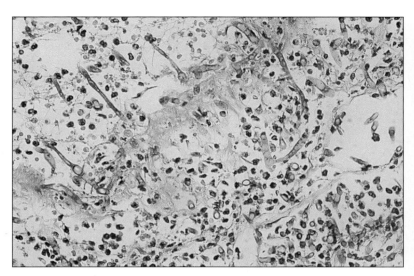

FIGURE 7-21 Tissue section showing *Aspergillus* with septate hyphae and branching. The organism in tissue is characterized by having septate hyphae and 45° angle (dichotomous) branching. Note that the organism is within the vessel wall. (Hematoxylin-eosin stain; × 400.)

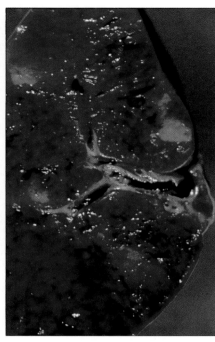

FIGURE 7-22 Gross specimen showing multiple nodules of aspergillosis in the spleen. Multiple white nodules can be seen on the surface of the spleen. On histopathologic section, these proved to be hematogenous foci of aspergillosis. The patient had died of invasive aspergillosis complicating prolonged neutropenia. (*Courtesy of* S.F. Davies, MD, and G.A. Sarosi, MD.)

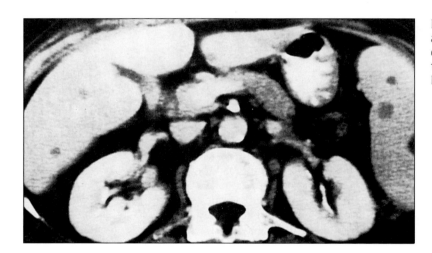

FIGURE 7-23 Abdominal computed tomography scan showing liver and spleen involvement in disseminated aspergillosis. Multiple low-density lesions can be seen in the spleen and liver. This is the typical radiographic presentation of hematogenous aspergillosis lesions. (*From* Lee *et al.* [3]; with permission.)

PARACOCCIDIOIDOMYCOSIS

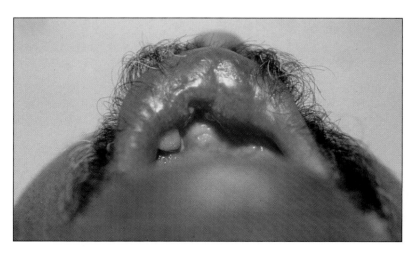

FIGURE 7-24 Mucocutaneous paracoccidioidomycosis affecting the upper lip. Paracoccidioidomycosis is the most prevalent of the deep mycoses in Latin America, with Brazil, Colombia, and Venezuela having the greatest number of cases. The organism lives in the soil, but not much is known about its natural habitat. The mold from the soil is inhaled and then in tissue it converts to a multiple budding yeast. This form is the characteristic form of this organism. The disease is thought to be a primary pulmonary one that spreads to the mucosa of the mouth, nose, and occasionally the gastrointestinal tract. This patient shows marked edema of the upper lip, with dermal papules and nodules and loss of teeth. (*Courtesy of* G.J. Raugi, MD.)

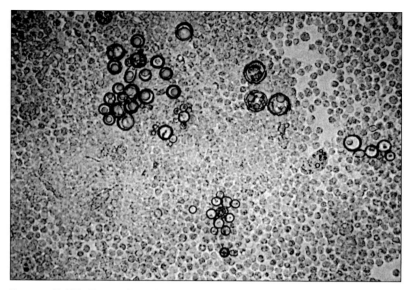

FIGURE 7-25 Potassium hydroxide preparation of *Paracoccidioides brasiliensis* from pus smear. Yeast cells with multiple buds and variations in cell size are apparent. (× 200.) (*From* Restrepo [7]; with permission.)

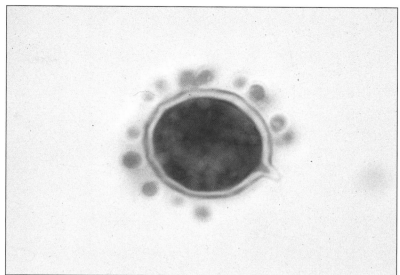

FIGURE 7-26 Lactophenol blue stain of yeast form of *Paracoccidioides brasiliensis* grown in culture at 37° C on blood agar. The larger yeast cell is reproducing by the formation of multiple buds. (× 400.)

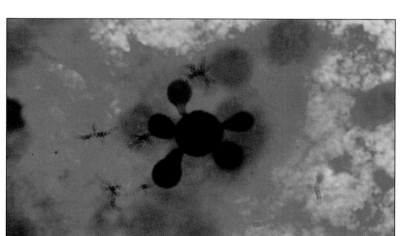

FIGURE 7-27 Characteristic "pilot-wheel" yeast form of *Paracoccidioides brasiliensis*. *P. brasiliensis* is a large yeast, 8 to 15 μm in diameter. It has characteristic thin-necked buds that are distributed around the periphery of the organism, giving the budding yeast the appearance of a pilot wheel on a ship. (Grocott's silver stain; × 1000.) (*From* Salfelder *et al.* [8]; with permission.)

REFERENCES

1. Washburn RG, Bennett JE: Deep mycoses. *In* Blaser MJ, Ravdin JI, Smith PD, *et al* (eds.): *Infections of the Gastrointestinal Tract*. New York: Raven Press; 1995:957–967.

2. Polis M: Esophagitis. *In* Mandell GL, Bennett JE, Dolin R (eds.): *Principles and Practice of Infectious Diseases*, 4th ed. New York: Churchill Livingstone; 1995:962–965.

3. Lee JK, Sagel SS, Stanley RJ (eds.): *Computed Body Tomography with MRI Correlation*, 2nd ed. New York: Raven Press; 1989.

4. Morgan DE, Koehler RE: Role of radiological procedures in the diagnosis of gastrointestinal infections. *In* Blaser MJ, Ravdin JI, Smith PD, *et al*. (eds.): *Infections of the Gastrointestinal Tract*. New York: Raven Press; 1995:1315–1328.

5. Young H, Swanson K, Slosberg E, Cello J: Role of endoscopy in the diagnosis of gastrointestinal infections. *In* Blaser MJ, Ravdin JI, Smith PD, *et al*. (eds.): *Infections of the Gastrointestinal Tract*. New York: Raven Press; 1995:1291–1315.

6. Wheat LJ: *Histoplasma capsulatum*. *In* Gorbach SL, Bartlett JG, Blacklow NR (eds.): *Infectious Diseases*. Philadelphia: WB Saunders; 1992:1905–1912.

7. Restrepo A: *Paracoccidioides brasiliensis*. *In* Mandell GL, Bennett JE, Dolin R (eds.): *Principles and Practice of Infectious Diseases*, 4th ed. New York: Churchill Livingstone; 1995:2386–2389.

8. Salfelder K, deLiscano TR, Sauerteig E: *Atlas of Fungal Pathology*, vol 17. Boston: Kluwer Academic Publishers; 1990:118.

SELECTED BIBLIOGRAPHY

Kwon-Chung KJ, Bennett JG: *Medical Mycology*. Philadelphia: Lea & Febiger, 1992.

Larone DH: *Medically Important Fungi*, 3rd ed. Washington, DC: American Society for Microbiology Press, 1995.

Wheat J: Endemic mycoses in AIDS: A clinical review. *Clin Microbiol Rev* 1995, 8:146–159.

CHAPTER 8

Diagnostic Imaging

Robert A. Gatenby

ESOPHAGUS

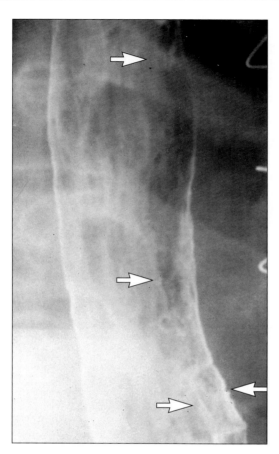

FIGURE 8-1 Herpes simplex esophagitis. A double-contrast esophagogram in a patient following heart transplantation shows multiple shallow ulcers (some of which are linear) in the distal esophagus (*arrows*) with intervening normal mucosa. Biopsies demonstrated herpes virus.

STOMACH

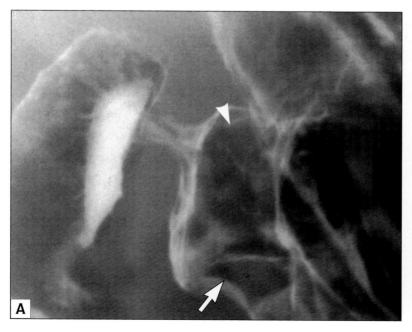 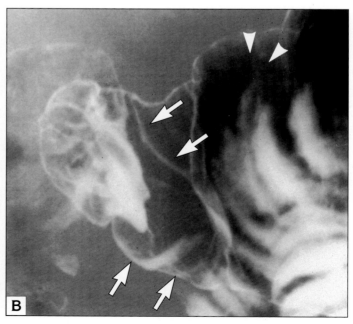

FIGURE 8-2 Gastric ulcers due to *Helicobacter pylori* infection. **A** and **B**, Films from a double-contrast upper gastrointestinal series show very thickened folds (*arrows*) in the antrum and body of the stomach with shallow ulcers (*arrowheads*) indicating gastritis. Although this ulceration might represent gastritis due to many etiologies (including peptic and medication-induced), the presence of the very thick folds suggest *H. pylori* infection, which was demonstrated at endoscopy.

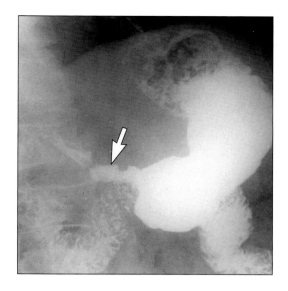

FIGURE 8-3 Antral syphilis. A barium examination of the stomach demonstrates thickening and narrowing (*arrow*) of the antrum. This appearance and location are typical of gastrointestinal involvement by syphilis, now rarely seen.

SMALL INTESTINE

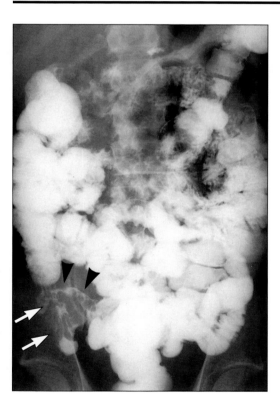

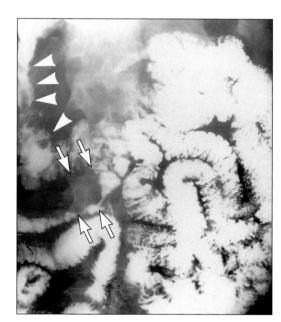

FIGURE 8-4 Ileocecal tuberculosis. A barium examination of the small bowel shows marked narrowing and irregularity of the terminal ileum (*arrowheads*) and cecum (*arrows*). This appearance and location are characteristic of tuberculosis involving the gastrointestinal tract. Radiographically, Crohn's disease and lymphoma must be considered in the differential diagnosis.

FIGURE 8-5 Giardiasis. A barium small bowel examination demonstrates marked thickening of the folds in the duodenum and proximal small bowel (*arrowheads*), with thickening of the bowel wall demonstrated by the separation of bowel loops (*arrows*). These are typical findings of giardiasis.

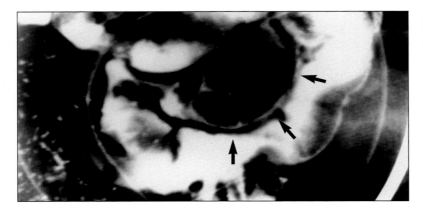

FIGURE 8-6 Ascariasis of the small bowel. A barium small bowel examination demonstrates a tubular filling defect within the small bowel lumen (*arrows*), which represents ascariasis.

COLON

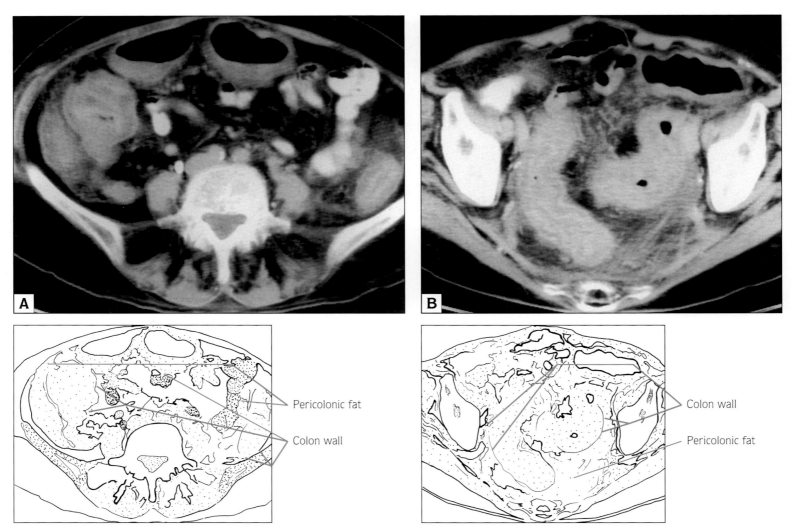

Pericolonic fat

Colon wall

Colon wall

Pericolonic fat

FIGURE 8-7 Pseudomembranous colitis. **A** and **B**, Computed tomography scans of the abdomen show marked thickening of the wall of the entire colon. There is evidence of intense inflammation with spiculated increased soft tissue in the pericolonic fat. This presentation is the characteristic appearance of *Clostridium difficle* colitis in a patient who previously had received clindamycin therapy.

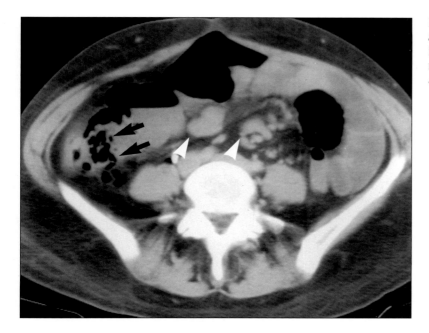

FIGURE 8-8 Colonic necrosis. Computed tomography scan of the abdomen demonstrates pneumatosis in the right colon extending into the pericolonic fat (*arrows*) and enlarged mesenteric lymph nodes (*arrowheads*). This patient with AIDS had *Mycobacterium avium intracellulare* infection.

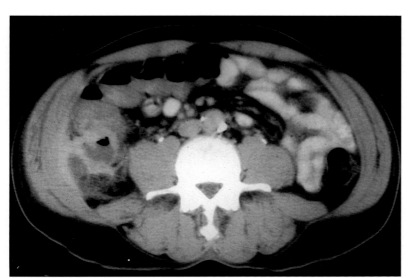

FIGURE 8-9 Right-sided diverticulitis with abscess formation. A computed tomography scan shows a thick-walled fluid collection adjacent to the right colon. There is associated thickening of the colonic wall as well as marked inflammatory changes in the retroperitoneal fat. Differential diagnostic considerations include perforated colonic carcinoma, abscess due to a retrocecal appendicitis, and ameboma.

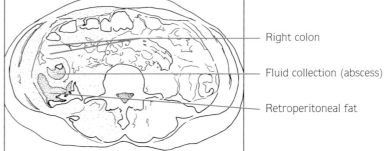

Right colon

Fluid collection (abscess)

Retroperitoneal fat

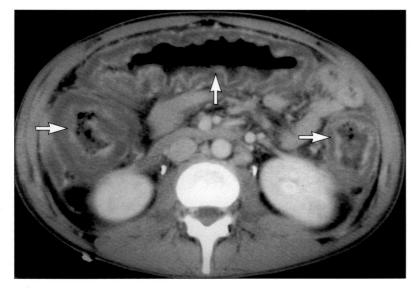

FIGURE 8-10 Cytomegalovirus colitis. A computed tomography scan of the abdomen demonstrates marked thickening of the wall of the entire colon (*arrows*) in a patient with severe diarrhea and AIDS. Biopsy done via colonoscopy demonstrated cytomegalovirus.

LIVER

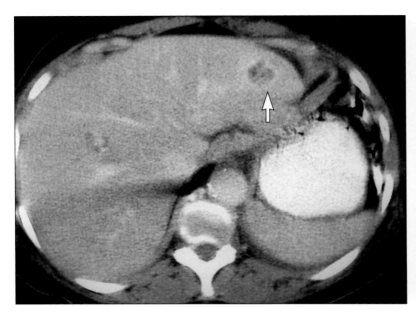

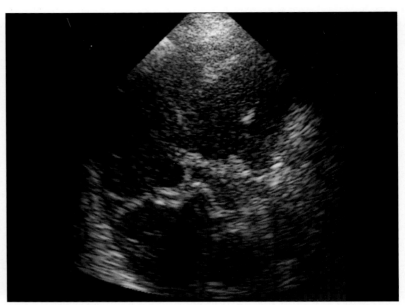

FIGURE 8-11 Hepatic abscess. A computed tomography scan with oral and intravenous contrast material demonstrates a low-density lesion in the left lobe of the liver with an enhancing edge (*arrow*). This lesion proved to be a polymicrobial abscess in this patient with diverticulitis. Enhancement in the periphery of the abscess after intravenous injection of contrast material is a common finding in hepatic abscess, distinguishing it from a simple cyst or hepatic tumor.

FIGURE 8-12 Liver ultrasound showing periportal fibrosis from schistosomiasis. Ultrasound examination of the liver demonstrates intense echogenicity in the periportal region due to periportal fibrosis in a patient with schistosomiasis. *Schistosoma japonicum* and *S. mansoni* typically migrate into the inferior mesenteric vein or superior mesenteric vein, and from there, they discharge their ova into the portal venous system, impacting the liver. The presence of these ova causes considerable irritation and inflammatory reaction, ultimately resulting in periportal fibrosis.

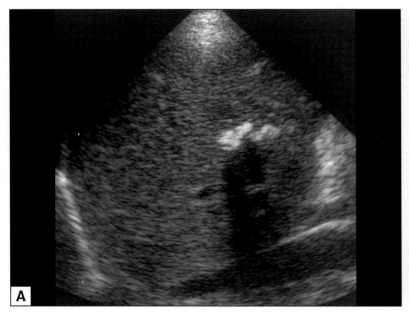

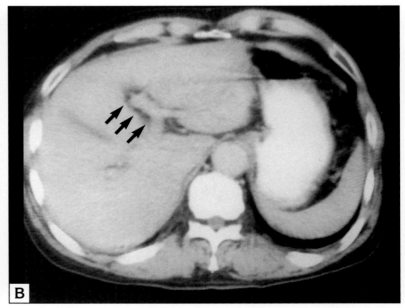

FIGURE 8-13 Severe periportal fibrosis from schistosomiasis. Ultrasound and computed tomography (CT) scans of the liver demonstrate severe periportal fibrosis. **A**, The ultrasound scan demonstrates intense echogenicity in the periportal region, which causes considerable sonic dropout (shadowing). **B**, In the CT scan, the periportal fibrosis is manifested as the low-density thickening of soft tissues around the portal vein (*arrows*). Both patients developed periportal fibrosis due to infection with *Schistosoma mansoni*.

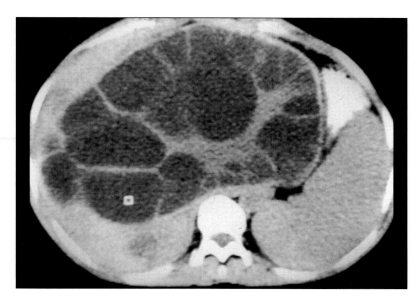

FIGURE 8-14 Liver cyst due to echinococcus granulosus infection. Computed tomography scan demonstrates a large multilocular cystic mass in the liver with distinctive internal daughter cysts characteristic of *Echinococcus* infection. Approximately 40% of echinococcal (hydatid) cysts will demonstrate some crescentic or curvilinear calcification.

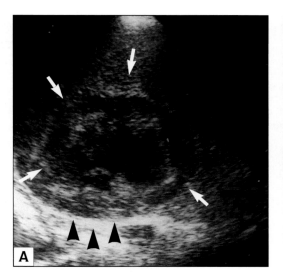

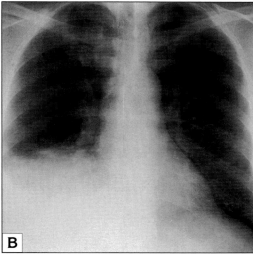

FIGURE 8-15 Amebic abscess of liver. **A**, Ultrasound shows a thick-walled cystic mass (*arrows*) with heterogeneous internal echoes in the periphery of the right lobe of the liver adjacent to the diaphragm (*arrowheads*). This presentation is the characteristic appearance and location of an amebic abscess in the liver. **B**, A chest radiograph demonstrates an associated right pleural effusion, which suggests rupture through the diaphragm into the right pleural space.

GALLBLADDER

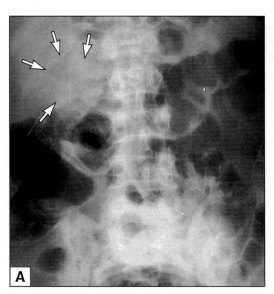

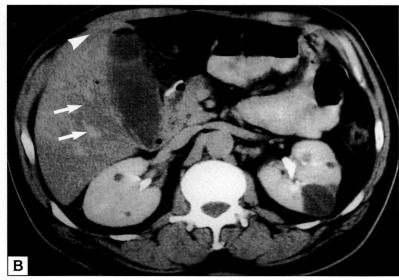

FIGURE 8-16 Emphysematous cholecystitis. **A**, Plain film of the abdomen shows a rounded air collection in the right upper quadrant (*arrows*). **B**, A computed tomography scan of the abdomen demonstrates irregularity of the gallbladder wall (*arrows*) and air within the lumen of the gallbladder (*arrowhead*), indicating emphysematous cholecystitis.

PANCREAS

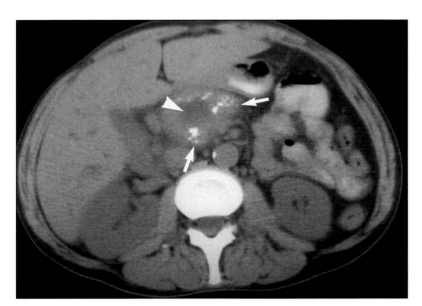

FIGURE 8-17 Abscess superimposed on chronic pancreatitis. A computed tomography scan of the abdomen shows multiple areas of calcification (*arrows*) in the head of the pancreas, indicating chronic pancreatitis. Within this area is a low-density lesion (*arrowhead*), which represents a superimposed pancreatic abscess.

SPLEEN

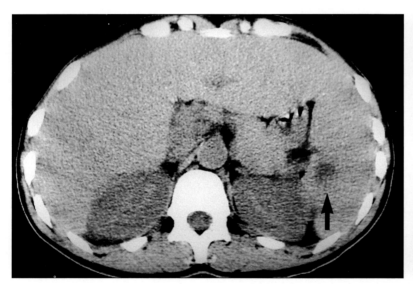

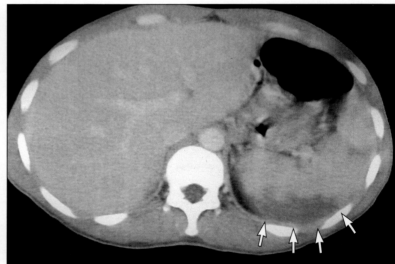

FIGURE 8-18 Splenic abscess. Computed tomography scan through the upper abdomen shows a low-density area (*arrow*) in the spleen with irregular ill-defined borders. This lesion proved to be a *Staphylococcus aureus* abscess in this intravenous drug abuser. The presence of ill-defined borders with internal debris or septations is frequent in splenic abscesses. Gas may be seen within the abscess but is not common.

FIGURE 8-19 Infected splenic infarct. Computed tomography scan of the abdomen shows a classic peripheral, low-density (*arrows*) lesion in the spleen due to septic emboli in a patient with bacterial endocarditis.

INTRA-ABDOMINAL SPACE

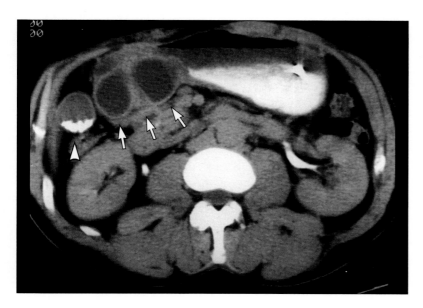

FIGURE 8-20 Lesser sac abscess. A computed tomography scan of the abdomen with oral and intravenous contrast demonstrates a loculated, thick-walled fluid collection posterior to the duodenal bulb and antrum (*arrows*). This lesion represents an abscess due to a penetrating duodenal ulcer. The abscess compressed the antrum of the stomach, producing partial gastric outlet obstruction. Calcified gallstones are incidentally noted, layering in the dependent portion of the gallbladder just lateral to the abscess (*arrowhead*).

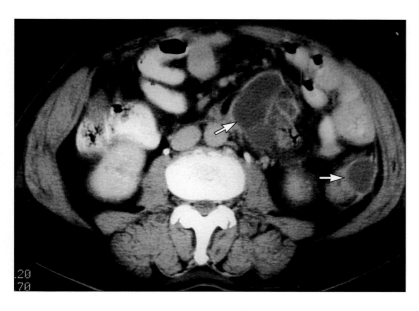

FIGURE 8-21 Intraperitoneal abscesses following cholecystitis. A computed tomography scan of the abdomen demonstrates an irregular fluid collection in the left pericolonic gutter and in the central abdomen (*arrows*). This patient proved to have multiple intraperitoneal abscesses apparently due to peritoneal dissemination of infection following cholecystitis.

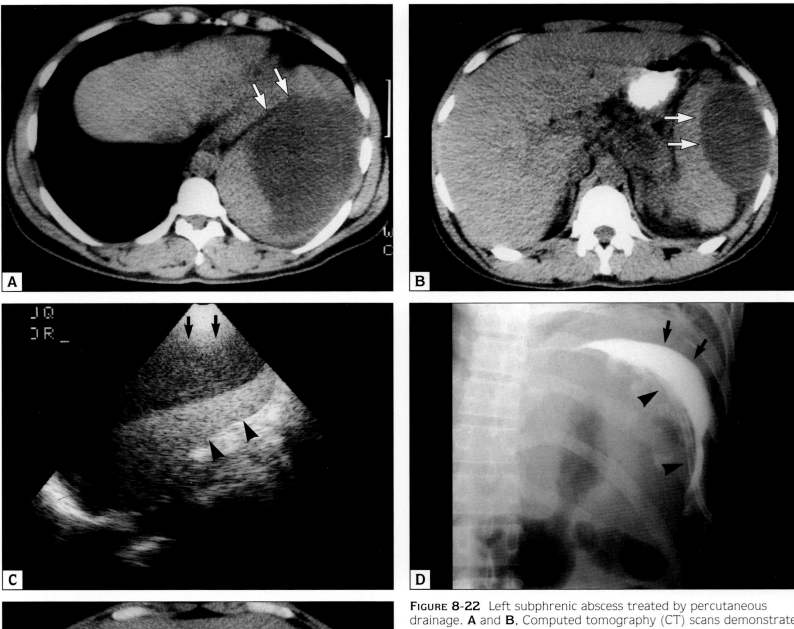

FIGURE 8-22 Left subphrenic abscess treated by percutaneous drainage. **A** and **B**, Computed tomography (CT) scans demonstrate a perisplenic fluid collection extending into the left subphrenic space (*arrows*). **C**, Separation from the spleen is evident on the CT scans and is confirmed by ultrasound, which also demonstrates the echo texture of the abscess (*arrows*) to be distinct from the more echogenic splenic parenchyma (*arrowheads*). **D**, A 10-French catheter was placed into the abscess under combined CT and fluoroscopic guidance, successfully avoiding surgery. A plain film demonstrates the catheter (*arrowheads*) in the left subphrenic space, with contrast injected through the catheter outlining the collapsed abscess cavity (*arrows*). **E**, A postdrainage CT scan shows successful evacuation of the perisplenic fluid with the catheter still in place (*arrow*).

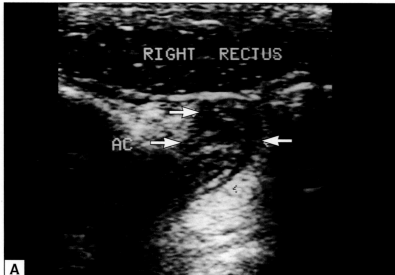

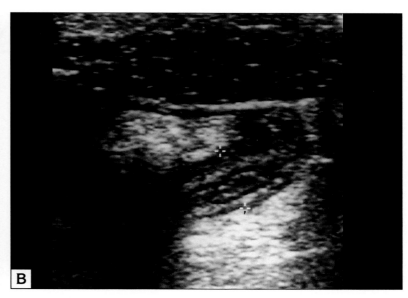

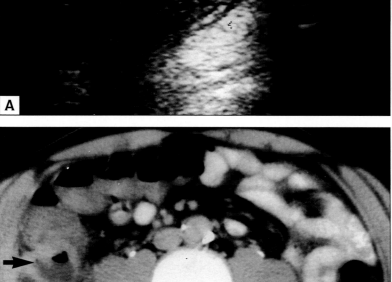

FIGURE 8-23 Appendicitis. **A,** Ultrasound of the appendix is accomplished by compressing the rectus muscle against the psoas muscle, entrapping the appendix (*arrows*) between them. **B,** An appendiceal diameter > 6 mm is diagnostic of appendicitis. **C,** Computed tomography (CT) scans are equally accurate in the diagnosis. Characteristic findings include spiculation of pericecal fat, appendicolith, and thickening of the appendix (although the appendix is frequently not visible). This CT scan demonstrates spiculation in the pericecal fat (*arrowheads*) with a thick-walled, air–fluid collection (*arrow*), indicating a periappendiceal abscess.

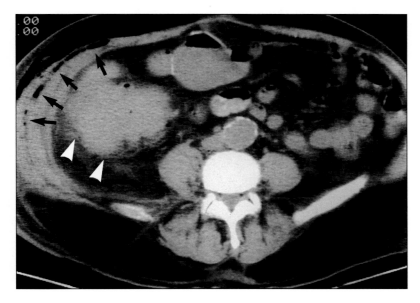

FIGURE 8-24 Necrotizing fasciitis. Computed tomography scan of a patient presenting with extensive edema demonstrates air in the subcutaneous tissues (*arrows*) along the right flank due to necrotizing fasciitis. The scan also demonstrates an unsuspected mass in the right colon (*arrowheads*), which extends into the pericolonic fat; it was found to be a primary adenocarcinoma of the cecum.

GENITOURINARY TRACT

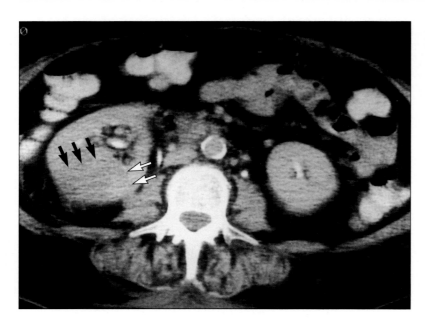

FIGURE 8-25 Computed tomography scan through the kidneys demonstrates diffuse swelling of the right kidney, with a wedge-shaped, vague area of diminished contrast enhancement (*black arrows*) that represents a discrete area of parenchymal inflammation (lobar nephronia). Note the inflammatory changes in the perinephric fat adjacent to the region of parenchymal inflammation (*white arrows*).

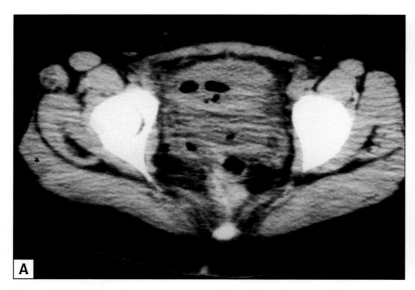

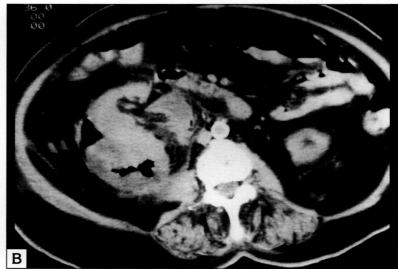

FIGURE 8-26 Emphysematous cystitis and pyelonephritis. **A** and **B**, Computed tomography scans through the pelvis and abdomen show air in the bladder and right kidney, demonstrating emphysematous cystitis and pyelonephritis in this diabetic patient.

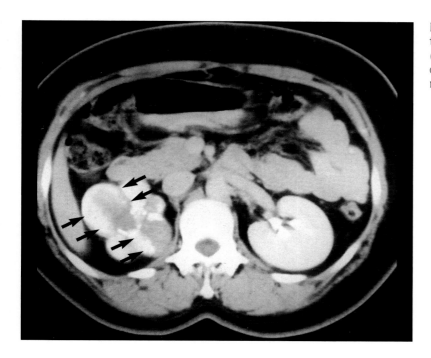

FIGURE 8-27 Renal abscesses. Computed tomography scan through the kidneys shows two well-defined right renal masses (*arrows*) with thick irregular walls surrounding central areas of diminished density. This appearance is characteristic of renal abscesses.

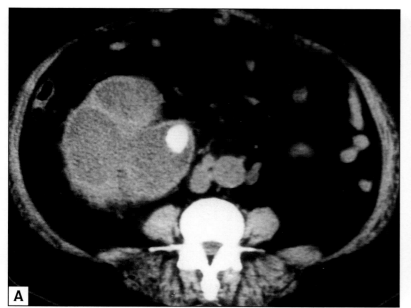

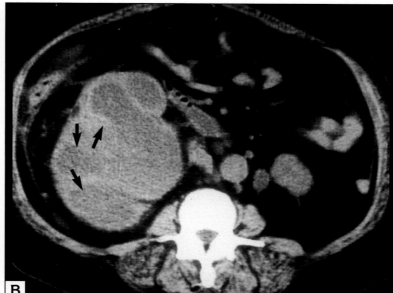

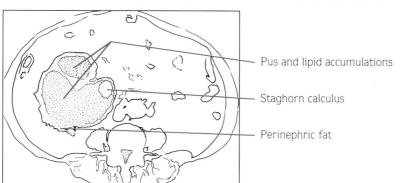

Pus and lipid accumulations

Staghorn calculus

Perinephric fat

FIGURE 8-28 Xanthogranulomatous pyelonephritis. **A** and **B**, Computed tomography scans through the right kidney demonstrate no excretion. A staghorn calculus can be seen. The renal parenchyma is replaced with multiple low-density masses (*panel 28B; arrows*), which represent collections of pus and lipid accumulating xanthoma cells. There is some spiculation in the perinephric fat and thickening of Gerota's fascia.

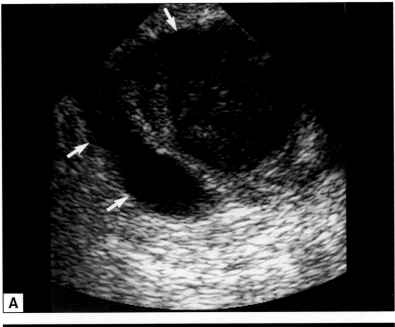

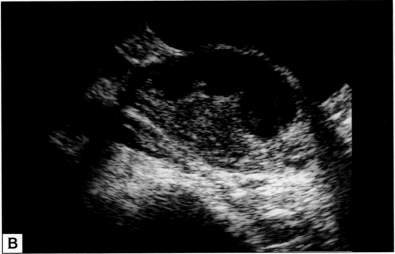

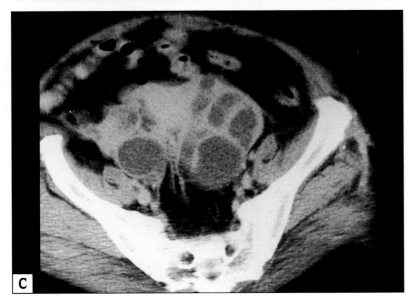

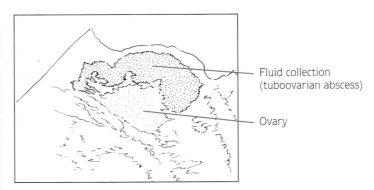

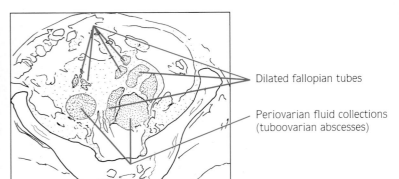

FIGURE 8-29 Pelvic inflammatory disease and tuboovarian abscess. **A**, Transabdominal ultrasound demonstrates dilatation of the fallopian tube (*arrows*) to the level of the ovary, as typically seen in pelvic inflammatory disease. **B**, Ultrasound of the ovary demonstrates a fluid collection adjacent to the ovary, indicating a tuboovarian abscess. **C**, A computed tomography scan confirms bilateral fallopian tube dilatation and periovarian fluid collections, diagnostic of pelvic inflammatory disease and tuboovarian abscesses.

Fluid collection (tuboovarian abscess)

Ovary

Dilated fallopian tubes

Periovarian fluid collections (tuboovarian abscesses)

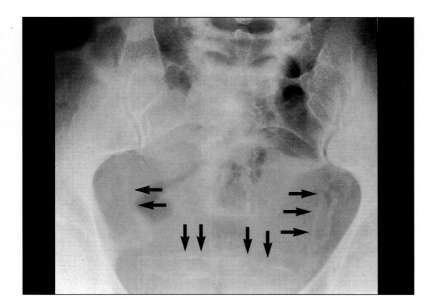

FIGURE 8-30 Schistosomiasis of the urinary tract. Plain film of the pelvis shows dense calcification in the distal ureter and bladder (*arrows*) typical of urinary tract infection by *Schistosoma haematobium*.

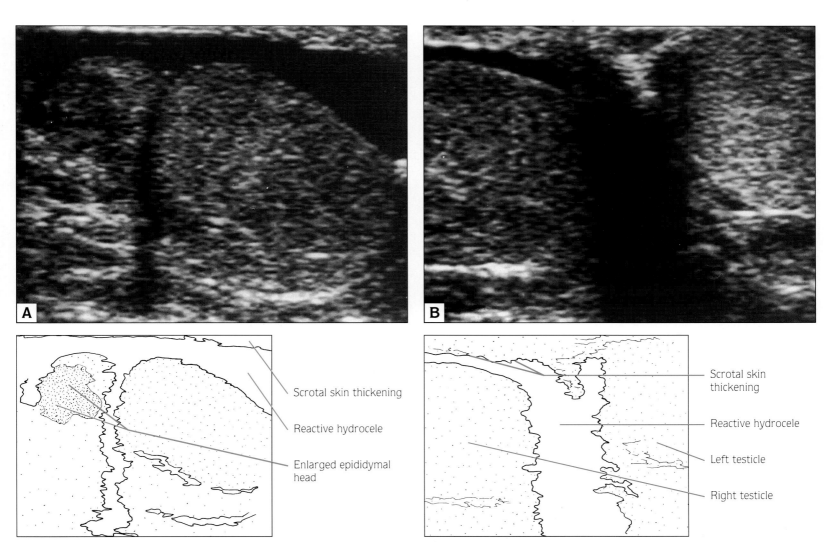

FIGURE 8-31 Epididymo-orchitis on scrotal ultrasound. **A.** Longitudinal ultrasound of the right testicle demonstrates marked enlargement of the epididymal head associated with a reactive hydrocele. **B.** On axial scans, the right testicle is enlarged and hypoechoic when compared with the left testicle, and there is scrotal skin thickening. These findings are characteristic of epididymitis with associated inflammatory changes in the testicle (orchitis).

SELECTED BIBLIOGRAPHY

Balthazar EJ (ed.): Imaging the acute abdomen. *Radiol Clin North Am* 1994, 32:829–950.

Builtrago-Tellez CH, Boos S, Heinemann F, *et al.*: Non-traumatic acute abdomen in the adult: A critical review of imaging modalities. *Eur Radiol* 1992, 2:174–179.

Goldstein HM, Bova JB: Esophagitis. *In* Taveras JM, Ferrucci JT (eds.): *Radiology: Diagnosis—Imaging—Intervention*. Philadelphia: J.B. Lippincott; 1995:13.

Kuhlman JE, Fishman EK: Acute abdomen in AIDS: CT diagnosis and triage. *Radiographics* 1990, 10:621–628.

Reeder MM: Infectious colitis. *In* Taveras JM, Ferrucci JT (eds.): *Radiology: Diagnosis—Imaging—Intervention*. Philadelphia: J.B. Lippincott; 1995:484–498.

Taourel P, Baron MP, Pradel J, *et al.*: Acute abdomen of unknown origin: Impact of CT on diagnosis and management. *Gastrointest Radiol* 1992, 17:287–293.

INDEX